ATLAS OF
SURFACE PALPATION: ANATOMY OF THE NECK, TRUNK, UPPER AND LOWER LIMBS

For Elsevier
Senior Content Strategist: Rita Demetriou-Swanwick
Content Development Specialist: Nicola Lally
Project Manager: Louisa Talbott
Designer/Design Direction: Miles Hitchen

ATLAS OF SURFACE PALPATION

Anatomy of the Neck, Trunk, Upper and Lower Limbs

Third Edition

Serge Tixa

Instructor in Anatomy and Palpatory Anatomy at the School of Osteopathy (ATSA) in Lyon,
at the Institute of Osteopathy (IFKO), and at the Institute of Massage and Physical Therapy (IFMK) in Montpellier

Translated by
Louis Honoré and Elaine Richards

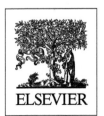

ELSEVIER

Edinburgh   London   New York   Oxford   Philadelphia   St Louis   Sydney   Toronto   2016

ELSEVIER

This English language edition is produced from two French language Works originally published as:
Atlas d'anatomie palpatoire. Tome 1: Cou, tronc, membre supérieur, 2012, Elsevier Masson SAS. All rights reserved.
Atlas d'anatomie palpatoire. Tome 1: Membre inférieur, 2012, Elsevier Masson SAS. All rights reserved.

ISBN 978-0-7020-6225-4

The author arranged the sets to be photographed, and the photography was done by Charles Menge and Laurent Dabosville.

The illustrated plates were produced by Hélène Fournie and Marie Schmitt.

Notices

your source for books,
journals and multimedia
in the health sciences
www.elsevierhealth.com

Working together
to grow libraries in
developing countries

www.elsevier.com • www.bookaid.org

The publisher's policy is to use paper manufactured from sustainable forests

Printed in Great Britain.
Last digit is the print number: 10 9 8 7 6

Table of Contents

Table of Contents

Table of Contents

Table of Contents

Acknowledgements

For all the photographs in the various editions of my work, I wish to express heartfelt thanks to the many students who agreed to volunteer their time and energy by posing in photography sessions that were often very long and very tedious.

They are too numerous to mention by name here, but I must pay tribute to them all. To them all I wish to express my most profound gratitude. I am anxious for them to know that I remember them all and will never forget them, since without them this book would not be what it is.

And for this new edition, I offer my sincere thanks to my students, in particular Gabrielle Galais, Julie Garcia, Francky Roullier, and Lucile Sarrailh, who devoted themselves dependably and wholeheartedly to the various stages of the work required to produce this book.

Finally, very particular thanks go to Francky Roullier, who had the demanding and time-consuming task of coordinating and organizing the participation of all those involved.

Introduction

This book presents a method of palpatory anatomy, which we have called Manual Exploration of Surface Anatomy (MESA). This is a method of locating anatomical structures (bones, ligaments, tendons, muscles, and neurovascular bundles). It is highly visual, as each structure studied is illustrated with a photograph; it also provides practical instruction, since each photograph is accompanied by a section of text describing a method of approach (MA) to the structure concerned.

Who is the book intended for?
It is aimed at all who need a method of applied anatomy in their professional practice.

How is the book organized?
This atlas consists of over 800 photographs of the neck, trunk, and upper and lower limbs. There are twelve chapters (The Neck, The Trunk and the Sacrum, The Shoulder, The Arm, The Elbow, The Forearm, The Wrist and the Hand, The Hip, The Thigh, The Knee, The Leg, and The Ankle and the Foot). Each has up to four subsections, as appropriate, treating the various aspects of that region. These cover osteology, myology (musculotendinous structures), arthrology (joints and ligaments), and, lastly, nerves and blood vessels.

The nomenclature used is the most recent anatomical terminology.

The two types of photograph
- Descriptive photographs include:
- An overall photograph at the start of each chapter (The Neck, The Trunk and the Sacrum, The Shoulder, The Arm, The Elbow, The Forearm, The Wrist and the Hand, The Hip, The Thigh, The Knee, The Leg, The Ankle and the Foot).
- Topographical photographs showing a body region with its group of notable structures accessible to palpation (e.g., anterior region of the neck or the thoracolumbar spine; the lateral inguinofemoral region or the lateral border of the foot).
- Structural photographs illustrating, wherever possible, an anatomical structure and its relationships with the adjacent structures. These are mainly photographs of muscles or muscle groups (e.g., pectoralis major; quadriceps femoris).
- The MESA photographs constitute the main body of the book. Each displays a structure to be studied. A descriptive note on the **method of approach (MA)** accompanies each photograph.
- For every photograph showing an anatomical structure accessible to palpation, a subject whose physique shows the structure very clearly has been carefully selected. When students have actually seen a structure on a living body, they know it exists and can be palpated, whatever the patient's body type. To assist palpation, the method of approach is described.
- Finally, the photographs are in black and white, a very definite decision that allows anatomical details to stand out better, thus making the method of approach even clearer.

How is the book intended to be used?
There are two possible methods:
- To explore a particular region in its entirety (e.g., the neck or the knee) or part of a region (e.g., the lateral region of the neck, the lateral border of the foot), simply turn to the relevant chapter or subsection, as indicated in the list of contents.

- To look at a specific structure in all its possible aspects, consult the index for a list of all the photographs that cover that topic (e.g., scapula; sartorius muscle, which is dealt with in the chapter on the thigh as well as in the chapters on the hip and the knee).

What is new in this edition?

- New methods of approach, illustrated by new photographs.
- Anatomical dissection plates specially made for this new edition use visual illustration to enhance the instructional material by showing the location of a given muscle, its relationship to neighboring muscles, and the visualization of its sites of origin and insertion. In the same way it aids the localization of bony structures, joint cavities, nerves and blood vessels.
- Information on the attachments of muscles is contained in notes following the description of the corresponding technique of approach. They are presented clearly and distinctly for easy reference and use. Practitioners and students alike are well aware of how easy it is to learn and forget anatomy many times before finally mastering it. It is primarily to address this concern that the information on muscle attachments has been included in this new edition. It is impossible to master palpatory anatomy without a thorough knowledge of theoretical anatomy.
- Information on the actions of muscles. In this new edition, these headings appear on each page on which a muscle or muscle group is presented, as always in order to help the student master palpatory anatomy.
- A new feature enhances this edition, as ever with the aim of improving the student's mastery of anatomic palpation: description of nerve trunks and their branches. A few cases of clinical anatomy closely connected to palpatory anatomy show how ever-present this subject is for every hands-on approach to diagnosis.

Note: *The boundaries of each region studied in each of the ensuing chapters must not be viewed as strictly defined. When studying certain muscles, it is inevitable that the area under consideration will extend beyond the region under discussion. The reason for this lies in the approach being taken. Each is viewed both in terms of a "transverse" approach that localizes it with respect to adjacent structures, and in terms of a "longitudinal" approach that looks at its proximal part, its main body, and its distal part.*

The terms "proximal" and "distal," occasionally used in presenting methods of approach, need to be clarified. These terms apply to the therapist's hand or grip/contact, as seen in the illustrations. "Proximal" and "distal" refer respectively to the hand that is closer to the site of attachment of the patient's lower limb and to the hand that is farther away from that attachment site.

1
The neck

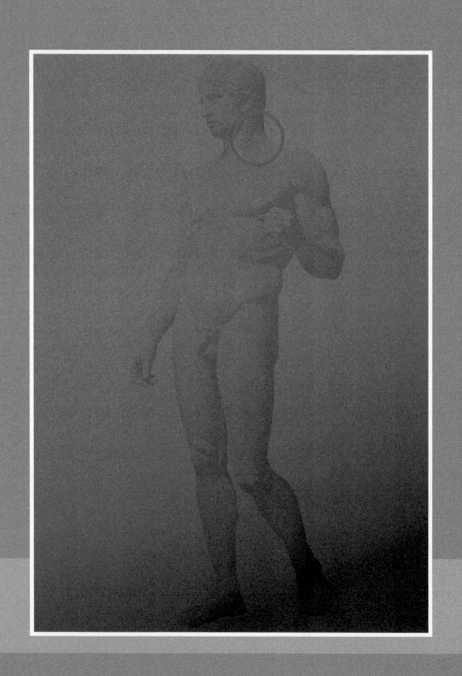

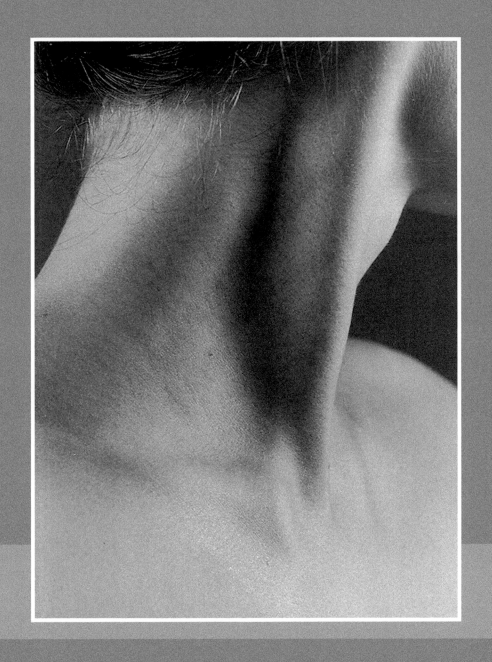

OSTEOLOGY

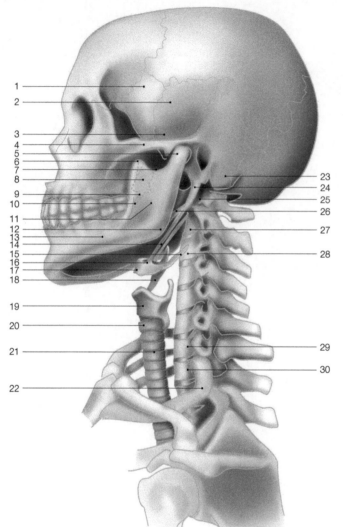

Osteology of the neck

1. Sphenoid
2. Temporal bone
3. Temporal fossa
4. Zygomatic arch
5. Condylar process of mandible
6. Coronoid process of mandible
7. Mandibular notch
8. Lateral pterygoid plate *(dotted line)*
9. Pterygoid hamulus *(dotted line)*
10. Pterygomandibular raphe *(dotted line)*
11. Ramus of mandible
12. Angle of mandible
13. Body of mandible
14. Stylohyoid ligament
15. Greater horn of hyoid
16. Lesser horn of hyoid
17. Body of hyoid
18. Epiglottis
19. Thyroid cartilage
20. Cricoid cartilage
21. Trachea
22. First rib
23. Mastoid process
24. Styloid process
25. Atlas (C1)
26. Stylomandibular ligament
27. Axis (C2)
28. Vertebra C3
29. Vertebra C7
30. Vertebra T1

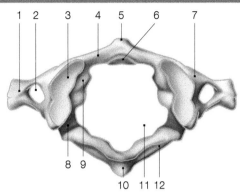

Atlas (C1) superior view

1. Transverse process	8. Groove for vertebral artery
2. Foramen transversarium	9. Tubercle for transverse
3. Superior articular facet	ligament of the atlas
4. Anterior arch	10. Posterior tubercle
5. Anterior tubercle	11. Vertebral foramen
6. Facet for dens	12. Posterior arch
7. Lateral part	

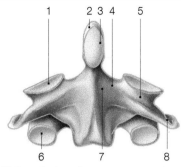

Axis (C2) anterior view

1. Articular facet for atlas
2. Dens
3. Superior articular facet
4. Pedicle
5. Articular process
6. Inferior articular facet
7. Body
8. Transverse process

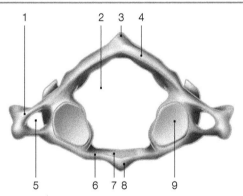

Atlas (C1) inferior view

1. Transverse process	6. Anterior arch
2. Vertebral foramen	7. Facet for the dens
3. Posterior tubercle	8. Anterior tubercle
4. Posterior arch	9. Inferior articular process of
5. Foramen transversarium	the lateral mass for the axis

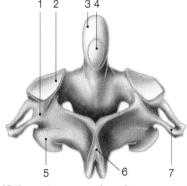

Axis (C2) posterosuperior view

1. Articular process
2. Superior articular facet
3. Dens
4. Posterior articular facet
5. Inferior articular process
6. Spinous process
7. Transverse process

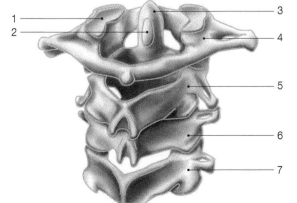

Superior cervical vertebrae, articulated (posterosuperior view)

1. Superior articular facet
2. Posterior articular facet
3. Dens
4. Atlas (C1)
5. Axis (C2)
6. C3
7. C4

Vertebra C4, superior view

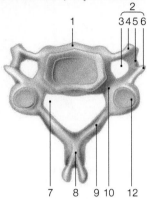

Vertebra C7, superior view

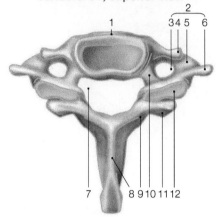

1. Body	7. Vertebral foramen
2. Transverse process	8. Spinous process
3. Foramen transversarium	9. Lamina
4. Anterior tubercle	10. Pedicle
5. Groove for spinal nerve	11. Inferior articular process
6. Posterior tubercle	12. Superior articular facet

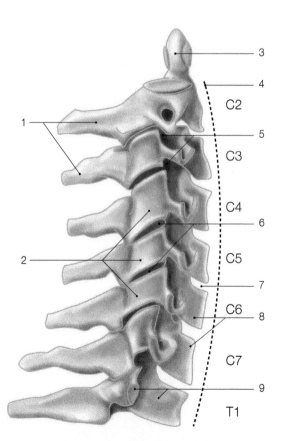

Vertebrae C2–T1, lateral view, from the right

1. Spinous process
2. Articular column formed by articular processes and interarticular parts
3. Dens
4. Cervical curvature
5. Intervertebral foramina for spinal nerves
6. Zygapophysial joints
7. Intervertebral joint
8. Vertebral body
9. Costal facets for first rib

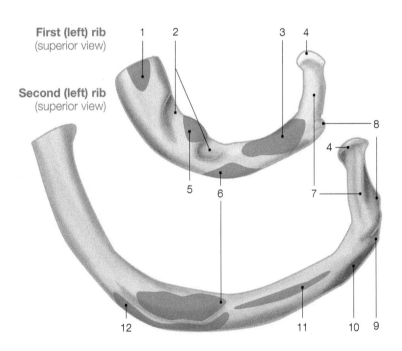

First (left) rib
(superior view)

Second (left) rib
(superior view)

1. Subclavian muscle	7. Neck
2. Grooves for subclavian artery and vein	8. Costal tubercle
3. Scalenus medius	9. Costal angle
4. Head	10. Serratus posterior superior
5. Scalenus anterior	11. Scalenus posterior
6. Serratus anterior (first digitation)	12. Serratus anterior (second digitation)

THE ANTERIOR CERVICAL REGION

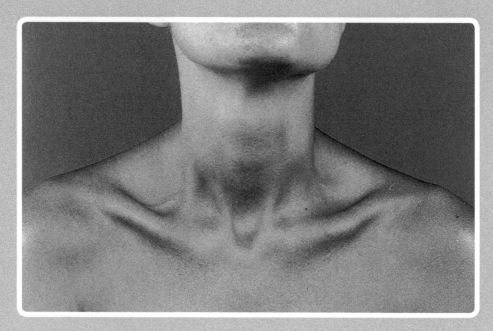

Fig. 1.2 Anterior view of the neck region

The notable structures that can be detected by palpation are:
- Thyroid cartilage (Figs. 1.3–1.6)
- Superior thyroid notch (Figs. 1.5 and 1.6)
- Hyoid:
  - Body of hyoid (Fig. 1.3; Figs. 1.6 and 1.7)
  - Median tubercle of hyoid (Fig. 1.7)
  - Lesser horn (Fig. 1.8)
  - Greater horn (Fig. 1.9)
- Cricoid cartilage (Fig. 1.10)
- Trachea (Fig. 1.11).

Fig. 1.3 Display of the osseocartilaginous elements belonging to the larynx

MA: The larynx, the essential organ of voice, is situated in the median anterior part of the neck. It opens superiorly into the laryngopharynx, the inferior part of the pharynx. It lies below the hyoid bone and above the trachea, and can be palpated between the hyoid above, and the superior border of the sternal manubrium. It is mobile, rising by approximately the height of one vertebra, when the subject is speaking, breathing, and especially swallowing. The larynx is composed of a number of cartilages. The only ones discussed here are those providing support: the thyroid and cricoid cartilages.

Note: Although the hyoid is attached to the thyroid cartilage by the thyrohyoid membrane, it does not form part of the skeleton of the larynx.

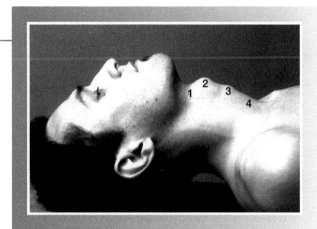

1. Position of hyoid
2. Thyroid cartilage
3. Cricoid cartilage
4. Trachea

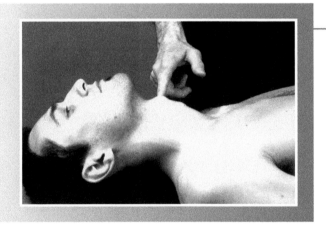

Fig. 1.4 Thyroid cartilage

MA: This can best be displayed if the subject's head is hyperextended. The thyroid cartilage is situated between the hyoid above and the cricoid cartilage below. The thyroid cartilage (indicated by the practitioner's index finger) is the largest of the cartilages of the larynx. Its name (from the Greek for a "shield") refers to both its shape and its position, since it covers or shields the other elements of the larynx anteriorly. It is much more prominent in males than in females.

Note: Three of the eleven cartilages constituting the larynx are unpaired, median structures: the thyroid cartilage (which tends to ossify in adults and the elderly), the cricoid cartilage, and the epiglottis.

Fig. 1.5 Superior thyroid notch, lateral view

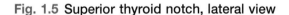

MA: The superior thyroid notch can be palpated at the point where the two lobes of the body of the thyroid join, above the prominence. In the adjacent figure it is very marked. The practitioner's index finger indicates the notch, which is situated in the median line, on the superior border of the thyroid cartilage, at the Adam's apple.

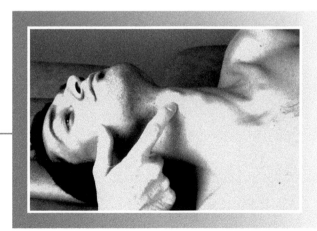

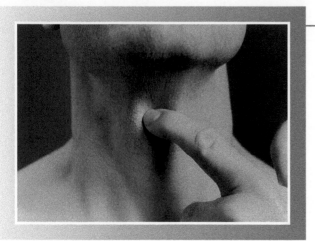

Fig. 1.6 Body of the hyoid, step 1

MA: Place your index finger on the superior thyroid notch, on the superior border of the thyroid cartilage. This is the first stage in locating the body of the hyoid, which is situated immediately above.

Fig. 1.7 Body of the hyoid, step 2, and median tubercle of the hyoid

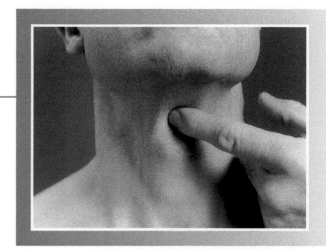

MA: When you have completed the first step in locating the hyoid, move your index finger upward to make contact with the body of the hyoid. You will find it one finger's breadth above, in the direction of the mandible, when the subject's neck is slightly extended. The median tubercle of the hyoid forms a bony projection that can be felt directly beneath the skin.

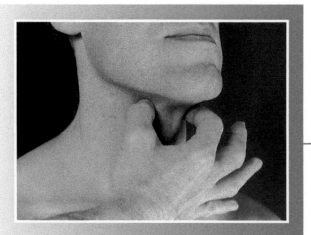

Fig. 1.8 Body of the hyoid: lesser horn

MA: Once you have located the superior border of the thyroid cartilage, body of the hyoid, and median tubercle of the hyoid, gently shift your contact slightly to each side, using your thumb and index finger; continue to follow the line of the body of the hyoid. You will then make contact with two small raised bony projections – tiny upwardly oriented horns.

Fig. 1.9 Body of the hyoid: greater horn and posterior tubercle of the greater horn

MA: Having located the body of the hyoid and the lesser horns, simply shift your thumb and finger laterally, using the same contact, to find the greater horns. These extend upward, posteriorly and laterally to the body of the hyoid, and end posteriorly in a tubercle that you can also feel beneath your fingers. Position the subject's head in extension to perceive these structures more clearly.

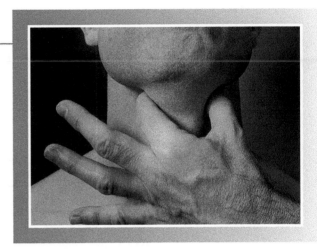

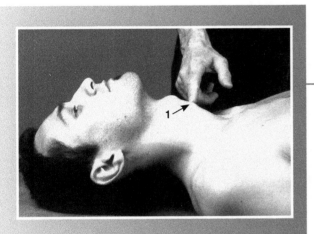

Fig. 1.10 Cricoid cartilage

MA: This is the most inferiorly situated of the cartilages of the larynx. In this figure, the practitioner's index finger indicates the cricoid cartilage, which lies two finger-breadths below the laryngeal prominence (1). The cricoid cartilage forms the base of the laryngeal pyramid and creates the transition between the larynx and the first tracheal cartilage.

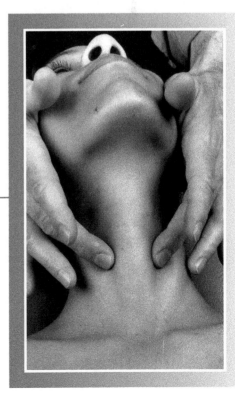

Fig. 1.11 Trachea

MA: The subject's head should be hyperextended to isolate this structure clearly.

The trachea extends from the inferior border of the sixth cervical vertebra to the fifth thoracic vertebra or a little beyond. It has the shape of a cylindrical tube which is flattened posteriorly. The cylindrical part has rings of cartilage, separated by spaces or interannular depressions, and can easily be palpated.

The trachea follows an oblique course running down from above and from anterior to posterior. The cervical portion of the trachea extends from the inferior border of the cricoid cartilage (level with intervertebral disc C6–C7) to the superior border of the sternum. It has an overall length of around 12 cm (5 inches), varying according to the position of the larynx (which rises and descends in the living adult male). Its diameter is approximately 12 mm (½ inch).

THE DORSAL AND LATERAL CERVICAL REGION

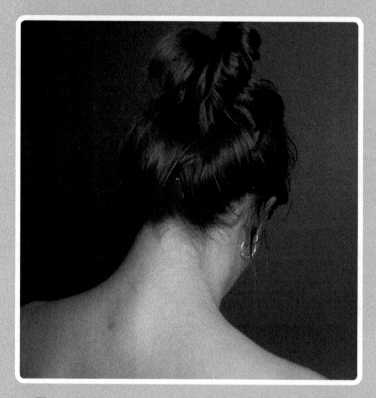

Fig. 1.12 The dorsal cervical region (nuchal region)

The notable structures that can be detected by palpation are:
- Cervical spine (Fig. 1.13)
- Spinous process of the seventh cervical vertebra (Fig. 1.14)
- Spinous process of the sixth cervical vertebra (Fig. 1.15)
- Posterior tubercle of the atlas (Fig. 1.16)
- Spinous process of the axis (Fig. 1.17)
- Transverse process of the atlas (Fig. 1.18)
- Transverse process of the axis (Fig. 1.19)
- Transverse processes of the third to seventh cervical vertebrae (Fig. 1.20)
- Articular processes of the cervical vertebrae (Figs. 1.21 and 1.22)
- Spinous process of a cervical vertebra (Figs. 1.23 and 1.28)
- Lamina of a cervical vertebra (Figs. 1.24 and 1.28)
- Articular processes (Figs. 1.25, 1.27, and 1.28)
- Transverse processes (Figs. 1.26–1.28)
- Cervicothoracic transition (Figs. 1.29–1.36)
- Spinous process of C5 (Figs. 1.37 and 1.43)
- Spinous process of C4 (Figs. 1.38 and 1.42)
- Posterior tubercle of C1 (Fig. 1.39)
- Spinous process of C2 (Fig. 1.40)
- Spinous process of C3 (Fig. 1.41).

Fig. 1.13 The cervical spine

MA: The practitioner is indicating the general topographical location of the cervical spine, between the occipital bone and the first thoracic vertebra. It consists of seven cervical vertebrae arranged one above the other and each articulating with the next.

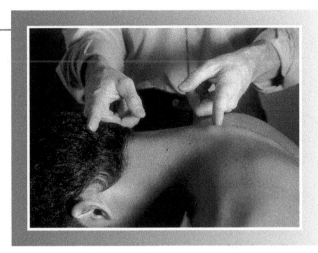

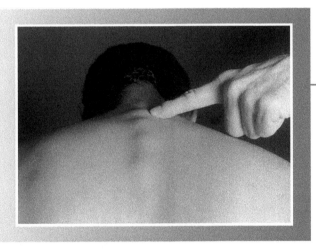

Fig. 1.14 Spinous process of the seventh cervical vertebra

MA: This process is distinguished by its length and prominence and by having a single tubercle at its extremity. However, it is easy to confuse with the first thoracic vertebra. Identification of C6 requires various other tests (see Figs. 1.33–1.36).

Note: As a general rule, the spinous process of C7 is the most prominent of the spinous processes of the cervicothoracic transition (C6–C7–T1).

Fig. 1.15 Spinous process of the sixth cervical vertebra

MA: This structure is easy to find once you have clearly identified the spinous process of the seventh cervical vertebra; the sixth is situated immediately above it. Identification can be confirmed by asking the subject to rotate his head repeatedly to the left and right, when the process of C6 can distinctly be felt to shift beneath your fingers relative to the spinous process of C7.

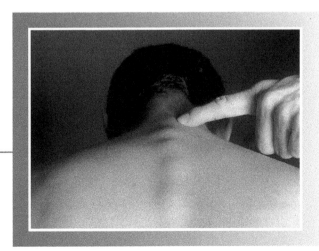

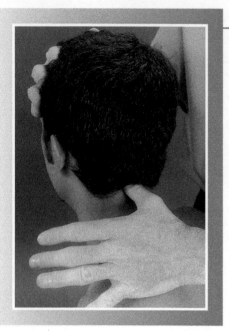

Fig. 1.16 Posterior tubercle of the atlas

MA: This can be found in the extension of the external occipital crest (on the exocranial surface of the occipital bone). The posterior border of the foramen magnum can be felt beneath your fingers, and just beneath this (in the caudal direction), you will detect a small depression. Within this depression the practitioner's thumb can be seen making contact with the posterior tubercle of the atlas.

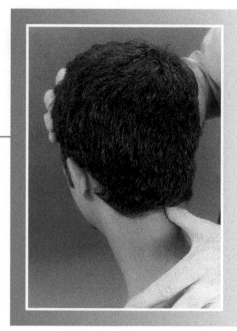

Fig. 1.17 Spinous process of the axis

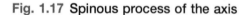

MA: Below the small depression mentioned above (Fig. 1.16) (within which the posterior tubercle of the atlas is found) you can detect a bony structure beneath your fingers. This is the spinous process of the axis. It is very prominent, and can be revealed distinctly by slightly flexing and extending the subject's head; this should be done by a gentle movement using your fingers on his forehead.

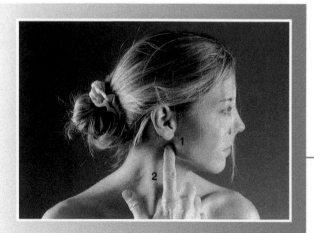

Fig. 1.18 Transverse process of the atlas

MA: Begin by locating the ramus of the mandible (1) and the sternocleidomastoid (2). The practitioner's index finger indicates the space between the two, and it is here that it is possible to palpate the transverse process of the atlas with its single tubercle. It is very prominent laterally.

Fig. 1.19 Transverse process of the axis

MA: The point of reference in the approach to this structure is the angle of the mandible (1). The transverse process of the axis can be palpated either behind or in front of the sternocleidomastoid (2). It differs from the transverse process of the atlas in that it is very small.

Note: Great care should be taken in the approach to this structure. This need for caution applies to all the structures of the neck region.

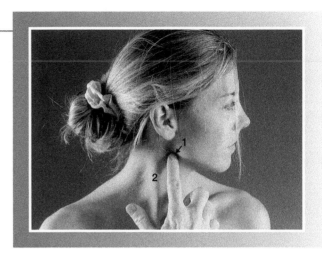

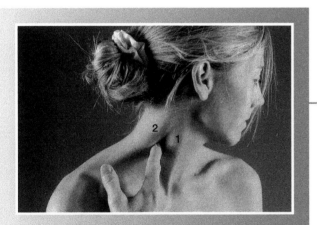

Fig. 1.20 Transverse processes of the third to seventh cervical vertebrae

MA: In the illustration opposite, the practitioner's index finger indicates the region between sternocleidomastoid (1) and trapezius (2) muscles. These transverse processes can be located by sliding your contact into this region.

Fig. 1.21 The articular processes of the cervical vertebrae, global approach

MA: The practitioner has adopted a global approach, using a broad contact with his thumb and next three fingers to ease the cervical portion of the trapezius muscle forward, so as to make contact with the articular processes of the cervical vertebrae. Place your other hand on the subject's forehead, and use this to bring about side-bending of the head to each side alternately. This causes the articular processes to appear distinctly beneath your fingers.

Note: Once the lateral border of the cervical portion of trapezius has been located, ensure that the muscle is thoroughly relaxed before beginning the palpation of the articular processes.

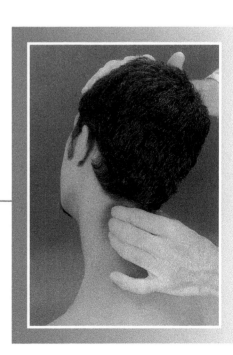

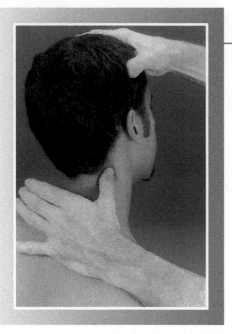

Fig. 1.22 The articular processes of the cervical vertebrae, global approach

MA: The contact is identical to that described in Figure 1.21. This photograph illustrates the position of the practitioner's thumb in the contact shown there.

Fig. 1.23 Spinous process of a cervical vertebra

MA: The spinous process of C2 is the largest of the upper cervical spine. The other very large spinous process is that of C7 (important for the method of approach to the different cervical vertebrae). The nuchal ligament can hinder palpation of the upper cervical spine (C0, C1, and C2).

Note: C0 corresponds to the cranium.

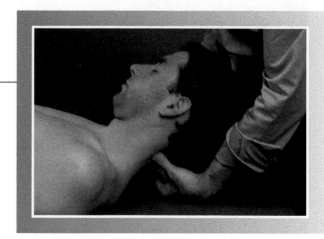

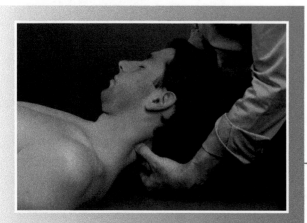

Fig. 1.24 Lamina of a cervical vertebra

MA: First locate the spinous process. The practitioner's thumb is seen extending the contact anteriorly to encounter the lamina, which runs from the spinous process to the column of articular processes.

Fig. 1.25 Analytical palpation of the articular processes

MA: Begin by locating the column of articular processes as a whole. Proceed in the same way along each vertebral segment in turn.

Note: The column of articular processes is situated immediately anterior to the laminae. Lateroflexion of the subject's head and neck to the left and right can be a helpful way of locating the laminae, as this movement brings the structures you are seeking into contact beneath your fingers.

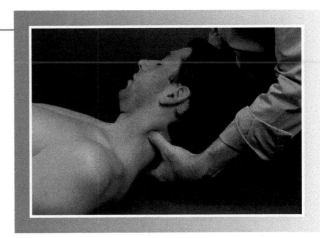

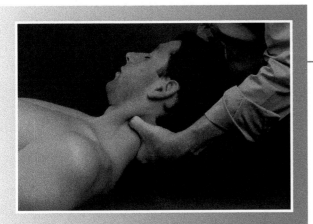

Fig. 1.26 Analytical palpation of the transverse processes

MA: Begin by locating the column of transverse processes as a whole. Proceed in the same way along each vertebral segment in turn.

Note: The column of transverse processes is situated in the cervical spine, immediately anterior to the articular processes. Lateroflexion of the subject's head and neck to the left and right can be a helpful way of locating the articular processes; as the subject's neck bends laterally, this brings the structures you are seeking into contact beneath your fingers.

Fig. 1.27 The column of articular processes and transverse processes

MA: You can palpate the length of this column from below the mastoid process down to the supraclavicular fossa. This photograph shows the practitioner's thumb on the posterior part of the articular processes and his index finger on the transverse processes. These are anterior to the column of articular processes.

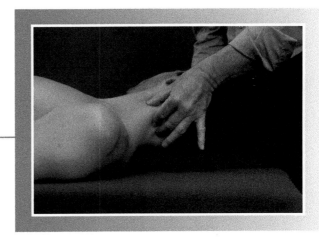

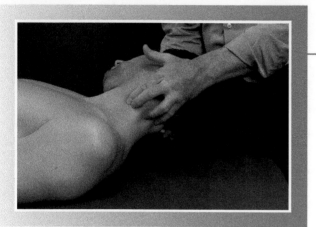

Fig. 1.28 Global approach, using a single contact on the different structures of a vertebral segment that can be palpated

MA: The subject is supine. Support his head with one hand, then bring it into rotation to the right. The other hand is positioned as follows:

• little finger on the spinous process;
• ring finger on the lamina;
• middle finger on the articular process;
• index finger on the transverse process.

Fig. 1.29 Display of the cervicothoracic transition (C6–C7–T1)

MA: With the subject lying on his side, bring his head into flexion, followed by flexion of the upper thoracic spine. The spinous processes of the vertebrae you seek, C7–T1, will then appear.

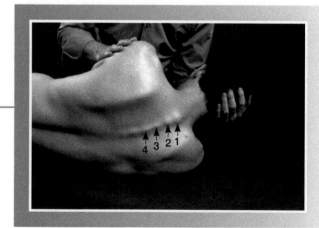

1. C7
2. T1
3. T2
4. T3

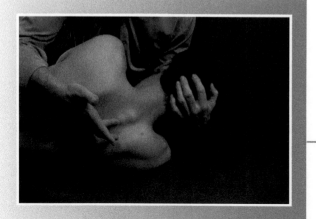

Fig. 1.30 The C6–C7–T1 transition (stage 1)

MA: The subject lies on his side; the practitioner stands facing him. Support his head with one hand, and then draw his head and neck into flexion. This causes the spinous processes of T1 and C7 to become prominent. Place the ring finger of your other hand on what appears to be the spinous process of T1.

Fig. 1.31 The C6–C7–T1 transition (stage 2)

MA: Subject and practitioner adopt the same positions as for stage 1. Maintain the contact of your ring finger with the spinous process of T1. You can then place your middle finger on what appears to be the spinous process of C7.

> **CLINICAL NOTE**
>
> If palpation of the transverse processes of C7 finds tenderness to pressure, you should suspect irritation of the C8 root. In that case, this technique may also cause or exacerbate pain at the medial border of the arm and forearm. There may also be pain and/or disturbances of sensation (paresthesia) in the ring finger and little finger.

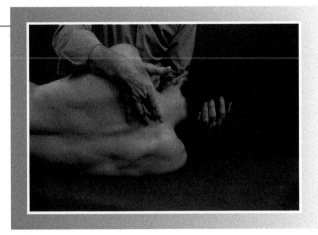

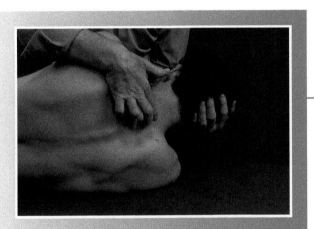

Fig. 1.32 The C6–C7–T1 transition (stage 3)

MA: Subject and practitioner adopt the same positions as for stage 2. Maintain the contact of your ring finger and middle finger with the spinous processes of T1 and C7. Then place your index finger on what appears to be the spinous process of C6.

Fig. 1.33 The C6–C7–T1 transition. Test in flexion/ extension (stage 4)

MA: Subject and practitioner adopt the same positions as for the previous stages, and the positioning of the practitioner's hands also remains the same. Then bring the subject's head and neck into flexion.

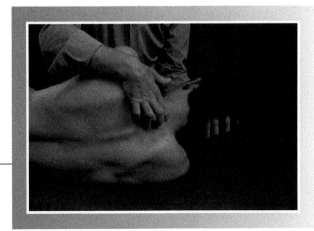

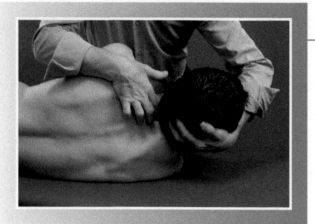

Fig. 1.34 The C6–C7–T1 transition. Test in flexion/ extension (stage 5)

MA: Subject and practitioner adopt the same positions as for the previous stages, and the positioning of the practitioner's hands also remains the same. Now bring the subject's head and neck into extension. If the spinous process of what appears to be C6 disappears under your index finger, this confirms the identification; it is the spinous process of C6.

> **CLINICAL NOTE**
>
> If palpation produces tenderness to pressure at the transverse processes of C6 and C7, this should cause you to suspect irritation of the C7 root. If so, this technique may also cause or exacerbate pain at the craniolateral part of the scapula and the posterolateral surface of the arm and forearm. There may also be pain and/or disturbances of sensation (paresthesia) in the index finger and middle finger.

Fig. 1.35 The C6–C7–T1 transition. Test in right rotation (stage 6)

MA: Subject and practitioner adopt the same positions as for the previous stages, and the positioning of the practitioner's hands also remains the same. Now rotate the subject's head and neck to the right. The spinous process of C6 is very mobile as compared with that of T1. (This is a way of locating C6.)

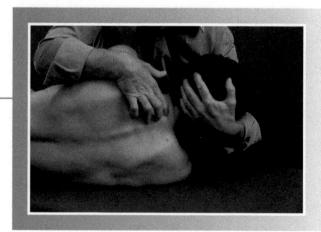

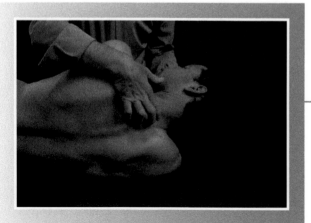

Fig. 1.36 The C6–C7–T1 transition. Test in left rotation (stage 6, repeat)

MA: The transition may be restricted on one side but not the other. The test should therefore be performed in rotation to the left as well as the right. Subject and practitioner adopt the same positions as for the previous stages, and the positioning of the practitioner's hands also remains the same. With the subject's head and neck rotated to the left, the spinous process of C6 is very mobile as compared with that of T1. (This is a way of locating C6.)

Fig. 1.37 Spinous process of C5: caudal approach

MA: Location of the spinous process of C5 is easily achieved once that of C6 has been found (see previous figure). Move approximately one finger's breadth in the cranial direction (toward C0) to make contact with the structure you are seeking.

> **CLINICAL NOTE**
>
> Tenderness of the transverse processes of C5 and C6 on palpation should lead you to suspect **irritation of the C6 root.** If so, this technique may also cause or exacerbate pain at the cranial border of the scapula and the lateral border of the arm and forearm. There may also be pain and/or disturbances of sensation in the thumb.

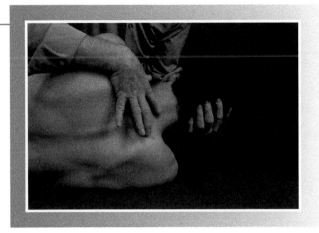

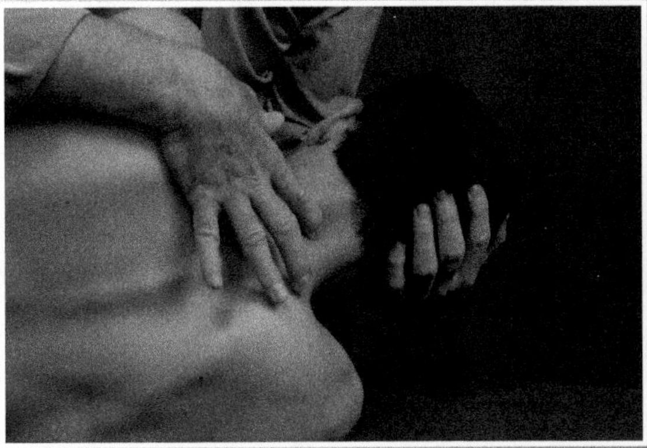

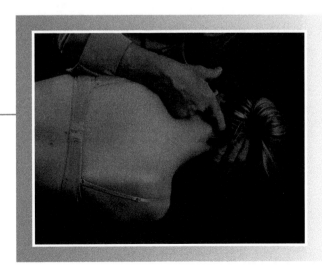

Fig. 1.38 Spinous process of C4: caudal approach

MA: Once you have located C5, start from the spinous process and move approximately one finger's breadth in a cranial direction to contact the structure you are seeking.

Note: It is more difficult to palpate this structure in subjects with cervical hyperlordosis.

> **CLINICAL NOTE**
>
> Tenderness of the transverse processes of C4 and C5 on palpation should lead you to suspect **irritation of the C5 root.** If so, this technique may also cause or exacerbate pain at the cranial border of the scapula and the anterolateral part of the arm. There may also be pain and/or disturbances of sensation in the anterolateral part of the arm.

Fig. 1.39 The posterior tubercle of C1

MA: Begin by locating C2, which has a very prominent process. Then move toward C0 (the cranium). Now apply passive mobilization of the head by bringing it into flexion and extension. With your index finger, palpate the depression between C0 and C1, opposite the posterior tubercle of C1.

Note: It is better to maintain the subject's head in extension so as to keep the nuchal ligament relaxed.

Reminder: The first cervical root has its exit point between C0 and C1, and the second cervical root between C1 and C2.

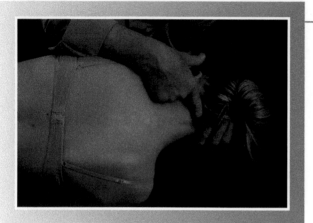

Fig. 1.40 The spinous process of C2

MA: This is very prominent. Passive mobilization of the subject's head in the sagittal plane will help you to see this structure more clearly.

Reminder: The third cervical root has its exit point between C2 and C3.

Fig. 1.41 The spinous process of C3

MA: This lies one finger's breadth below the spinous process of C2. Together with that of C4, this is the most difficult of the cervical spinous processes to palpate. These two are not very prominent and are situated quite deeply in the normal cervical lordosis. In subjects lacking this lordosis, it is quite easy to palpate.

Reminder: The fourth cervical root has its exit point between C3 and C4.

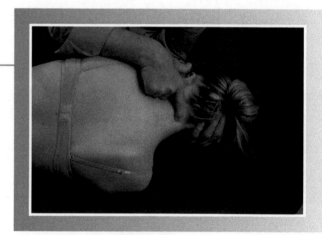

Fig. 1.42 The spinous process of C4

MA: This lies one finger's breadth below the spinous process of C3. To perceive it more clearly, put your fingers together, and place your:
- index finger on C2;
- middle finger on C3;
- ring finger on C4.

Reminder: The fifth cervical root has its exit point between C4 and C5.

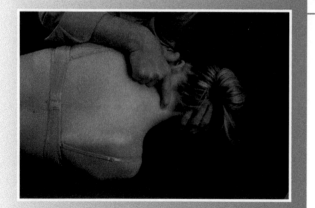

Fig. 1.43 The spinous process of C5

MA: Start from C6 (see Figs. 1.29–1.36), and move one finger's breadth upward.

Reminder: The sixth cervical root has its exit point between C5 and C6.

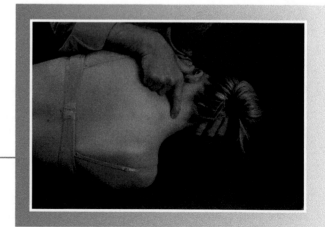

MYOLOGY

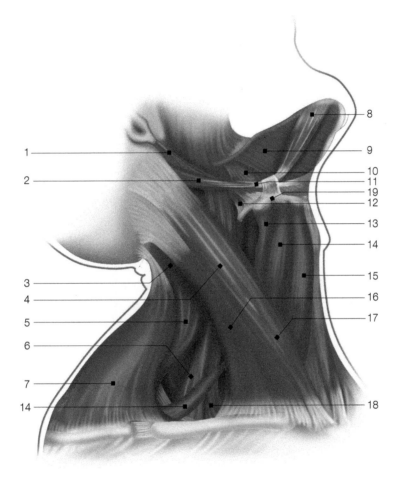

The muscles of the neck, anterolateral view

1. Stylohyoid
2. Posterior belly of digastric
3. Splenius capitis
4. Sternocleidomastoid
5. Levator scapulae
6. Scalenus medius
7. Trapezius
8. Anterior belly of digastric
9. Mylohyoid
10. Hyoglossus

11. Intermediate tendon of digastric
12. Middle constrictor of pharynx
13. Thyrohyoid
14. Omohyoid
15. Sternohyoid
16. Clavicular portion of sternocleidomastoid
17. Sternal portion of sternocleidomastoid
18. Scalenus anterior
19. Hyoid bone

THE LATERAL CERVICAL REGION

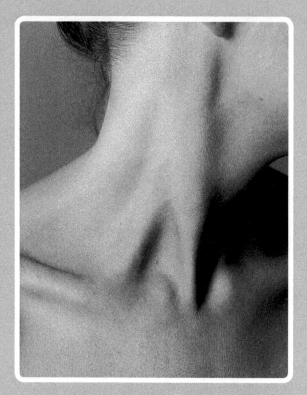

Fig. 1.44 Anterolateral view of the neck

The notable structures that can be detected by palpation are:
- Sternocleidomastoid (SCM) (Figs. 1.45, 1.46, 1.50, and 1.56–1.62)
- Trapezius (Figs. 1.45, 1.47, 1.54, and 1.56)
- Levator scapulae (Figs. 1.45, 1.48, 1.49, 1.52, 1.54, and 1.56)
- Scalenus anterior (anterior scalene) (Figs. 1.50–1.52, and 1.56)
- Scalenus medius (middle scalene) (Figs. 1.45, 1.52, and 1.53)
- Scalenus posterior (posterior scalene) (Figs. 1.45 and 1.53)
- Splenius (Figs. 1.45 and 1.54)
- Omohyoid (Figs. 1.45 and 1.55).

ACTIONS

- Sternocleidomastoid:
  - When both sternocleidomastoid muscles work together in concert, they flex the head and neck.
  - When one sternocleidomastoid muscle acts alone, this brings about rotation of the head and neck to the opposite side and lateroflexion.
- Trapezius (superior part):
  - When the fixed end is caudal, lateroflexion of head and neck.
  - When the fixed end is cranial, this elevates the shoulder.

- Levator scapulae:
  - When the fixed end is caudal, lateroflexion of the head and neck.
  - When the fixed end is cranial, the superomedial angle of the scapula moves upward and outward, causing the shoulder to dip down and the bone to swing medially.
- Posterior, middle, and anterior scalene muscles:
  - When the fixed end is the cervical vertebral column, these act as accessory inspiratory muscles.
  - When the fixed end is on the thorax, these muscles bring about lateroflexion (side-bending) to the same side together with slight rotation to the opposite side.
- Splenius:
  - Extension, lateroflexion, and ipsilateral rotation of the neck.
- Omohyoid (posterior belly):
  - When the fixed point is on the superior border of the scapula, this brings about ipsilateral inclination.
  - This muscle also appears to play a role in venous return.

INNERVATIONS

- SCM: cervical plexus (C2–C3) and accessory nerve (CN XI)
- Anterior scalene: cervical plexus (C5–C6–C7)
- Middle scalene: cervical plexus (C6–C7–C8)
- Posterior scalene: cervical plexus (C7–C8)
- Splenius cervicis: posterior branches of cervical nerves (C1–T1)
- Omohyoid (superior belly): ansa cervicalis of cervical plexus

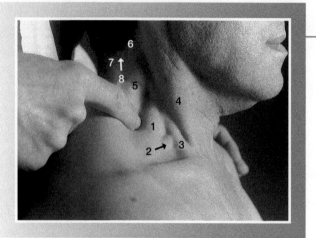

Fig. 1.45 Overall view of the muscles of the lateral cervical region

MA: Scalene muscles are classically described as being three in number; however, they can also be considered as proximally constituting a single muscle mass. The muscular mass (1) indicated by the practitioner's index finger is made up of the bodies of scalenus posterior and medius muscles; the more posteriorly situated part can be considered as scalenus posterior. To make this muscle mass appear, ask the subject to take several short, repeated in-breaths with the upper part of his thorax. This accessory inspiratory action is one of the actions of scalenus muscles when the fixed end is on the cervical vertebral column.

Note: Scalenus posterior is inserted into the superolateral surface of the second rib. Scalenus medius is inserted into the superior surface of the first rib, behind the scalene tubercle and posterior to the groove for the subclavian artery.

1. Muscle mass made up of the bodies of scalenus medius and scalenus posterior
2. Omohyoid, inferior belly
3. Sternocleidomastoid (clavicular head)
4. Sternocleidomastoid (sternal head)
5. Levator scapulae
6. Sternocleidomastoid (cleido-occipital head, proximal part)
7. Trapezius (cervical portion)
8. Splenius cervicis

Fig. 1.46 Step 1: location of sternocleidomastoid

MA: The subject is supine with her head turned to the left to cause the right sternocleidomastoid to become prominent. The practitioner takes up a position at the subject's head. Place one hand on the lateral surface of her cranium, above the right ear, to cause the muscle to become prominent.

ATTACHMENTS

Sternocleidomastoid can be described in terms of four heads: sterno-occipital, sternomastoid, cleido-occipital, and cleidomastoid.

- Inferiorly, the muscle arises from the pectoral girdle at two points; there is a clavicular and a sternal head.
  - The clavicular head arises from the medial one third of the superior surface of the clavicle, close to its posterior border. (The cleido-occipital head occupies a more superficial position than the cleidomastoid head, and lies closer to the anterior border of the clavicle.)
  - The sternal head is attached inferiorly to the anterior surface of the sternal manubrium, below the sternoclavicular joint, by a strong tendon. In some cases this head is divided into two; in such cases this tendon is common to the sterno-occipital and the sternomastoid heads.
- At the insertion, these four heads terminate in two occipital and two mastoid heads.
  - The two occipital heads are inserted into the lateral part of the superior nuchal line (superior curved line of the occipital bone): the cleido-occipital head medially and the sterno-occipital head laterally.
  - The two mastoid heads – cleidomastoid and sternomastoid – are inserted into the mastoid process of the temporal bone.

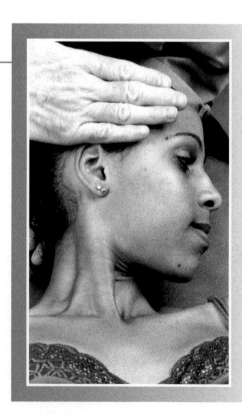

Fig. 1.47 Step 2: location of trapezius

MA: The subject should lie on her right side. Hold her left shoulder down with your right hand, while using your left hand on the inferolateral part of her cranium to resist left side-bending of the head. This causes the clavicular portion of trapezius (1), on the posterolateral part of the neck, to become prominent.

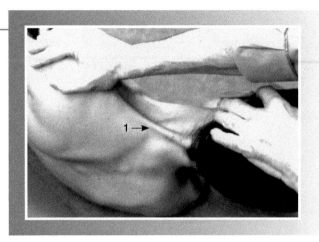

Fig. 1.48 Step 3: location of levator scapulae, posterior view

MA: One method (not shown in the adjacent figure) of causing this muscle to become prominent, or to appear beneath your fingers, is to place one hand on the lateral surface of the subject's head to resist side-bending. This method calls for a starting position with the subject's head resting on the abdominal wall of the practitioner. Ask the subject to contract and relax the muscle repeatedly. This starting position enables you to control the period of relaxation between each set of alternating contraction and relaxation.

Another method (shown here) is to ask the subject to perform side-bending of her head and neck. (In this case, the weight of the head provides all the resistance required.) This frees both your hands to take hold of the muscle to be investigated.

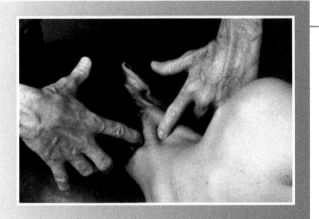

Fig. 1.49 Step 3: Another (anterior) view of levator scapulae

MA: In the adjacent figure, the practitioner is holding the body of levator scapulae (1) between his two index fingers.

ATTACHMENTS

- The origin of levator scapulae is by means of four tendons, from the posterior tubercles of the transverse processes of cervical vertebrae C1–C4.
- Its insertion is into the medial border of the scapula, above the spine of the scapula.

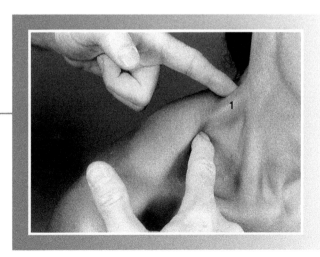

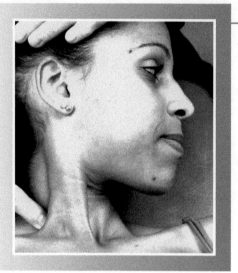

Fig. 1.50 Step 4

MA: The subject is supine, with her head turned to the left to make the right SCM appear prominently. The practitioner takes up a position at the subject's head. Place your left hand on the lateral surface of her cranium, above the right ear. This is to make prominent the posterior border of the clavicular head of SCM. Locating this is important to enable the next step, in which you locate scalenus anterior. This lies behind SCM. Its position is indicated on the adjacent figure by the practitioner's index finger.

Fig. 1.51 Step 5: location of scalenus anterior (anterior scalene)

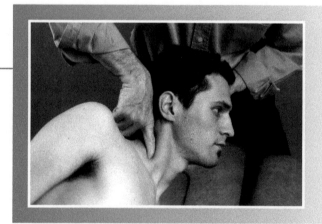

MA: The subject lies on the contralateral side. The practitioner's left hand supports his head. Slide the index finger (perhaps also the middle finger) of your other hand behind the clavicular head of SCM, so as to be able to palpate scalenus anterior. This is more easily done if you also carry out passive side-bending of the subject's head and cervical spine. You can also ask him to take repeated short in-breaths to mobilize the upper part of the thoracic cage and so facilitate the perception of this muscle. This is one of the actions of scalenus anterior when its fixed end is superior (on the cervical spine).

ATTACHMENTS

• Scalenus anterior arises superiorly, from the anterior tubercle of the transverse processes of vertebrae C3–C6.
• It inserts into the superior surface of the first rib (I), on the scalene tubercle behind the subclavian vein, and anterior to the subclavian artery. The phrenic nerve lies on its anterior surface.

Note: The phrenic nerve is situated in the sheath of scalenus anterior, and connects with the subclavian nerve. It enters the thorax between the subclavian artery and vein.

CLINICAL NOTE

The phrenic nerve and the way to stop the hiccups

The expulsion of air produced by a brief but energetic contraction of the diaphragm is sufficiently violent to make the vocal cords vibrate, producing the familiar sound. The phrenic nerve is the motor nerve of the diaphragm, and passes over the body of scalenus anterior. This nerve can be felt beneath the fingers as a very fine, solid cylinder, which can be palpated and therefore compressed. This combination of palpation and pressure can, if maintained for a few seconds, stop the hiccups. However, this technique calls for an expert hand.

Another method of stopping the hiccups is this: the person affected should first exhale completely, drawing the stomach area in, then breathe in deeply using the diaphragm and letting the stomach area expand, and hold the breath for several seconds until the hiccups stop.

Hiccups is a reflex response. It can be secondary to:

- peripheral irritation with a thoracic or mediastinal origin (such as myocardial infarction or tumor of the esophagus);

- a problem of the central nervous system (meningitis or cranial trauma);

- a general problem (such as infection);

- an emotional shock.

Fig. 1.52 Step 6: location of scalenus medius (middle scalene)

MA: Begin by locating levator scapulae. Shift your contact anterior to that muscle. Your fingers roll into contact with a muscle mass of considerable volume; it lies directly beneath your fingers in the supraclavicular fossa. The adjacent figure shows the practitioner taking hold of this muscle from each side, using two fingertips of each hand. Ask the subject to flex her head and neck ipsilaterally, while you resist the side-bending action with one hand. The muscle is easier to detect beneath your fingers if you ask her to take repeated short in-breaths. (The subject should lie on the contralateral side, with her head resting on the practitioner's abdomen.)

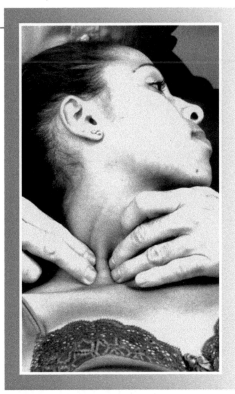

Note regarding scalenus medius:

• The dorsal scapular nerve (the nerve of rhomboids and elevator scapulae) passes from C5 and C6 across scalenus medius, which is a region at risk.
• The long thoracic nerve is in contact with scalenus medius, so that any muscular problem affecting that muscle and the region immediately around it can also affect the nerve.

ATTACHMENTS

• Scalenus medius arises superiorly:
  – from the transverse process of the axis;
  – from the anterior tubercles of the transverse processes of cervical vertebrae C3–C6;
  – from the transverse process of C7.
• Its insertion is into the superior surface of the first rib, posterior to the scalene tubercle and posterior to the subclavian artery.

> **CLINICAL NOTE**
>
> **Scalene syndrome (compression of the brachial plexus)**
>
> The following are typical:
>
> - hypertrophy of scalenus anterior;
>
> - a connection between scalenus anterior and scalenus medius;
>
> - the existence of a supernumerary scalene muscle between scalenus medius (near the brachial plexus) and scalenus anterior (near the blood vessels);
>
> - spasms associated with psychological tension.

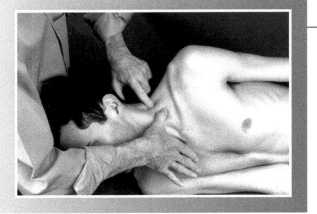

Fig. 1.53 Step 7: location of scalenus posterior (posterior scalene)

MA: The method is the same as that for scalenus medius. The adjacent figure shows the scalenus posterior between the practitioner's thumb and the index finger of the other hand. The bodies of scalenus medius and scalenus posterior sometimes fuse proximally so as to form a single muscle. In those cases where this has not happened, a depression can be felt between the two muscles.

ATTACHMENTS

• Scalenus posterior arises from the posterior tubercle of the transverse processes of cervical vertebrae C4–C6.
• Inferiorly, it is inserted into the superolateral surface of the second rib.

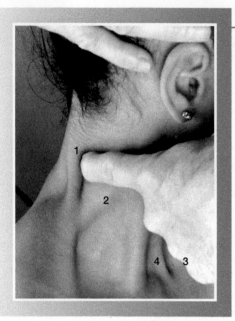

Fig. 1.54 Step 8: location of splenius

MA: This muscle is easy to locate once levator scapulae has been found. A position posterior to this muscle enables you to make contact with splenius; it is surrounded anteriorly and superiorly by SCM, anteriorly and inferiorly by levator scapulae, and posteriorly by trapezius (1).

ATTACHMENTS

Splenius arises inferiorly from the spinous processes of the middle cervical vertebrae and the inferior cervical and superior thoracic vertebrae (C4–T5). It then divides into two parts:

- *splenius capitis,* with its insertion into the squama of the occipital bone and superior nuchal line, anterior to SCM and on the mastoid process of the temporal bone;
- *splenius cervicis,* which is inserted into the transverse processes of the atlas and axis and sometimes also the transverse processes of the third cervical vertebra (C3).

1. Trapezius (superior part)
2. Levator scapulae
3. SCM, clavicular head
4. SCM, sternal head

Fig. 1.55 Step 9: location of omohyoid

MA: This muscle has two bellies and stretches from the hyoid to the superior border of the scapula. The practitioner's index finger indicates the inferior belly, at the inferior and lateral part of the supraclavicular fossa.

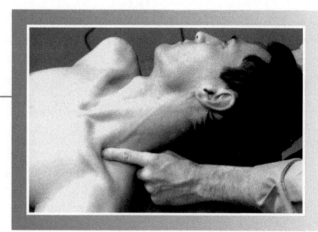

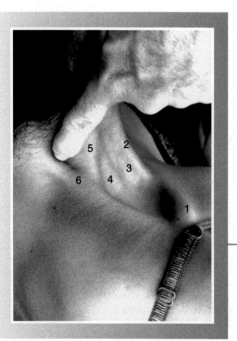

Fig. 1.56 Step 10: display and relations between the different muscles of the supraclavicular region

MA: In the adjacent figure, the practitioner's index finger indicates the position of splenius. It is also possible to visualize from this figure the relative positions of the muscles of the suprascapular region and the clavicle (1), SCM (2), scalenus anterior (3), and scalenus medius (4) – sometimes fused together in its proximal part with scalenus posterior – levator scapulae (5), and trapezius (superior part) (6).

Fig. 1.57 Frontal view of sternocleidomastoid

1. Sternal head of sternocleidomastoid
2. Occipital head of sternocleidomastoid
3. Clavicular head of sternocleidomastoid

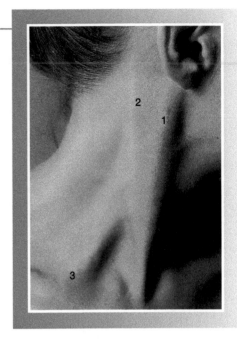

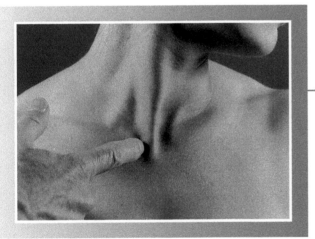

Fig. 1.58 Distal attachment of the sternal head of sternocleidomastoid

MA: The practitioner's index finger indicates the origin of this head, which is by means of a strong tendon attached to the sternal manubrium, medial to the sternoclavicular joint space. It can be made to protrude by asking the subject to rotate her head contralaterally (relative to the muscle concerned), slightly flexing it ipsilaterally.

Fig. 1.59 Division of the sternal head of sternocleidomastoid

MA: The sternal head is sometimes divided into two sets of fibers: sternomastoid and sterno-occipital. Where this is the case, these two sets of fibers attach to the sternum by two quite distinct tendons. The tendon of the sterno-occipital head is lateral to that of the sternomastoid head. The action required is exactly the same as that described above. Where two heads exist, the practitioner's index finger can slide between them as shown in the adjacent figure.

Note: Do not confuse the interstitium between the two heads with the triangular space that is easily palpable when the muscle is contracted (contralateral rotation with head inclined ipsilaterally), distinguishing the clavicular head from the sternal head.

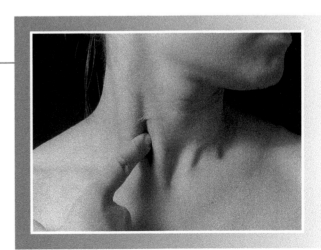

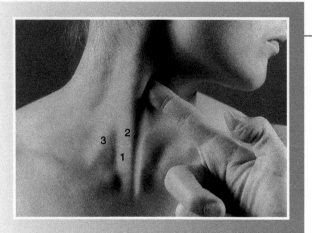

Fig. 1.60 Body of the sternal head of sternocleidomastoid

MA: The body of the muscle takes shape a little above the sternoclavicular joint, and runs in a cranio-posterolateral direction. Ask the subject to perform the same muscular action as that described for Figure 1.45.

Note: The number (1) indicates the triangular space between the sternal (2) and clavicular (3) heads of the sternocleidomastoid when the subject is asked to rotate her head and neck contralaterally.

Fig. 1.61 Clavicular head of sternocleidomastoid

MA: The practitioner's index finger indicates the cleido-occipital head, which is a superficial, oblique head arising distally on the medial third of the superior surface of the clavicle. It overlies the cleidomastoid head, which is aligned in a vertical direction. The muscular action requested of the subject is the same as that described for Figure 1.45. However, ask her this time to perform a more marked ipsilateral inclination of her head, and to flex her head slightly.

Note: In the illustration opposite, the practitioner's index finger rests in an enclosed triangular space whose base lies inferiorly, separating the sternal (1) and clavicular (2) portions, the two main sets of fibers of sternocleidomastoid.

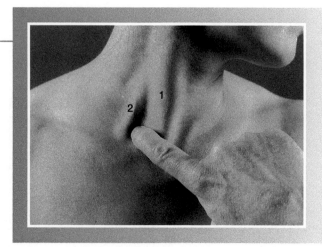

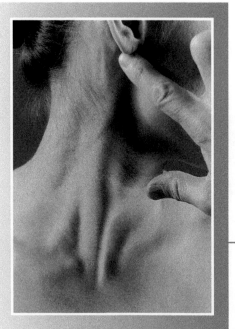

Fig. 1.62 The mastoid insertion of sternocleidomastoid

MA: Sternocleidomastoid terminates on the cranium by means of four heads:
- two occipital, with their insertion into the lateral part of the superior nuchal line (not shown on the adjacent figure);
- two mastoid, which are inserted into the mastoid process of the temporal bone (the structure indicated by the practitioner's index finger). The cleidomastoid head is inserted into the lateral surface of the mastoid process, and the sternomastoid on its apex.

THE ANTERIOR CERVICAL REGION

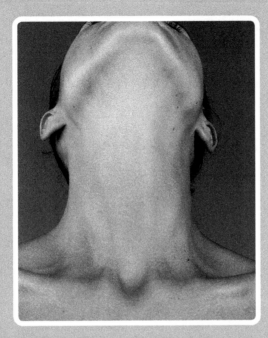

Fig. 1.63 The anterior cervical region

The notable structures that can be detected by palpation are:
- Platysma (Fig. 1.64)
- Mylohyoid (Fig. 1.65)
- Anterior belly of digastric (Fig. 1.66)
- Sternohyoid (topographical display) (Fig. 1.67)
- Body of sternohyoid (Fig. 1.68)
- Body of the superior (i.e., anterior) belly of omohyoid (Fig. 1.69)
- Sternothyroid (Fig. 1.70).

ACTIONS

- Suprahyoid muscles:
  - The geniohyoid and mylohyoid muscles and anterior belly of the digastric depress the mandible or elevate the hyoid. The action depends on which of these two bones is fixed.
  - The posterior belly of digastric, and stylohyoid, elevate the hyoid.
- Infrahyoid muscles: these depress the hyoid bone.
- All of the muscles acting on the hyoid also participate in lowering the mandible by fixing the inferior insertion of the suprahyoid muscles.

INNERVATIONS

- Platysma: facial nerve (CN VII)
- Mylohyoid: trigeminal nerve (CN V)
- Digastric (anterior belly): trigeminal nerve (CN V)
- Sternohyoid: ansa cervicalis of the cervical plexus
- Omohyoid (superior belly): ansa cervicalis of the cervical plexus
- Sternothyroid: ansa cervicalis of the cervical plexus

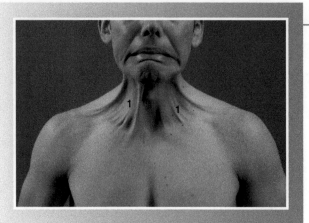

Fig. 1.64 Platysma

MA: This structure (1) can be made to appear if you ask the subject to turn down the corners of her mouth, at the same time pulling them outward (laterally) and backward. Platysma stretches between the labial commissure and the inferior border of the mandible superiorly, and the skin of the pectoral and deltoid regions inferiorly. Platysma creates ridges in the deep layer of the skin.

ATTACHMENTS

• This is a very broad, thin, quadrate muscle, covering the anterolateral region of the neck and the inferior part of the face. It extends from the thorax to the mandible and cheek.

Fig. 1.65 Mylohyoid

MA: This is the principal muscle of the floor of the mouth. Its inferior aspect is lined by the anterior belly of digastric and its superior aspect by geniohyoid. Ask the subject to lower her mandible, or open her mouth, or swallow. This will enable you to sense contraction below and inside the free border of the mandible. (This action elevates the hyoid bone when the fixed end is on the mandible.)

ATTACHMENTS

• Superiorly, this muscle arises along the full length of the mylohyoid line of the mandible by means of tendinous fibers.
• Inferiorly, it is inserted into the body of the hyoid.

The two mylohyoid muscles intersect on the median line to form a median raphe.

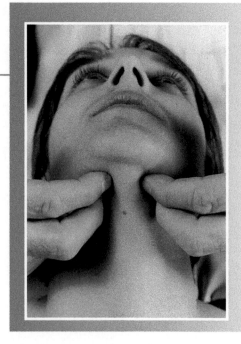

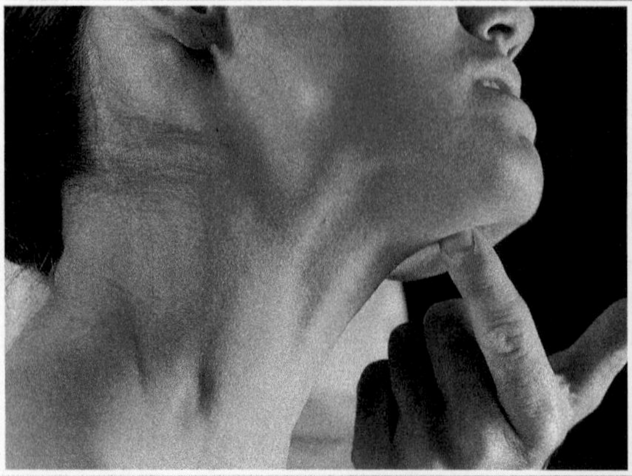

Fig. 1.66 Anterior belly of digastric

MA: This muscle is situated superior to the hyoid bone (Figs. 1.6–1.9); together with mylohyoid it forms part of the muscles of the floor of the mouth. Place your index finger in the interstitium between these two paired, symmetrical muscles, in contact with the raphe uniting the two mylohyoid muscles. The anterior bellies of the digastric muscles line the inferior surface of the mylohyoid muscles. The contraction can clearly be sensed if you ask the subject to lower her mandible.

Digastric is an elongated muscle made up of two bodies (the anterior and the posterior belly), which are joined by an intermediate tendon. It is situated in the superior, lateral part of the neck, and extends from the mastoid process to the mandibular symphysis.

Fig. 1.67 Sternohyoid (1), topographical display and attachments

MA: This muscle arises from the posterior surface of the sternoclavicular joint and adjacent parts of the clavicle and manubrium. It is inserted into the inferior border of the body of the hyoid bone, near the median line. These two muscles run superiorly and slightly medially (inward) in an oblique direction.

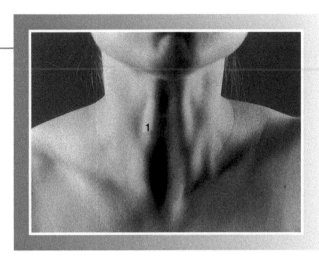

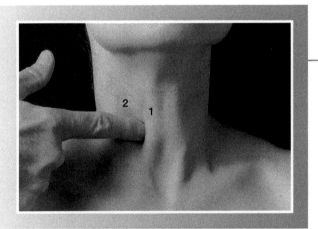

Fig. 1.68 Body of sternohyoid

MA: In the adjacent figure the practitioner's index finger is separating the body of sternohyoid (1) from sternocleidomastoid (2).

Topographical relations: This is a thin muscle extending from the clavicle to the hyoid, anterior to the sternothyroid and thyrohyoid muscles.

Note: In some subjects, the muscle bodies are less easy to identify.

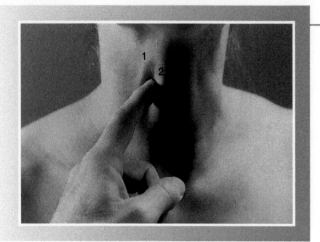

Fig. 1.69 Body of the superior belly of omohyoid

MA: This muscle (1) runs in a slightly oblique inferior and lateral (downward and outward) direction between the hyoid bone and the superior border of the scapula. The superior belly runs along the lateral border of sternohyoid (2) and then continues via an intermediate tendon into the inferior belly. The tendon marks the change in direction of the muscle, and lies at the same depth as the internal jugular vein. The inferior belly arises from the anterior surface of the body of the scapula, close to the superior border and medial to the suprascapular notch.

Note: Contraction of the omohyoid may possibly affect the blood flow of the internal jugular vein.

ATTACHMENTS

• The insertion of this muscle is by means of tendinous fibers on the inferior border of the body of the hyoid bone, lateral to sternohyoid.

Fig. 1.70 Sternothyroid

MA: Push aside the sternohyoid muscle laterally (1) with your index finger to access sternothyroid. It is not always possible to detect this muscle as such beneath your fingers in all subjects.

ATTACHMENTS

• This is a flattened, elongated muscle, extending from the sternum to the thyroid gland, anterior to the larynx and thyroid.

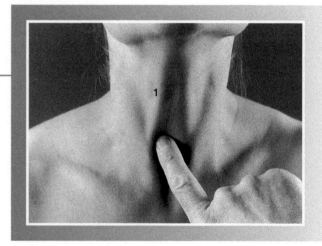

NERVES AND BLOOD VESSELS

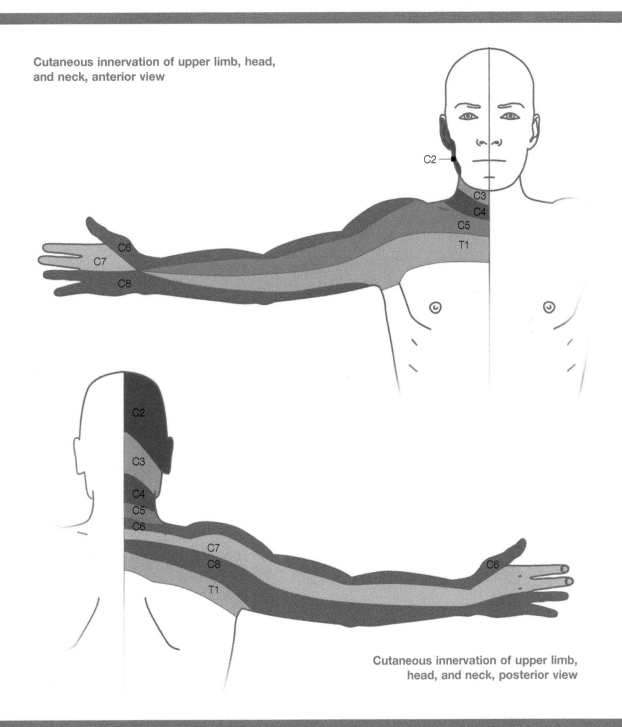

Cutaneous innervation of upper limb, head, and neck, anterior view

C2
C3
C4
C5
T1
C6
C7
C8

C2
C3
C4
C5
C6
C7
C8
T1
C6

Cutaneous innervation of upper limb, head, and neck, posterior view

THE PRINCIPAL NERVES AND BLOOD VESSELS

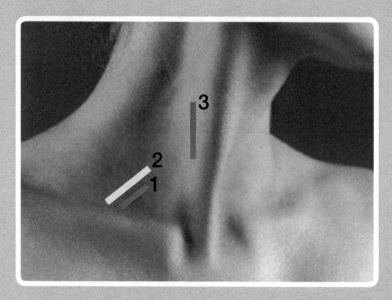

Fig. 1.71 The nerves and blood vessels of the neck
1. Subclavian artery
2. Brachial plexus
3. Carotid artery

The notable structures that can be detected by palpation are:
- Subclavian artery (Fig. 1.72)
- Brachial plexus (Fig. 1.73)
- Internal carotid artery. Taking the pulse (Fig. 1.74).

Fig. 1.72 Subclavian artery, taking the pulse

MA: Begin by locating the clavicular head of sternocleidomastoid. This can be done by contralateral rotation of the subject's head; ask her to turn her head to the opposite side. Place a broad contact with your fingers on the medial third of the clavicle, across the cleido-occipital head of the muscle; beneath your fingers you will detect the pulse of this artery.

Note: The subclavian artery passes just behind scalenus anterior.

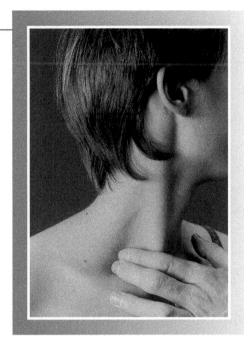

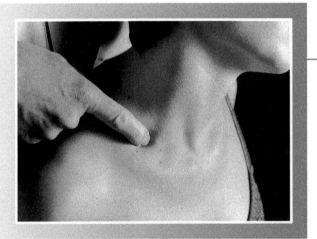

Fig. 1.73 Brachial plexus

MA: The approach is the same as that described above (Fig. 1.72). Through the cleido-occipital head, you will detect a full, cylindrical cord. This is the brachial plexus, indicated here by the practitioner's index finger. Ask the subject to rotate and incline her head to the opposite side; at the same time, extend and externally rotate her arm. This has the effect of stretching the structure and making it more easily perceptible.

Note: The brachial plexus passes between the scalenus anterior and scalenus medius muscles, together with the subclavian artery.

Fig. 1.74 Internal carotid artery, taking the pulse

The carotid pulse can be taken either anteriorly and medially to the sternal head of sternocleidomastoid (1), as in the adjacent figure, or posteriorly and laterally to it.

Note: The carotid pulse is only ever taken on one side at a time, so as not to arrest cerebral circulation completely. Great care should be taken when applying pressure to the carotid artery, because, if there are any atheromatous plaques present, they could become detached and cause a cerebral embolism. The carotid pulse is extremely useful in an emergency situation, as it can be detected at low blood pressure (around 60 mmHg). This level is just sufficient to keep the brain from hypoxia.

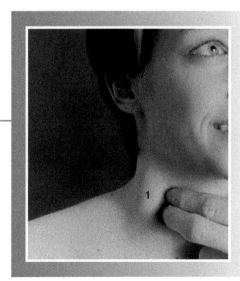

2
The trunk and sacrum

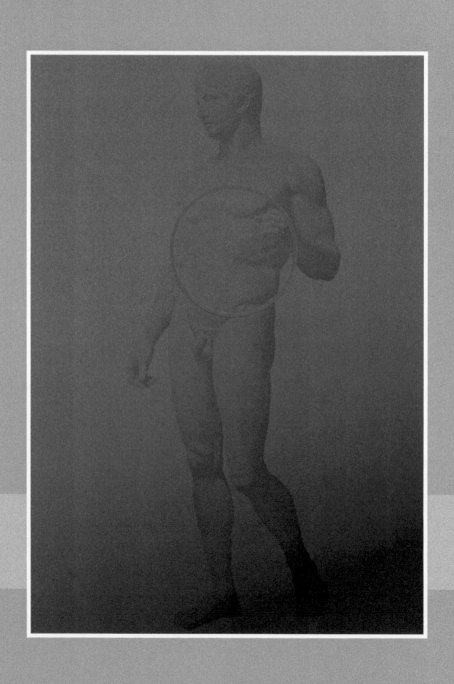

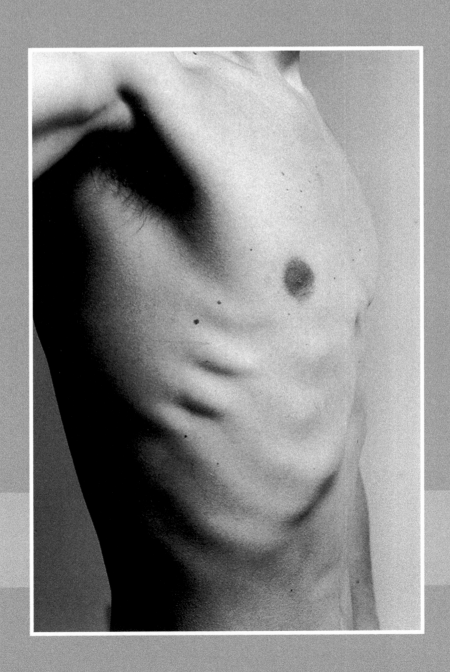

OSTEOLOGY

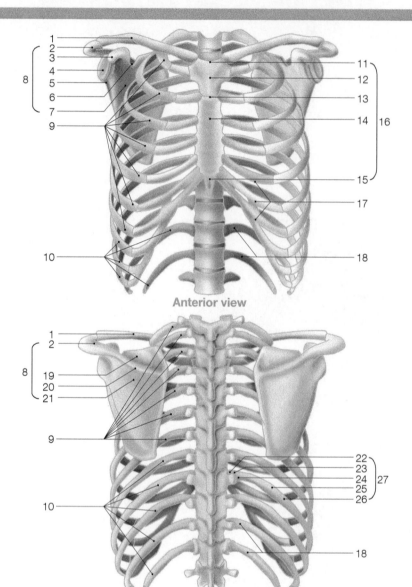

Anterior view

Posterior view

The bones of the thoracic cage

1. Clavicle	8. Scapula	15. Xiphoid process	22. Head
2. Acromion	9. True ribs	16. Sternum	23. Neck
3. Coracoid process	10. False ribs	17. Costal cartilages	24. Tubercle
4. Glenoid cavity	11. Jugular notch	18. Floating ribs	25. Angle
5. Neck	12. Manubrium	19. Supraspinous fossa	26. Shaft
6. Suprascapular notch	13. Sternal angle	20. Spine	27. Rib
7. Subscapular fossa	14. Body	21. Infraspinous fossa	

Vertebra T6

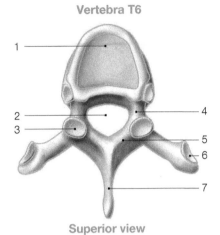

1
2
3
4
5
6
7

Superior view

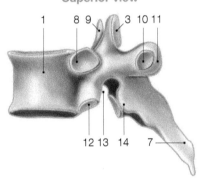

1 8 9 3 10 11

12 13 14 7

1. Body
2. Vertebral foramen
3. Superior articular facet
4. Pedicle
5. Lamina
6. Transverse costal facet
7. Spinous process
8. Superior costal facet
9. Superior articular process
10. Transverse costal facet
11. Transverse process
12. Inferior costal facet
13. Inferior vertebral notch
14. Inferior articular process
15. Costal facet

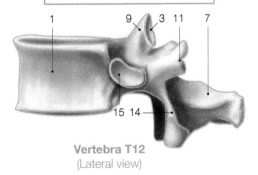

9 3 11 7
1
15 14

Vertebra T12
(Lateral view)

A typical rib
(superior view)

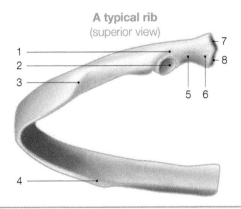

1
2
3
7
8
5 6
4

1. Tubercle
2. Articular facet for transverse process of vertebra
3. Angle
4. Costal groove
5. Neck
6. Head
7. Superior articular facet of head of rib
8. Inferior articular facet of head of rib

Vertebrae T7, T8, T9
(posterior view)

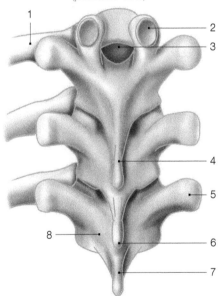

1
2
3
4
5
8
6
7

1. Seventh rib
2. Superior articular process and facet
3. Vertebral canal
4. Spinous process of T7
5. Transverse process of T9
6. Inferior articular process of T9
7. Spinous process of T9
8. Lamina

Vertebral column

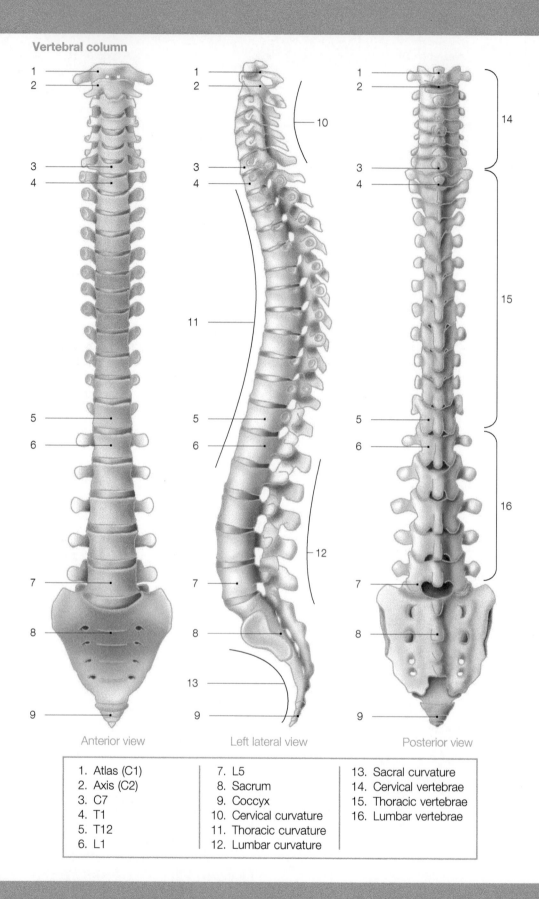

Anterior view

Left lateral view

Posterior view

1. Atlas (C1)	7. L5	13. Sacral curvature
2. Axis (C2)	8. Sacrum	14. Cervical vertebrae
3. C7	9. Coccyx	15. Thoracic vertebrae
4. T1	10. Cervical curvature	16. Lumbar vertebrae
5. T12	11. Thoracic curvature	
6. L1	12. Lumbar curvature	

Vertebra L2
Superior view

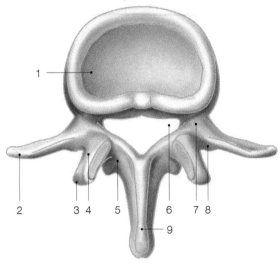

1. Body
2. Transverse process
3. Mammillary process
4. Superior articular process
5. Lamina
6. Vertebral foramen
7. Pedicle
8. Accessory process
9. Spinous process
10. Vertebral canal
11. Inferior articular process

Vertebrae L3 and L4
Posterior view

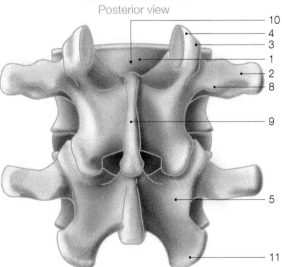

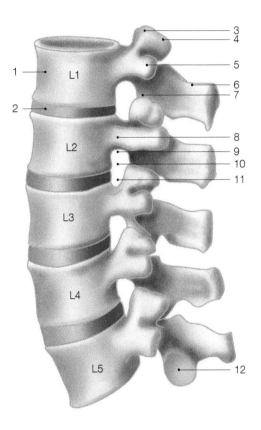

Lumbar vertebrae (left lateral view)

1. Body
2. Intervertebral disk
3. Superior articular process
4. Mammillary process
5. Transverse process
6. Spinous process
7. Inferior articular process
8. Pedicle
9. Inferior vertebral notch
10. Intervertebral foramen
11. Superior vertebral notch
12. Articular facet for the sacrum

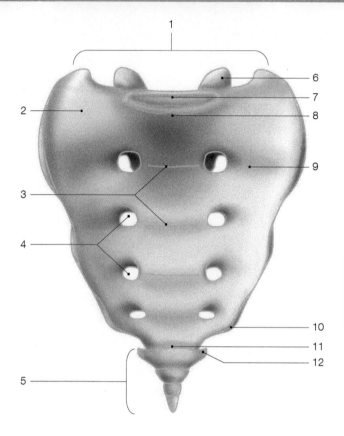

Sacrum
(anteroinferior view)

1. Base of sacrum
2. Ala (wing)
3. Transverse ridges
4. Anterior sacral foramina
5. Coccyx
6. Superior articular process
7. Lumbosacral articular facet
8. Promontory
9. Sacral part of pelvic inlet
10. Inferolateral angle (ILA)
11. Apex of sacrum
12. Transverse process of coccyx

Sacrum
(posterosuperior view)

1. Auricular surface
2. Sacral tuberosity
3. Lateral sacral crest
4. Median sacral crest
5. Posterior sacral foramina
6. Sacral hiatus
7. Articular facet of superior articular process
8. Lateral sacral horn (cornu)
9. Coccygeal horn (cornu)
10. Transverse process of coccyx

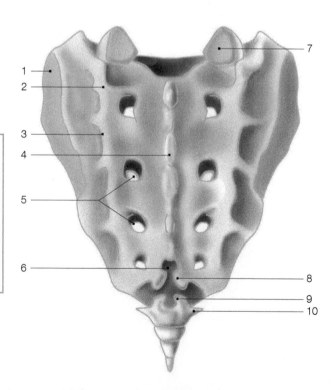

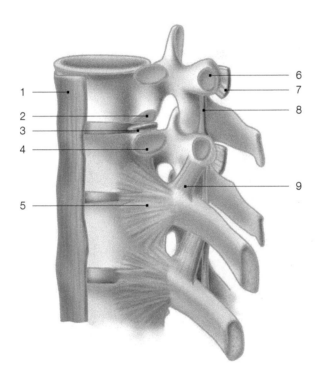

Costovertebral joints
(left lateral view)

1. Anterior longitudinal ligament
2. Inferior costal facet
3. Intra-articular ligament of costal head
4. Superior costal facet
5. Radial ligament of costal head
6. Costal facet of transverse process
7. Lateral costotransverse ligament
8. Intertransverse ligament
9. Superior costotransverse ligament

THE THORAX

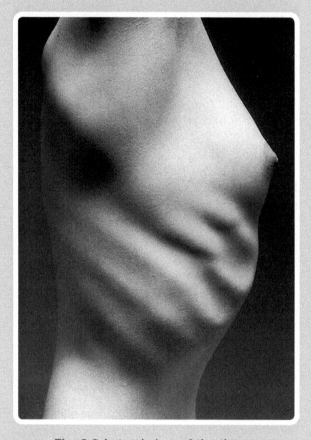

Fig. 2.2 Lateral view of the thorax

The notable structures that can be detected by palpation are:
- Sternum: general view (Fig. 2.3)
- Manubrium of the sternum (Fig. 2.4)
- Jugular (suprasternal) notch (Fig. 2.5)
- Sternal angle (Fig. 2.6)
- Body of sternum (Fig. 2.7)
- Xiphoid process (Fig. 2.8)
- Superior thoracic aperture (Fig. 2.9)
- First costal cartilage (Fig. 2.10)
- First rib: shaft above the clavicle (Fig. 2.11)
- Posterior extremity of the shaft of the first rib (Figs. 2.12 and 2.13)
- Tubercle of scalenus anterior muscle (Fig. 2.14)
- Anterior extremity of the shaft of the second rib (Fig. 2.15)
- Shaft of the second rib in the anterior part of the thorax (Fig. 2.16)
- The second rib in the lateral cervical region (Fig. 2.17)
- Posterior extremity of the shaft of the second rib (Fig. 2.18)
- True ribs (see Note to Fig. 2.11) (Fig. 2.19)
- False ribs (Fig. 2.20)
- Inferior thoracic aperture (Fig. 2.21)
- Notches of the costal margin (seventh, eighth, ninth, and tenth costal cartilages) (Fig. 2.22)
- Eleventh rib (Fig. 2.23): anterior extremity (Fig. 2.24)
- Twelfth rib (Fig. 2.25)
- Twelfth rib (Fig. 2.26): anterior extremity (Fig. 2.27)
- Tenth rib (Fig. 2.28)
- Angle of rib (Fig. 2.29).

Fig. 2.3 Sternum, general view

MA: This is a flat, unpaired bone occupying the median ventral part of the thorax, the area between the practitioner's index fingers in the adjacent figure. It is made up of three parts: the cranial part or manubrium (Fig. 2.4); a middle part, the body of the sternum (or mesosternum) (Fig. 2.7); and a caudal part, the xiphoid process (Fig. 2.8).

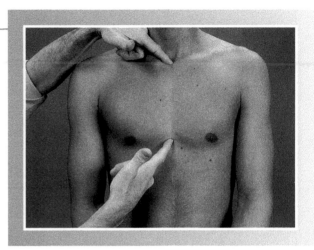

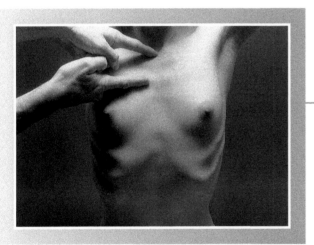

Fig. 2.4 Manubrium of the sternum

MA: The manubrium lies in the position indicated here between the practitioner's index fingers. It accounts for about one third of the total length of the sternum. The junction with the body of the sternum (Fig. 2.7) is at the level of the second rib.

Fig. 2.5 Jugular (suprasternal) notch

MA: This is situated on the base or superior (cranial) border of the sternum, as indicated by the practitioner's index finger. It can be felt beneath the index finger as an upward-facing concave notch.

Note: There are two other notches on this segment of the sternum: the clavicular notches. These receive the medial extremity of the clavicles. They are concave in the transverse direction and flat anteriorly and posteriorly, and they face upward and outward.

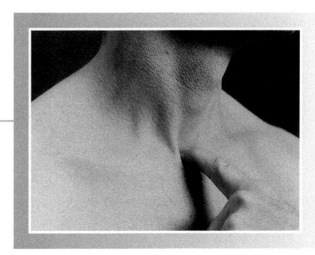

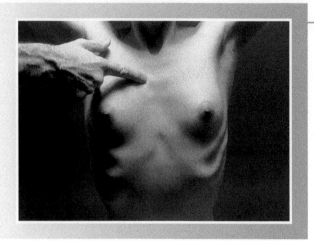

Fig. 2.6 Sternal angle

MA: This structure, indicated by the practitioner's index finger, represents the line of union between the manubrium (Fig. 2.4) and body (Fig. 2.7) of the sternum. This junction is at the level of the second rib, and forms the anteriorly raised crest of a dihedral angle.

Fig. 2.7 Body of the sternum

MA: The practitioner's index fingers indicate the general position of this part of the sternum, situated between the sternal angle (Fig. 2.6) and the xiphoid process (Fig. 2.8). When you palpate the anterior part of this structure, you will find three or four transverse crests, which are the vestiges of the fusion of the sternebrae. You will also detect vertical ridges that provide attachment to the sternochondral parts of pectoralis major (see Chapter 3).

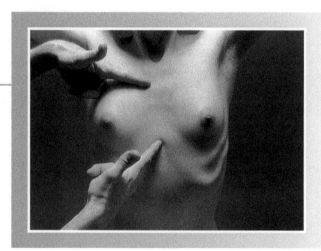

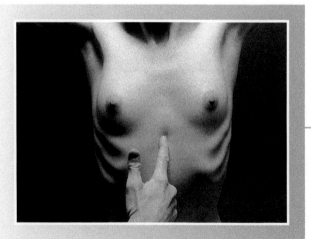

Fig. 2.8 Xiphoid process

MA: This is situated at the caudal extremity of the body of the sternum (Fig. 2.7), aligned as an extension of its posterior surface. Palpation of this structure therefore finds it to be slightly recessed. The tip of the xiphoid process is sometimes forked and may incline forward, backward, or to the side. Accessibility therefore varies between different subjects.

Note: This structure is almost always cartilaginous in adults.

Fig. 2.9 Superior thoracic aperture

MA: This aperture is elliptical in shape, the transverse diameter being the larger. It is inclined obliquely anteriorly and inferiorly. It is bounded anteriorly by the jugular notch (1) (see also Fig. 2.5), which aligns with the inferior border of the second thoracic vertebra. Laterally it is bounded by the first rib (2) and posteriorly by the superior border of the first thoracic vertebra.

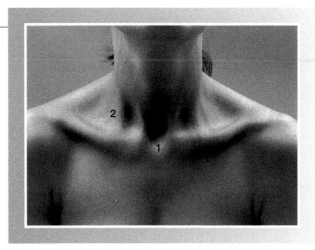

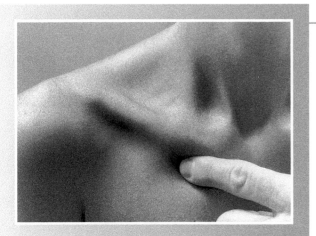

Fig. 2.10 The first costal cartilage

MA: To locate this structure, place your index finger immediately below the clavicle, in contact with the lateral border of the manubrium of the sternum. If this proves difficult, ask the subject to take rapid, repeated in-breaths. This makes it easier to sense the structure beneath your index finger.

CLINICAL NOTE

Costoclavicular syndrome

The point of compression is between the inferior surface of the clavicle and the superior part of the first rib. Here, the brachial plexus meets the subclavian artery and is in contact with the first rib. The compression is caused by the reduced angle created when the shoulders are lowered as they are pulled back, for example, when carrying a backpack. Closing of this angle can produce two possible scenarios:

- neurologic: pain, paresthesia, motor problems (of the upper limb);

- vascular: reduction or loss of the radial pulse, edema, or venous thrombosis.

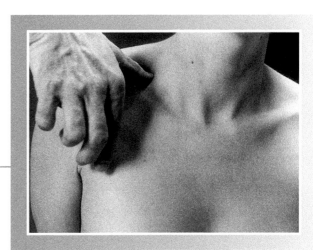

Fig. 2.11 First rib: shaft above the clavicle

MA: Place your contact above and behind the clavicle, where you will find a structure that feels dense. This is the first rib. It can be palpated along almost its entire length.

Note: The first rib is a true rib, i.e., a rib that is attached to the sternum by means of a costal cartilage.

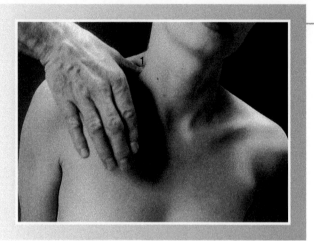

Fig. 2.12 Posterior extremity of the shaft of the first rib

MA: It is very easy to access the first rib at this point; push back the superior fibers of trapezius (1) in a posterior direction, as shown here, until you encounter it.

Fig. 2.13 Close-up of posterior extremity of the shaft of the first rib

MA: The adjacent figure shows the practitioner's thumb pushing back the superior fibers of trapezius (1) and resting on the posterior-most part of the cranial surface of the first rib.

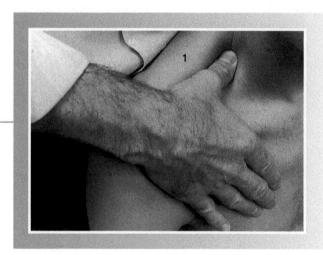

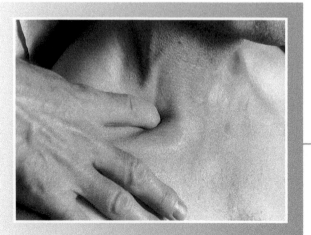

Fig. 2.14 Tubercle of scalenus anterior

MA: Beginning from a position above and behind the clavicle, loosen the musculature of the region; this will make it easier to locate the tubercle. The best way to do this is to ask the subject to turn and incline his head to the ipsilateral side. In some subjects, you will feel the tubercle through the thickness of the two clavicular heads of sternocleidomastoid.

Fig. 2.15 Anterior extremity of the shaft of the second rib

MA: This lies between the first rib and middle ribs, at the lateral extension of the sternal angle (1) (see also Fig. 2.6). In the adjacent figure, the practitioner's index finger is in the second intercostal space, lying in contact with the inferior part of the second rib.

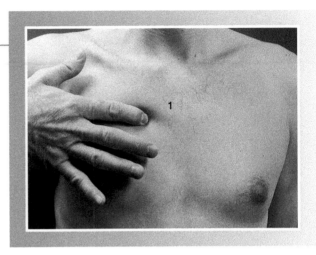

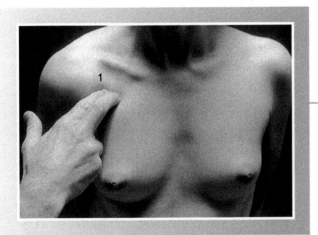

Fig. 2.16 Shaft of the second rib in the anterior part of the thorax

MA: As indicated in the adjacent figure, the second rib can be followed along its length, in the direction of the coracoid process (1), as far as the point where the rib passes under the clavicle.

Note: The second rib is a true rib (see Note to Fig. 2.11).

Fig. 2.17 Shaft of the second rib in the lateral cervical region (posterior triangle of the neck)

MA: In the lateral cervical region, behind the lateral extremity of the clavicle (1), there is a dense structure that can be felt beneath your fingers when you push aside trapezius (2) posteriorly. This bony structure is the second rib. It is easier to detect if you direct your contact downward and ask the subject to take short, repeated in-breaths using the upper part of the thoracic cage, so mobilizing the second rib.

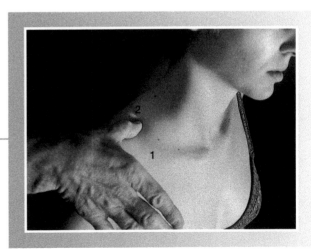

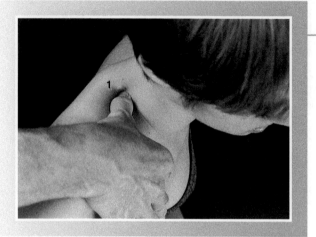

Fig. 2.18 Posterior extremity of the shaft of the second rib

MA: In the adjacent figure, the practitioner is palpating the spinal extremity of the second rib. Push aside trapezius (1) using a contact positioned posterior and inferior to the first rib (see Fig. 2.12).

Fig. 2.19 True ribs

MA: The sternal extremity of the true ribs (1) can clearly be seen down as far as the sixth rib in the adjacent figure. The seventh rib can be seen in Figure 2.20. The true ribs can be counted easily, starting from the sternal angle (see Fig. 2.6), which corresponds to the second rib. There are seven true ribs. (See Note to Fig. 2.11.)

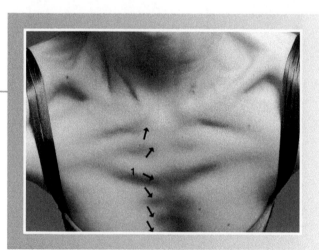

Fig. 2.20 False ribs (8, 9, and 10)

MA: The three false ribs (the eighth, ninth, and tenth), indicated by the practitioner's spread fingers in the adjacent figure, have the special feature that they are linked anteriorly by means of their cartilaginous ventral extremity, which extends and unites them to the costal cartilage above. Together with the cartilage of the seventh rib (7), they make up the costal margin (costal arch).

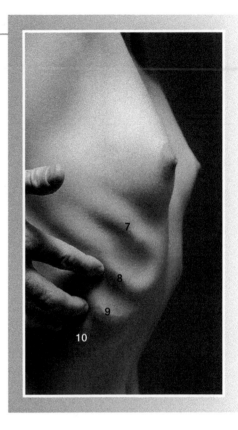

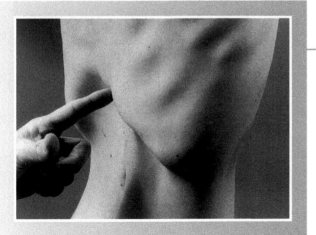

Fig. 2.21 Inferior thoracic aperture

MA: This is an elliptical aperture, whose larger diameter is transverse. It is approximately three times as large as the superior thoracic aperture (Fig. 2.9). It lies on a plane that is inclined downward and posteriorly. It is delimited ventrally (anteriorly) by the xiphoid process (Fig. 2.8), which is in line with the tenth thoracic vertebra, and dorsally (posteriorly) by the body of the twelfth thoracic vertebra. Laterally it is delimited by the costal margin (seventh, eighth, ninth, and tenth costal cartilages) and floating ribs. (See Figs. 2.23–2.27.)

Note: This aperture is filled by the diaphragm.

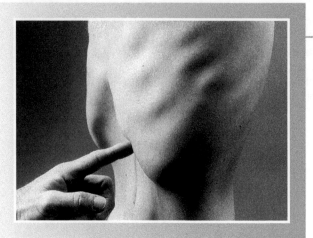

Fig. 2.22 The notches of the costal margin (seventh, eighth, ninth, and tenth costal cartilages)

MA: As you palpate along the inferior border of the costal margin from the xiphoid process, two notches are evident. The first (indicated in Fig. 2.21 by the practitioner's index finger) corresponds to the junction of the seventh and eighth costal cartilages. There is a second notch (indicated by the practitioner's index finger in the adjacent figure) corresponding to the junction of the ninth and tenth costal cartilages.

Note: These two notches are not always clearly marked.

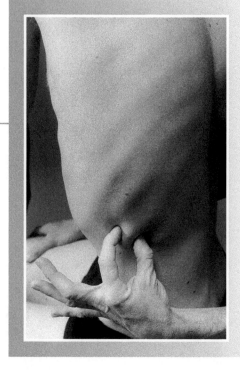

Fig. 2.23 Eleventh rib

MA: The adjacent figure shows the eleventh rib, held between the practitioner's thumb and index finger. The best approach is to stand behind the subject, placing your two hands on the inferior border of the costal margin (Fig. 2.20). Locate the inferior border of the tenth rib and place your contact here. Now shift your contact to a position level with the anterolateral abdominal wall, toward the iliac crest, feeling for a rib situated immediately below the caudal border of the costal margin, one that has a free ventral (anterior) extremity.

Note: The iliac crest is described in Chapter 8.

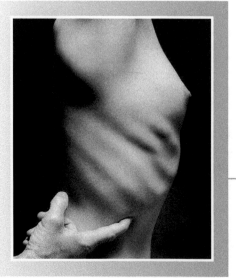

Fig. 2.24 Eleventh rib, anterior extremity

MA: In the adjacent figure, the practitioner's index finger indicates the ventral (anterior) extremity of the eleventh rib, with a tapered costal cartilage whose end is free. This is termed a floating rib.

Note: This rib has a length of around 20 cm (8 inches). Its ventral extremity is usually at some distance from the inferior border of the tenth rib. However, it can be close to it, or even fused with it.

Fig. 2.25 Twelfth rib

MA: The adjacent figure shows the twelfth rib, which the practitioner is grasping between thumb and index finger. Having located the eleventh rib (Figs. 2.23 and 2.24), shift your contact down the subject's side in the direction of the iliac crest, at the same time moving it posteriorly, since the twelfth rib is slightly shorter than the eleventh.

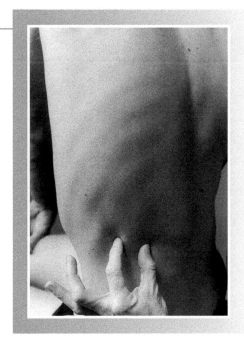

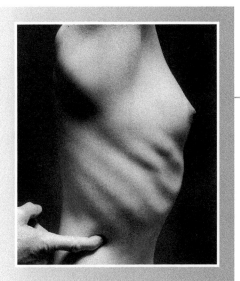

Fig. 2.26 Twelfth rib, anterior extremity – lateral view

MA: In the adjacent figure, the practitioner's index finger is positioned on the ventral (anterior) extremity of the twelfth rib. Like the eleventh, it ends in a tapered, free costal cartilage.

Note: The twelfth rib is also floating, and is usually (in about two thirds of cases) between 10 and 14 cm (4–5½ inches) long. However, it can be very short, measuring 3–6 cm (1½–2½ inches), in which case it can be confused with the transverse process of a lumbar vertebra.

Fig. 2.27 Twelfth rib, anterior extremity – anterolateral view

MA: In the adjacent figure, the practitioner's index finger is positioned on the ventral (anterior) extremity of the twelfth rib. This anterolateral view of the thorax shows the relationship between this structure and the eleventh rib (Figs. 2.23 and 2.24) and with the seventh, eighth, ninth, and tenth ribs, which make up the costal margin (Fig. 2.20).

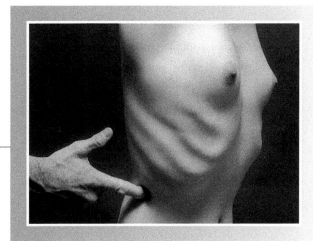

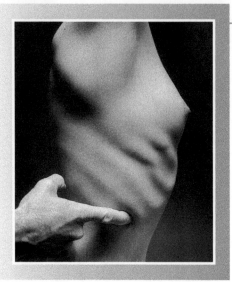

Fig. 2.28 Tenth rib

MA: The ventral (anterior) extremity of the tenth rib may be unattached to the cartilage of the ninth. In that case its anterior extremity remains free. The practitioner's index finger is on that extremity in this figure.

Fig. 2.29 The angle of the rib

MA: This angle represents the first change in direction of the rib on the dorsal part of the thorax. From this point on, it takes a downward, anterior direction.

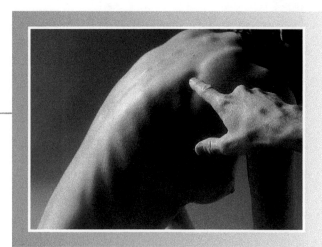

THE THORACOLUMBAR SPINE

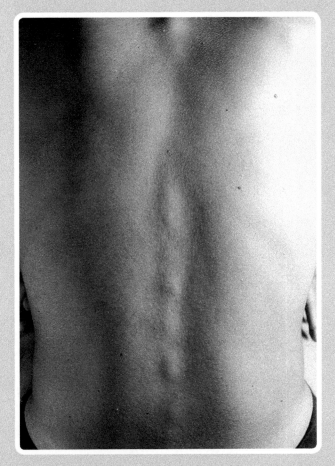

Fig. 2.30 Posterior view of the thoracolumbar spine in the forward flexed position

The notable structures that can be detected by palpation are:
- Thoracic spine: all the thoracic vertebrae from T1 to T12 (Fig. 2.31)
- Cervicothoracic transition (C6–C7–T1) (Fig. 2.32)
- Vertebrae C6, C7, and T1 (Figs. 2.33 and 2.34)
- Display of relations between the scapula and spinous processes of the vertebrae (Fig. 2.35)
- Spinous process of T1 (Fig. 2.36)
- Spinous process of T3 (Fig. 2.37)
- Spinous process of T7 (Fig. 2.38)
- Transverse process of the thoracic vertebrae (Fig. 2.39)
- Lumbar spine: all the lumbar vertebrae from L1 to L5 (Fig. 2.40)
- Fourth (L4) and fifth (L5) lumbar vertebrae (Figs. 2.41 and 2.42)
- Costal process of the lumbar vertebrae (Fig. 2.43).

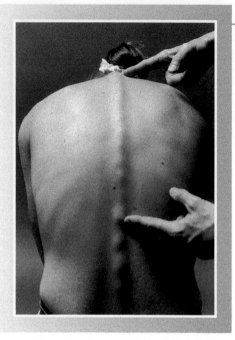

Fig. 2.31 Thoracic spine: all the thoracic vertebrae from T1 to T12

MA: The extent of the thoracic spine (all the thoracic vertebrae from T1 to T12) is shown here by the position of the practitioner's two index fingers.

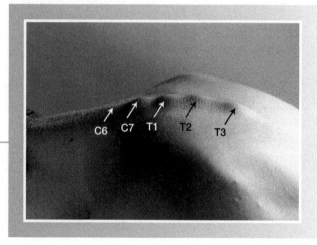

Fig. 2.32 The cervicothoracic transition C6–C7–T1

MA: The adjacent figure clearly shows the spinous processes of the last cervical vertebra, C7, and the first thoracic vertebrae, T1, T2, and T3.

Note: The subject is seated, with head bent forward.

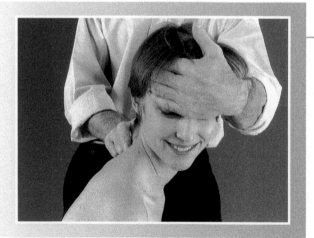

Fig. 2.33 Exploration of C6, C7, and T1, test while rotating the head

MA: The subject is seated with her head in a neutral position (or slightly bent). The practitioner should stand beside her. Place your index, middle, and ring fingers on the spinous processes of the sixth (C6) and seventh (C7) cervical vertebrae and first thoracic vertebra (T1) (Fig. 2.32). Then, with your other hand, take hold of the subject's head and ease it into rotation to the right and then to the left, several times if necessary. You will detect a slight movement at the level of C7; no movement occurs at T1, but there is marked movement at C6.

Note: The slight motion detected when the subject's head is turned can vary; it may be zero when the head is turned to the right, but more marked when turned the other way. That is why it is necessary to test both sides.

Fig. 2.34 Exploration of C6, C7, and T1, test with head extended

MA: The subject should be seated with her head in a neutral position (neither flexed nor extended). The practitioner stands beside the subject. Place the index, middle, and ring fingers of one hand on the spinous processes of the sixth and seventh cervical vertebrae (C6 and C7) and first thoracic vertebra (T1) (Fig. 2.32). Hold the subject's forehead in the palm of your other hand, and ease her head into hyperextension. The spinous process of C6 will "disappear" into the physiological cervical curvature, the spinous process of C7 will be "displaced" (the extent of this varies, depending on the subject), and the spinous process of T1 will remain immobile beneath your fingers.

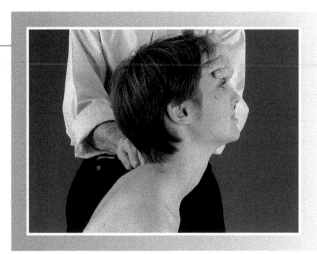

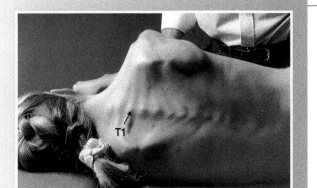

Fig. 2.35 Display of the relationship between the scapula and spinous processes

MA: In the adjacent figure, with the subject lying on her side, the craniomedial angle of the scapula is seen to be in line with the spinous process of the first thoracic vertebra, T1. The medial extremity of the spine of the scapula is in line with the spinous process of T3, and the inferior angle of the scapula with the spinous process of T7.

Note: You should regard the above approach as aiming to help initial rapid exploration of the spinous processes. The next stage is to "count" along from C7 (see Figs. 2.32–2.34) or from L5 (see Figs. 2.41 and 2.42). The positions described here should simply be taken as indicative. Various factors may significantly affect the topographical relationships between the scapula and vertebral column. For example: the position of the scapula on the thoracic cage (and its mobility), the position of the subject on the table, or a number of possible dysmorphisms (kyphosis, flat back, scoliosis, etc.).

Fig. 2.36 Locating the spinous process of T1

MA: In the adjacent figure, the practitioner's thumb and index finger demonstrate the relationship (see Fig. 2.35) between the craniomedial angle of the scapula (indicated by the practitioner's thumb) and the spinous process of the first thoracic vertebra (indicated by the practitioner's index finger).

Note: Figures 2.33 and 2.34 show the most reliable method of finding T1.

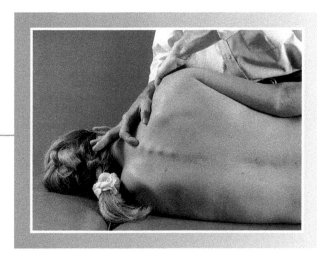

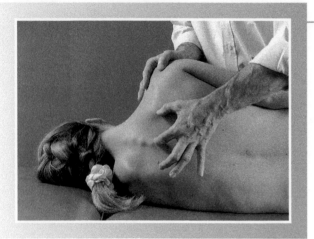

Fig. 2.37 Locating the spinous process of T3

MA: In the adjacent figure, the practitioner's thumb and index finger contact demonstrates the relationship (see also Fig. 2.35) between the medial extremity of the spine of the scapula (indicated by the practitioner's thumb) and the spinous process of the third thoracic vertebra (T3, indicated by the practitioner's index finger).

Note: The most reliable method of locating this structure is by counting from vertebra C7 (Figs. 2.32–2.34).

Fig. 2.38 Locating the spinous process of T7

MA: In the adjacent figure, the practitioner's thumb and index finger demonstrate the relationship (see also Fig. 2.35) between the inferior angle of the scapula and the spinous process of the seventh thoracic vertebra, T7 (indicated by the practitioner's index finger).

Note: The most reliable method of locating this structure is by counting from vertebra C7 (Figs. 2.32–2.34).

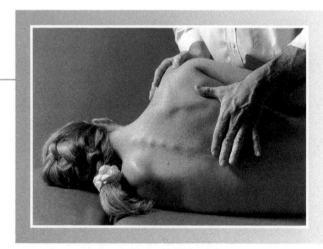

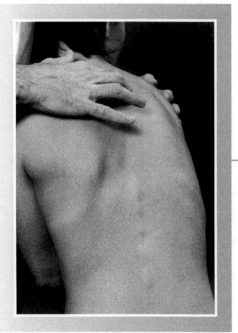

Fig. 2.39 Transverse process of the thoracic vertebrae

MA: The subject is seated, with the practitioner standing alongside. Cradle the anterior surface of her shoulders in the palms of your hands. Search medial to the costal angle and about two finger-breadths lateral to the spinous processes. The transverse process is felt as a dense entity, as it is a bony structure. Use of a cradling hold will enable you to induce rotation of the trunk, which makes it easier to locate the structure. It can be difficult to access in some subjects for reasons of morphology.

Note: The figure shown here demonstrates the method of approach, not the bony structure concerned. Rotation of the trunk makes the costal angle more prominent and easier to distinguish from the transverse process of the vertebra, two finger-breadths away from the spinous process.

Fig. 2.40 The lumbar spine: all the lumbar vertebrae from L1 to L5

MA: In the adjacent figure, the practitioner's index fingers indicate the lumbar spine (all the lumbar vertebrae from L1 to L5).

Note: The lumbar spine consists of five lumbar vertebrae. Their number may be increased by one if the first sacral vertebra, S1, appears as a lumbar vertebra, or decreased by one if the last lumbar vertebra, L5, takes the form of a sacral vertebra.

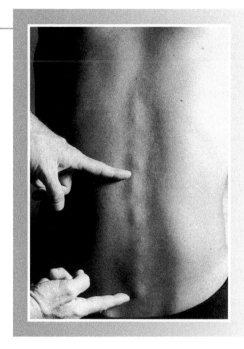

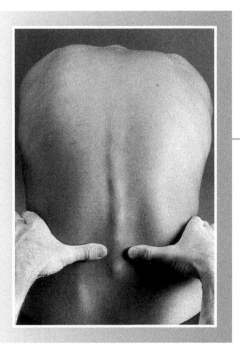

Fig. 2.41 Locating the fourth (L4) and fifth (L5) lumbar vertebrae

MA: In the adjacent figure, the practitioner's hands are resting on the iliac crest with his thumbs extended toward the lumbar spine. If you let your thumbs fall naturally, so that they are placed slightly ahead of your palms, they point toward the intervertebral disc (L4–L5, as in the figure here). If your thumbs are placed in the same plane as the palms of your hands, they point toward the spinous process of the fourth lumbar vertebra, L4.

Fig. 2.42 Locating the fifth (L5) lumbar vertebra

MA: Once you have located L4 (see Fig. 2.41), the spinous process of the vertebra below it can be contacted. This is the fifth lumbar vertebra, indicated in this figure by the practitioner's index finger.

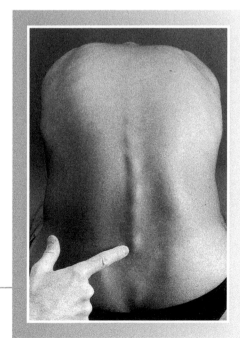

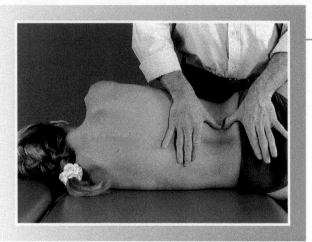

Fig. 2.43 Transverse or costal process of the lumbar vertebrae

MA: The subject should lie on the contralateral side. Place your thumbs lateral to the erector spinae muscles and direct your contact toward the lumbar spine until you make contact with a dense structure. This is the structure you are looking for.

Notes:

- When examining well-muscled subjects, you should locate this density using a posterior approach through the mass of the erector spinae muscles.
- The transverse (costal) process of the first lumbar vertebra is shorter than that of the other lumbar vertebrae. The costal process of the fifth lumbar vertebra is longer than that of the other lumbar vertebrae. If this process is more than usually developed, it may connect and fuse with the hip bone (coxal bone, pelvic bone). This has the effect of making L5 a sacral vertebra (see also note to Fig. 2.40).

THE SACRUM

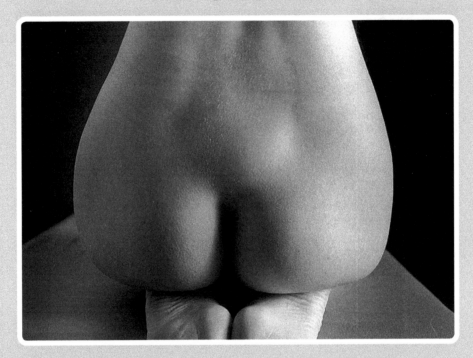

Fig. 2.44 Posterior view of the pelvis and sacrum

The notable structures that can be detected by palpation are:
- Posterolateral display of the sacrum (Fig. 2.45)
- Dorsal (posterior) and lateral part of the first sacral vertebra (S1) (Fig. 2.46)
- Spinous process of the first sacral vertebra (S1) (Fig. 2.47)
- Spinous process of the second sacral vertebra (S2) (Figs. 2.48–2.50)
- Median sacral crest (Fig. 2.51)
- Sacral cornua (sacral horns) (Fig. 2.52)
- Sacral hiatus (Fig. 2.53)
- Lateral border of the sacrum: posterolateral view (Fig. 2.54)
- Lateral border of the sacrum: posterior view (Fig. 2.55)
- The "base" of the sacrum (Fig. 2.56)
- Sacral sulci (Fig. 2.57)
- Median sacral crest (Fig. 2.58)
- The ipsilateral border (Fig. 2.59)
- Lateral borders (Fig. 2.60)
- The contralateral border (Fig. 2.61)
- Sacral cornua (sacral horns) (Fig. 2.62)
- The inferolateral angles (ILA) (Fig. 2.63)
- The inferolateral angles, another method of approach (Fig. 2.64).

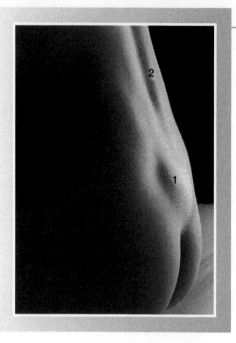

Fig. 2.45 Posterolateral display of the sacrum

MA: In the adjacent figure, the position of the sacrum (1) can be seen in relief below the lumbar spine (2).

Fig. 2.46 Dorsal (posterior) and lateral part of the first sacral vertebra (S1)

MA: The subject should lie face down. The practitioner should stand alongside the root of her lower limbs. Begin by placing your hands on either side of the lumbar spine, then move them down the lumbar spine, sliding the pressure along until (just below L5) you make contact with a ridge which you will feel beneath your fingers (as shown in the adjacent figure). This is the structure you are seeking.

Note: Beyond L5, the practitioner's hands have naturally come to rest on the sacrum, as its dorsal (or posterior) surface is oriented dorsally and cranially (backward and upward).

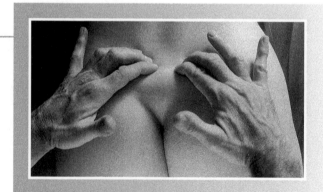

Fig. 2.47 Spinous process of the first sacral vertebra (S1)

MA: Begin by locating the spinous process of L5 (see Figs. 2.41 and 2.42). Then shift your contact caudally to find the first tubercle situated along the median sacral crest. This tubercle is the spinous process of S1.

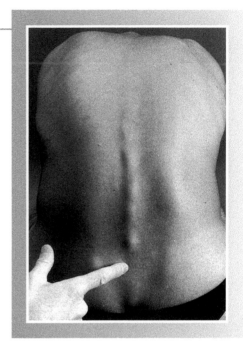

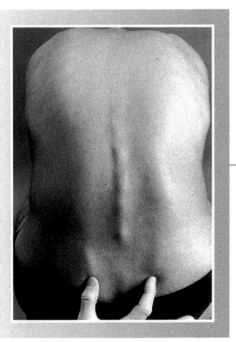

Fig. 2.48 Spinous process of the second sacral vertebra (S2), step 1

MA: In the adjacent figure, the subject is seated, leaning forward. The practitioner's thumb and index finger indicate the posterior superior iliac spine of each of the two hip bones.

Fig. 2.49 Spinous process of the second sacral vertebra (S2), step 1 – another approach

MA: In the adjacent figure, the practitioner's index finger indicates the depression (which varies in intensity from one subject to another) opposite the sacroiliac joint. This position on the skin corresponds approximately to the posterior superior iliac spine.

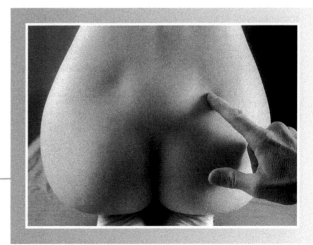

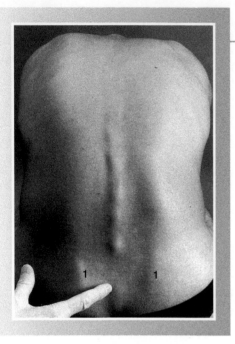

Fig. 2.50 Spinous process of the second sacral vertebra (S2), step 2

MA: Once you have located the posterior superior iliac spines (1), which may be clearly visible (as in Fig. 2.48) or not (as in Fig. 2.49), trace a hypothetical horizontal line between the two. The center of this line corresponds to the second tubercle of the median sacral crest. This is the structure you are seeking.

Fig. 2.51 Median sacral crest

MA: Broad fingertip contact in the middle of the dorsal surface of the sacrum, as shown in this figure, continuous with the spinous processes of the lumbar vertebrae, locates the median sacral crest. You will be better able to sense its anatomical structure if you rub your fingers across it, using the contact described, in a transverse direction.

Note: The median sacral crest is made up of three or four tubercles, created by the fusion of the spinous processes of the five sacral vertebrae. A slight depression separates each individual spinous process from the next.

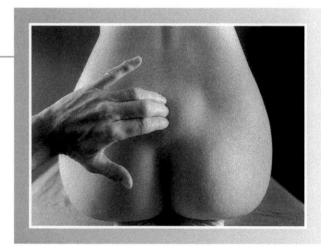

Fig. 2.52 Sacral cornua (sacral horns)

MA: These structures can be seen just above the intergluteal cleft, as two small bony columns either side of the depression that constitutes the sacral hiatus (Fig. 2.53), standing out slightly laterally relative to the median sacral crest (Fig. 2.51).

Note: The sacral crest divides in two at its caudal extremity, at the level of the third and fourth posterior sacral foramina, to form two small bony columns. These are the sacral cornua.

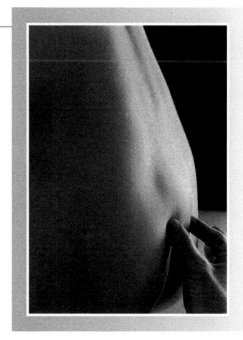

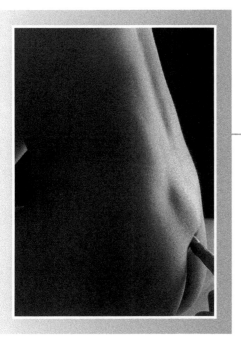

Fig. 2.53 Sacral hiatus

MA: A depression can be seen in the extension of the median sacral crest (Fig. 2.51), just above the intergluteal cleft, as shown here. This depression is formed by the divergence of the sacral cornua (sacral horns) (Fig. 2.52), in a caudal direction from superior (downward from above) and from medial outward. These mark the limits of the sacral hiatus. The top of the sacral hiatus marks the end of the sacral canal.

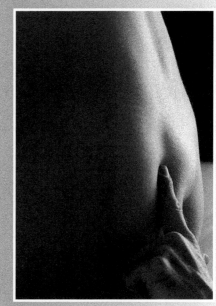

Fig. 2.54 Lateral border of the sacrum, posterolateral view
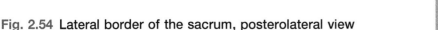

MA: In the adjacent figure, the practitioner's index finger is flat against the lateral border of the sacrum, which can be felt beneath your fingers as a thick, bubbly border.

Note: This border corresponds to the last three sacral vertebrae.

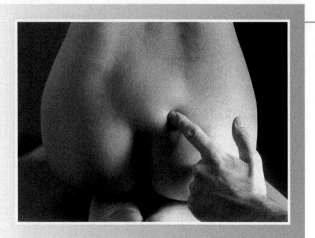

Fig. 2.55 Lateral border of the sacrum, posterior view

MA: This view shows the position of this border.

Note: Articulatory techniques for the sacroiliac joint often refer to a fulcrum operating on the "inferolateral angle" (ILA) of the sacrum. This is not an anatomical term, but refers simply to the most prominent part of the lateral border of the sacrum (indicated here by the practitioner's index finger).

Fig. 2.56 The "base" of the sacrum

MA: The subject lies face down. Take up the contact with both hands as shown. Slide your thumbs between the posterior part of the two iliac crests until they encounter the base of the sacrum (a hard stop).

Note: "Base" is a misleading term here. This is the posterior part of the base, formed by the first sacral vertebra.

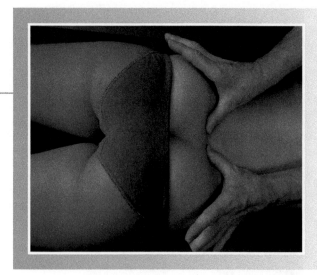

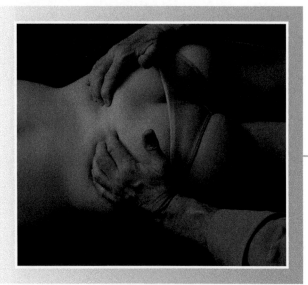

Fig. 2.57 Sacral sulci

MA: The sulci are palpable depressions between the posterior part of the sacrum and the left and right base of the sacrum. The subject lies face down. Place your hands between the posterior part of the iliac crest and the sacrum. Use the pads of your fingers to assess the depth of each sulcus, left and right. This may be asymmetrical: the depression may be filled to a greater or lesser extent, if the sacrum is rotated either left or right.

Note: In the case of right rotation, the left sulcus will be "filled."

Fig. 2.58 Median sacral crest

MA: The subject lies face down. Follow the extension of the line of the spinous processes, tracing the median sacral crest (in the middle of the sacrum) down to the sacral hiatus (between the two horns of the sacrum).

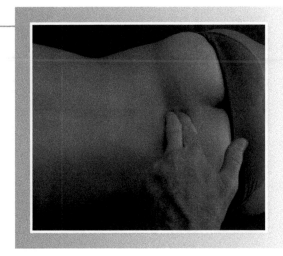

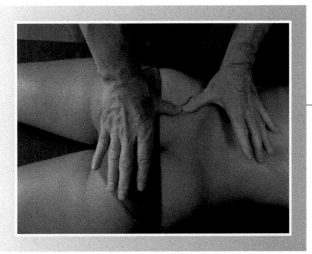

Fig. 2.59 The ipsilateral border of the sacrum

MA: The subject lies face down. Place your two thumbs on the lateral border of the sacrum, which can be palpated through the muscle mass of the gluteal region, being felt as a bony density (a hard stop).

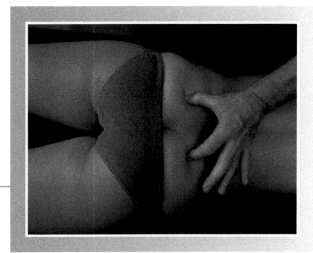

Fig. 2.60 Lateral borders of the sacrum

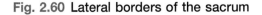

MA: The subject lies face down. Use your thumb and index finger to make contact with the two lateral borders of the sacrum, which can be sensed beneath your fingers as a bony density (a hard stop).

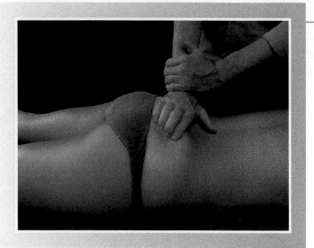

Fig. 2.61 The contralateral border of the sacrum

MA: The subject lies face down. Make contact by using all four fingers to grasp the contralateral border of the sacrum. You can sense this beneath your fingers as a bony density (hard stop). Place your other hand above your wrist, and use this to stabilize the contact.

Fig. 2.62 Sacral cornua (sacral horns)

MA: The subject lies face down. Make the contact using your thumb and index finger just above the intergluteal cleft, where you will sense two small raised points; these are extended to varying degrees, variously pronounced and various in symmetry. These horns "frame" the sacral hiatus, at the end of the filum terminale.

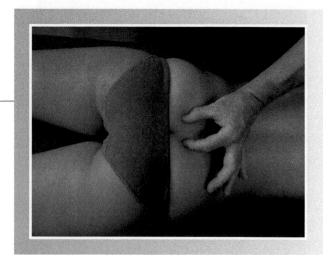

Fig. 2.63 The inferolateral angles of the sacrum (ILA)

MA: The subject lies face down. Begin by making contact using your thumb and index finger on the sacral horns (see Fig. 2.62). Then shift your contact a finger's breadth laterally to locate the structures you are seeking.

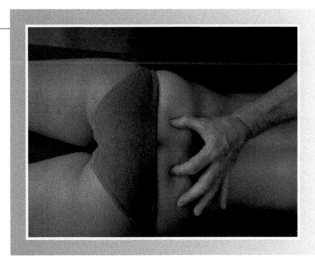

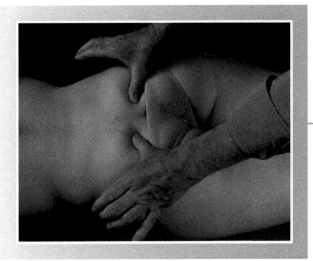

Fig. 2.64 The inferolateral angles of the sacrum, another method of approach

MA: The subject lies face down. The practitioner stands beside the subject. Place your thumbs on the ILAs using a distoproximal approach (your fingers encounter a hard stop).

MYOLOGY

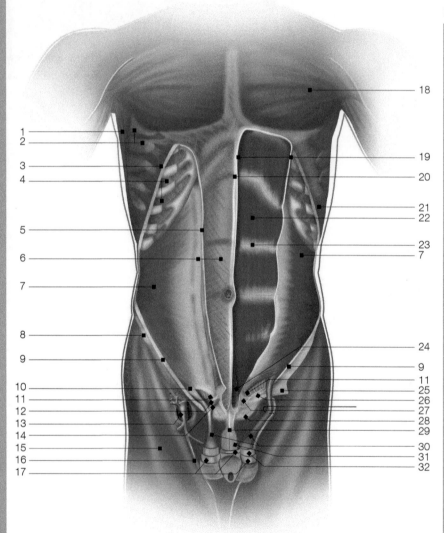

The anterior abdominal wall: intermediate dissection

1. Latissimus dorsi
2. Serratus anterior
3. External oblique (cut edge)
4. External intercostal muscles
5. External oblique aponeurosis (cut edge)
6. Rectus sheath
7. Internal oblique
8. Anterior superior iliac spine
9. Inguinal ligament (Poupart's ligament)
10. Cremaster muscle (lateral origin)
11. Inguinal falx (conjoint tendon)
12. Reflected inguinal ligament
13. Femoral vein
14. Cremaster muscle (medial origin)
15. Fascia lata
16. Great (long) saphenous vein
17. Dartos fascia; subcutaneous tissue of penis and superficial fascia of scrotum (cut away)
18. Pectoralis major
19. Anterior layer of rectus sheath (cut edges)
20. Linea alba
21. External oblique (cut away)
22. Rectus abdominis
23. Tendinous intersection
24. Pyramidalis
25. Fascia of external oblique (cut)
26. Lacunar ligament (Gimbernat's ligament)
27. Reflected inguinal ligament
28. Pubic tubercle
29. Suspensory ligament of penis
30. Cremaster muscles
31. Fascia of penis (Buck's fascia)
32. External spermatic fascia (cut away)

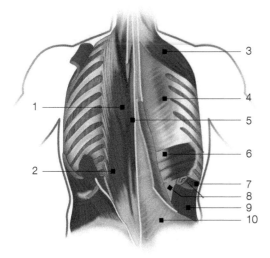

Muscles of the posterior region

Erector spinae muscles
1. Longissimus
2. Iliocostalis

Plane of the serratus posterior muscles
3. Serratus posterior superior
4. Intermediate fascia of serratus posterior
5. Spinalis
6. Serratus posterior inferior
7. External oblique
8. Grynfeltt's triangle
9. Internal oblique
10. Thoracolumbar fascia

Iliocostalis, longissimus, and spinalis muscles

1. Longissimus
2. Spinalis
3. Iliocostalis

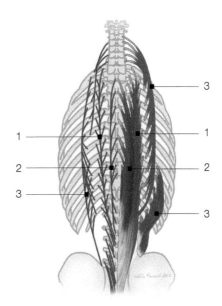

Posterior muscles of the trunk (Left: superficial layer. Right: plane of the rhomboid muscle)

1. Trapezius
2. Latissimus dorsi
3. External oblique
4. Levator scapulae
5. Rhomboid minor
6. Rhomboid major
7. Internal fascia of serratus muscles
8. Serratus posterior inferior
9. Thoracolumbar fascia

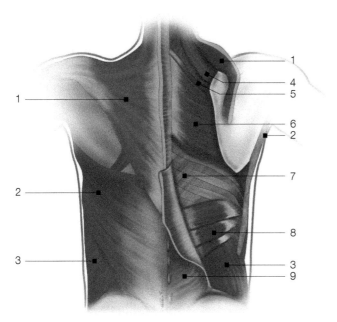

THE POSTERIOR MUSCLE GROUP

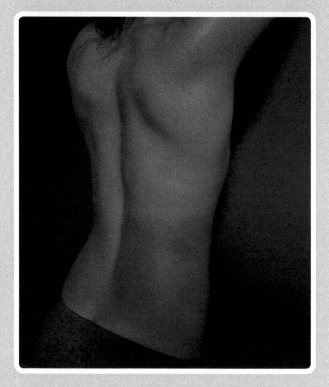

Fig. 2.65 Overall view of the posterior muscles of the trunk

The notable structures that can be detected by palpation are:

- Trapezius: overall display (Fig. 2.66)
- Trapezius: superior fibers (Fig. 2.67)
- Trapezius: intermediate fibers (Fig. 2.68)
- Trapezius: inferior fibers (Fig. 2.69)
- Latissimus dorsi (Figs. 2.70 and 2.71); cranial or superior part at the level of the thoracic vertebral column (Fig. 2.72)
- Rhomboid major (Fig. 2.73)
- Layer of the serratus posterior muscles (Fig. 2.74)
- Intermediate aponeurosis of the serratus posterior muscles (Fig. 2.75)
- Erector spinae muscles (Figs. 2.76 and 2.77)
- Lumbar part of iliocostalis lumborum and longissimus thoracis (Fig. 2.78)
- Thoracic part of iliocostalis lumborum and longissimus thoracis (Figs. 2.79 and 2.80)
- Quadratus lumborum in the superior lumbar triangle (Grynfeltt's/Lesshaft's triangle) (Fig. 2.81).

ACTIONS

Quadratus lumborum:

- When its fixed end is inferior: inclines the lumbar spine to the same side.
- It lowers the twelfth rib.
- When its fixed end is superior: inclines the pelvis to the same side.

Erector spinae:

- All extend the spine.
- Transversospinalis brings about contralateral rotation.
- Longissimus and iliocostalis lumborum bring about lateral flexion and ipsilateral rotation.

Trapezius, when the fixed end is on the vertebral column:

- The superior fibers move the shoulder upward and medially.
- The middle part draws the scapula medially.
- The inferior fibers draw the medial (vertebral) border of the scapula inward and downward and slightly raise the shoulder.

Trapezius, when the fixed end is on the shoulder girdle (pectoral girdle):

- The superior fibers bring about ipsilateral flexing and contralateral rotation of the head and neck.
- The two sets of inferior fibers help to elevate the trunk.

Latissimus dorsi, when the fixed end is inferior:

- It adducts the arm, rotates it medially, and moves it posteriorly.
- It lowers the shoulder and (jointly) laterally flexes the trunk.
- It is an accessory inspiratory muscle.
- These are also essential "climbing" muscles.

Serratus posterior superior:

- Raises the upper ribs: an inspiratory muscle.

Serratus posterior inferior:

- Draws the lower ribs downward: an expiratory muscle.

INNERVATIONS

- Quadratus lumborum: lumbar plexus (T12–L1–L2)
- Erector spinae: posterior rami of spinal nerves (T1–S3)
- Trapezius: accessory nerve; nerve of trapezius (C2–C3–C4)
- Latissimus dorsi: thoracodorsal nerve (C6–C7–C8)
- Serratus posterior: intercostal nerves
- Rhomboid major: dorsal scapular nerve (C4–C5)

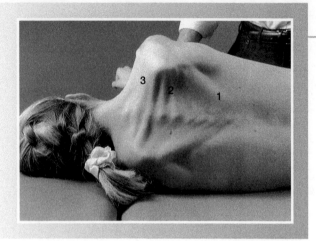

Fig. 2.66 Trapezius, overall display; occipital and vertebral origins

MA: The adjacent figure shows the topographical location of this muscle. Together with latissimus dorsi, it constitutes the most superficial layer of the muscles of the back. The intermediate (middle) and inferior fibers of this muscle belong to this region.

ATTACHMENTS

- This muscle arises from the cranium on the exocranial surface of the squama of the occipital bone, on the superior nuchal line.
- At the vertebral column, it arises from the posterior border of the nuchal ligament and the tip of the spinous processes of C7 to T11.

1. Inferior (ascending) part of trapezius
2. Middle (transverse) part of trapezius
3. Superior (descending) part of trapezius

Fig. 2.67 Trapezius, superior fibers

MA: The subject should lie on one side, facing the practitioner. Place a broad contact, using the palmar surface of one hand, on the lateral part of her head, and place the other hand on the body of her shoulder. Ask her to raise this shoulder while flexing her head to the same side. Resist both these movements. The trapezius (1) will appear in the lateral part of the neck.

ATTACHMENTS TO THE CLAVICLE

- The superior fibers run obliquely downward and laterally, and insert into the lateral third of the inferior border of the clavicle and on the adjacent part of the superior surface.
- The arrows (2) indicate the inferolateral limits of the trapezius. The origins (cranial attachments, and the attachments on the vertebral column) are described under Fig. 2.66.

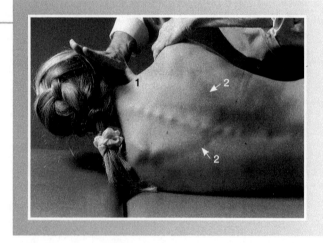

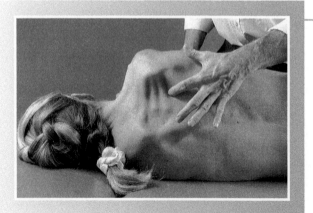

Fig. 2.68 Trapezius, intermediate fibers

MA: The subject should lie on one side, with both arms positioned to create 90° flexion of the shoulders. Apply resistance to the lateral surface of her arm, above the elbow, and ask her to abduct her shoulder horizontally against your resistance. In this figure, the practitioner's index finger indicates the intermediate fibers.

ATTACHMENTS ON THE SCAPULA AND VERTEBRAL COLUMN

- The intermediate (middle) fibers run transversely, inserting into the acromion and the superior side of the posterior border of the spine of the scapula. There is a particularly extensive insertion into the tubercle of the scapular spine, a prominence that is sometimes called the deltoid tubercle.
- At the vertebral column, these fibers arise from the spinous processes of the first five thoracic vertebrae.

Fig. 2.69 Trapezius, inferior fibers

MA: In the adjacent figure, the subject is shown lying on her side, with her shoulder and elbow flexed at 90°. Apply resistance to the lateral surface of her arm, above the elbow, and ask her to abduct her arm horizontally. The practitioner's thumb and index finger contact in this illustration shows the two muscles you are looking for.

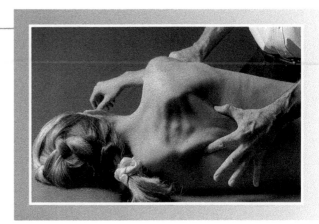

ATTACHMENTS ON THE SCAPULA AND VERTEBRAL COLUMN

- The fibers run obliquely upward and laterally and insert into the medial extremity of the spine of the scapula by means of a flattened aponeurosis.
- On the vertebral column, they arise from the spinous processes of the last six thoracic vertebrae.

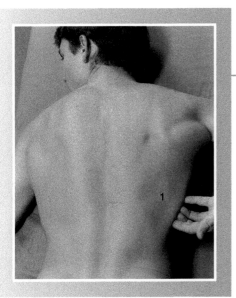

Fig. 2.70 Latissimus dorsi (1), global display and topographical location

MA: This muscle, together with trapezius, makes up the most superficial layer of the muscles of the back. Latissimus dorsi is large and flattened, and shaped like a triangle with a broad lateral base.

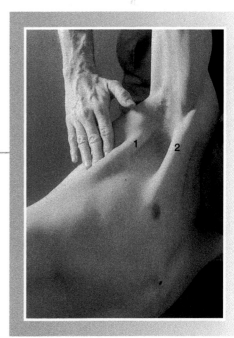

Fig. 2.71 Latissimus dorsi

MA: The adjacent figure shows an anterolateral view of this muscle. The subject is lying on one side, with his arm abducted at 90°. Apply resistance to the medial surface of his arm above the elbow. Ask him to adduct his arm against your resistance.

ATTACHMENTS

- The origin is via a tendinous aponeurosis (the thoracolumbar fascia) with attachments to:
  - the spinous processes of T7–L5 and corresponding interspinal ligaments;
  - the median sacral crest;
  - the outer lip of the iliac crest.
- Latissimus dorsi is also attached at the three or four last ribs and inferior angle of the scapula, by means of muscular digitations.
- Its insertion is by means of a flattened tendon passing around the teres major, into the crest of the lesser tubercle of the humerus. (A synovial bursa separates it from teres major.)

1. Latissimus dorsi
2. Pectoralis major

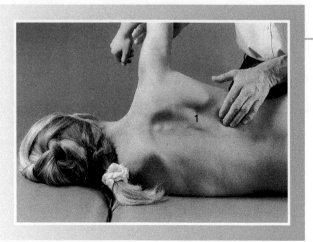

Fig. 2.72 Latissimus dorsi, cranial or superior part at the level of the thoracic spine

MA: Figure 2.69 describes the technique for making the inferior fibers of trapezius (1) more prominent. Begin by locating this muscle, then slide your fingertips underneath the most caudal part of the inferior fibers. This will bring them into contact with the most distal part of latissimus dorsi on the thoracic spine.

Fig. 2.73 Rhomboid major

MA: Begin by locating the inferior fibers of trapezius. Then rotate (i.e., swing) the scapula laterally sufficiently to free rhomboid major which is situated here, directly under trapezius. Palpate between the thoracic spine and the medial (vertebral) border of the scapula.

ATTACHMENTS

- Rhomboid major arises from the first five thoracic vertebrae.
- It inserts into the part of the medial border of the scapula below the spine of the scapula.

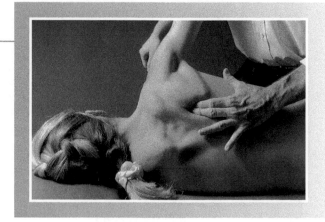

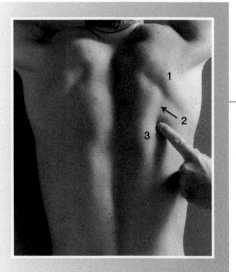

Fig. 2.74 Layer of the serratus posterior muscles

MA: These are two flattened, quadrilateral muscles, one situated superiorly and one inferiorly, and joined by an intermediate aponeurosis. In the adjacent figure, with the scapula (1) moved aside, the practitioner's index finger indicates the "point of penetration" (inside the posterior angle of the ribs) (2), which is the position you should palpate to approach the layer of the serratus posterior muscles. This is done through the fibers of latissimus dorsi, by slipping your contact under trapezius (3).

ATTACHMENTS

- The serratus posterior muscles arise from the line of the spinous processes of C7–L3.
- Their insertion is at the angle of all the ribs, slightly lateral to the angle.

Fig. 2.75 Intermediate aponeurosis of the serratus posterior muscles

MA: Between serratus posterior superior and serratus posterior inferior, the layer of the serratus posterior muscles consists of a thin intermediate aponeurosis stretched from the vertebral column to the ribs, bounded by the fourth and ninth ribs.

Note: This figure completes the method of approach described in Figure 2.74 (where the subject is lying prone rather than on one side, as here).

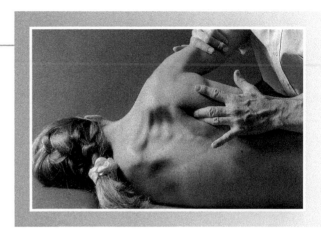

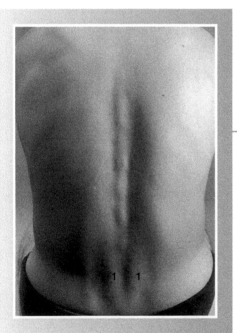

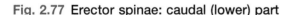

Fig. 2.76 Erector spinae muscles (1), topographical location

MA: These muscles make up the deep layer of the posterior muscles of the trunk. They are situated on either side of the spinous processes, on the posterior part of the laminae and transverse processes. They extend from the cervical region to the sacrum, and are composed of closely interwoven muscles which completely fill the vertebral grooves.

1. Common mass

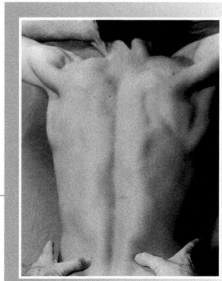

Fig. 2.77 Erector spinae: caudal (lower) part

MA: The subject should lie face down; then ask him to extend his trunk. A muscular mass will appear in the lumbar region, at the vertebral grooves.

Note: The erector spinae muscles consist of transversospinalis, spinalis thoracis, longissimus thoracis, and iliocostalis. Caudally, transversospinalis, spinalis, longissimus, and iliocostalis form an undifferentiated common muscle mass (see 1, on Fig. 2.76).

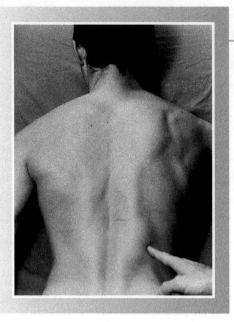

Fig. 2.78 Lumbar part of iliocostalis lumborum and longissimus thoracis

MA: These two muscles are closely interwoven and share the same caudal origin (iliac crest, tuberculum of iliac crest, and sacral crest). Ask the subject to extend his trunk, to make the desired muscles appear more prominently. The muscle mass is indicated by the practitioner's index finger in the illustration.

Note: The most recently agreed nomenclature does not assign a separate name to the lumbar part of longissimus; it is a division of longissimus thoracis. Also, iliocostalis lumborum has a lumbar and a thoracic part.

Fig. 2.79 Thoracic part of iliocostalis lumborum and longissimus thoracis, topographical location

MA: The adjacent figure shows the topographical location of these muscles. They are situated at the vertebral grooves, covered by the following muscle layers (listed here in succession from the deep to the superficial layer): the layer of serratus posterior, the layer of rhomboid major, opposite the scapula, and finally, more superficially, by trapezius cranially and latissimus dorsi caudally.

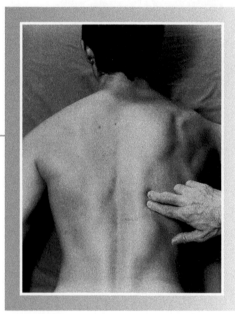

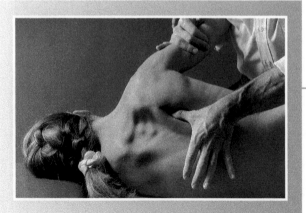

Fig. 2.80 Thoracic part of iliocostalis lumborum and longissimus thoracis

MA: Begin by locating the inferior fibers of trapezius. Then slide your contact (either of two fingers together, or the thumb, as shown in the adjacent figure) in the direction of the thoracic spine. The bundles of fleshy fibers may be seen to roll under your fingers. The fibers belong to the thoracic part of iliocostalis lumborum laterally and longissimus thoracis medially.

Note: This muscle may be very differently perceived in different subjects.

Fig. 2.81 Quadratus lumborum in the superior lumbar triangle

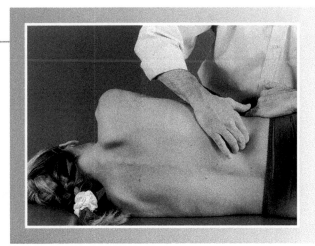

MA: The subject should lie on one side. Place one hand on the twelfth rib in the superior lumbar triangle (see Note below). (This is also variously known as the triangle of Grynfeltt, Lesshaft's space, Grynfeltt–Lesshaft triangle, lumbar tetragon, or superior quadrilateral lumbar space.) The other hand lies on the iliac crest. Ask the subject to draw the iliac crest toward her twelfth rib, and resist this motion. You will sense the contraction of the quadratus lumborum under your cranial hand.

Note: The **superior lumbar triangle** is formed of aponeuroses and bounded by the following muscles:

- medially by the common muscle mass of the erector spinae group;
- below and laterally by the posterior border of the internal oblique muscle of the abdomen;
- above and medially by serratus posterior inferior;
- above and laterally by the inferior border of the twelfth rib.

This layer of muscles is covered posteriorly by a layer containing the inferior lumbar triangle (triangle of Petit). This is bounded as follows:

- below, by the posterior part of the iliac crest;
- laterally and anteriorly, by the posterior border of the external oblique muscle of the abdomen;
- medially, by the lateral border of latissimus dorsi.

These two spaces, the superior and inferior lumbar triangles, are the two weak points of the posterior abdominal wall.

ATTACHMENTS

- Quadratus lumborum is flattened and quadrilateral in shape, and arises from the posterior part of the medial lip of the iliac crest.
- It inserts into the twelfth rib and lumbar spine. It is situated anterior to the erector spinae muscles, and separated from them by the fascia of the origin of transversus abdominis.

THE MUSCLES OF THE ANTEROLATERAL WALL OF THE THORAX AND ABDOMEN

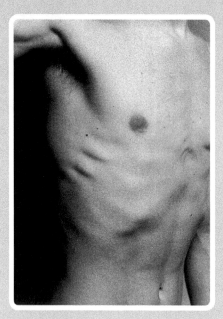

Fig. 2.82 Anterolateral view of the thorax and abdomen

The notable structures that can be detected by palpation are:

- The external intercostal muscles (Fig. 2.83)
- External oblique:
  - Costal attachments (Figs. 2.84, 2.85, 2.89, and 2.90)
  - Costal digitations (Figs. 2.84, 2.85, and 2.86)
  - Body of the muscle (Figs. 2.86, 2.87, and 2.88)
- The anterolateral muscles of the abdomen (Fig. 2.91)
- Psoas major (greater psoas muscle) (Figs. 2.92–2.94).

ACTIONS

- The external intercostal muscles:
  - Are inspiratory muscles.
  - Support the thoracic cage by resisting its expansion.
- The iliopsoas:
  - Flexes and laterally rotates the thigh on the pelvis.
  - If the fixed end is the femur, it flexes the trunk and rotates it contralaterally.

- The muscles of the anterolateral abdominal wall:
  - Contraction of these muscles compresses the abdominal viscera. They are therefore involved in micturition, defecation, vomiting, childbirth, and forced expiration.
  - If the fixed end is superior, they bring about retroversion of the pelvis.
  - Contraction of external oblique on one side draws the anterior surface of that half of the thorax toward the opposite side.
  - Contraction of internal oblique on one side draws the anterior surface of the other half of the thorax toward itself.
  - If the fixed end is on the thorax, these muscles of the anterolateral abdominal wall bring about retroversion of the pelvis.

Fig. 2.83 The external intercostal muscles

MA: These muscles lie in each of the intercostal spaces. They consist (working inward from the outside) of the external intercostal muscles, internal (i.e., middle) intercostal muscles, and innermost intercostal muscles. There are three per space, joining the adjacent borders of the ribs and cartilages. Small muscles are attached to them; these are the levatores costarum and subcostales.

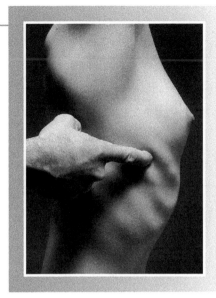

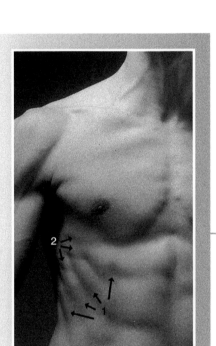

Fig. 2.84 External oblique, digitations

MA: The adjacent figure shows the fleshy fibers of external oblique (1), running in a diagonal direction toward the last seven or eight ribs to insert into the external surface of the ribs. The illustration also shows how this muscle interlinks with serratus anterior (2).

Fig. 2.85 External oblique and internal oblique

MA: External oblique lies over internal oblique. (Here, the practitioner's index finger indicates one of the costal digitations of external oblique.)

ATTACHMENTS OF INTERNAL OBLIQUE

- This muscle overlies transversus abdominis, covering it almost completely. It extends from the iliac crest to the last ribs, linea alba, and pubis.
- It arises:
  – from the three quarters of the iliac crest anterior to the interstitium and the one third external to the inguinal ligament;
  – via a tendinous aponeurosis interwoven with the thoracolumbar fascia, on the quarter posterior to the iliac crest and on the spinous process of L5.
- From here, the fibers fan out between the last ribs and the pubis, passing via the linea alba.
  – The posterior fibers (running obliquely upward and anteriorly) insert into the inferior border and tip of the last four costal cartilages.
  – The middle fibers continue by means of a broad tendinous aponeurosis which forms part of the linea alba.
  – The inferior fibers attach to the pubic symphysis, pubis, and pecten pubis.

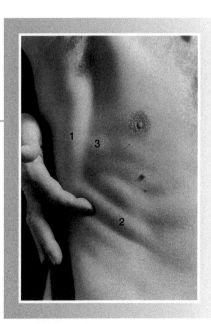

1. Latissimus dorsi
2. Digitations of external oblique
3. Digitations of serratus anterior

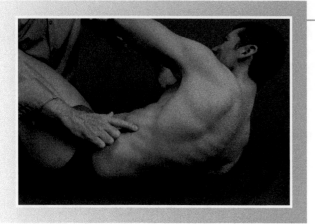

Fig. 2.86 Costal digitations of external oblique

MA: The subject lies with his shoulder and elbow both flexed at 90°. The practitioner should stand on the other side of the subject. Ask him to rise from the table, bringing the flexed elbow across toward his opposite knee. Resist this action, using your hand on his elbow. The adjacent figure shows how, with this method of approach, the cranial (costal) digitations of this muscle can clearly be seen. They insert into the lateral surface and inferior border of the last seven or eight ribs.

Note: This technique also reveals the body of external oblique.

Fig. 2.87 Body of external oblique

MA: The method shown here also displays the body of external oblique (in addition to the method described above). This involves simple lateral flexion of the trunk and slight flexion. The practitioner should stand at the subject's head. Instruct him to flex his trunk to the left, while you watch and control the movement. Resist as necessary with your left forearm, matching your resistance to the force of the lateral flexion. Take hold of the body of the muscle with your fingers.

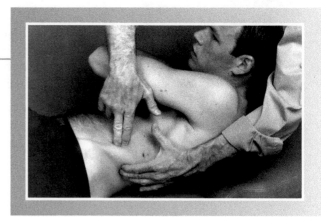

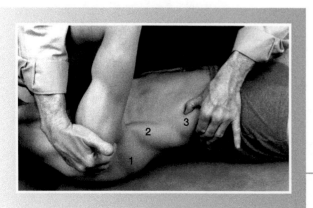

Fig. 2.88 Body of external oblique, another approach – relations with the other muscles of the region

MA: Note the relation between teres major (1), latissimus dorsi (2), and the body (3) of external oblique.

Fig. 2.89 External oblique, costal attachments – relations to serratus anterior

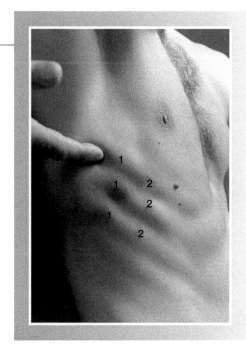

MA: In this figure, the practitioner's index finger indicates the digitations of serratus anterior (1) and its close relations with external oblique (2).

External oblique is a broad, thin muscle, fleshy posteriorly and tendinous anteriorly. It is the most superficial muscle of the anterolateral abdominal wall.

ATTACHMENTS OF EXTERNAL OBLIQUE

- The fibers arise from the thoracic wall (at the external surface and inferior border of the last seven to eight ribs; the last attaches to the cartilage of the twelfth rib). These interdigitate with the inferior fibers of serratus anterior and with latissimus dorsi below.
- These fleshy fibers give way to a broad tendinous portion, the aponeurosis of the external oblique, which forms part of the linea alba, and inserts inferiorly into the pubis and the inguinal ligament.
- The four posterior portions of external oblique arise from the last two or three ribs and insert into the anterior half of the lateral lip of the iliac crest.

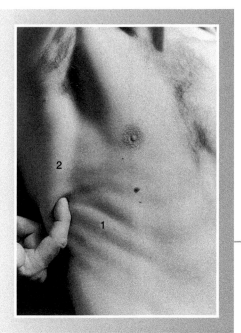

Fig. 2.90 External oblique

COSTAL ATTACHMENTS: RELATIONS TO LATISSIMUS DORSI

In the adjacent figure, the practitioner's index finger rests on one of the digitations of external oblique (1), and also on latissimus dorsi (2). This emphasizes the close relation between these two muscles. They are closely interwoven on the lateral surface of the last two or three ribs.

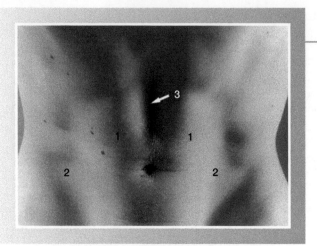

Fig. 2.91 The anterolateral muscles of the abdomen: rectus abdominis and transversus abdominis

MA: The adjacent figure shows the position of the two rectus abdominis muscles (1), separated by the linea alba (3). The bodies (2) of external oblique, internal oblique, and transversus abdominis can be found to either side of rectus abdominis. They are listed here in the order they occur, from superficial to deep.

Note: There are five muscles of the anterolateral abdominal wall: rectus abdominis, pyramidalis, transversus abdominis, external oblique, and internal oblique.

ATTACHMENTS

- Rectus abdominis is a long, flattened, thick muscle, stretching the length of the median line in the anteroinferior part of the abdomen.
  - It takes its origin inferiorly, on the anterior surface of the pubis, from the pubic tubercle on the pubic crest to the symphysis, and on the anterior surface of the symphysis.
  - It inserts into the external surface and the inferior border of the fifth, eighth, and seventh costal cartilages, via three digitations.
- Transversus abdominis is the deepest muscle of the anterolateral abdominal wall. The middle portion takes the form of the muscle body, and the two extremities terminate in a tendinous membrane. Its attachments are:
  - on the medial surface of the last six costal cartilages, via six digitations. These are interwoven with the digitations of the diaphragm at ribs 10–12;
  - on the tip of the transverse processes of the first four lumbar vertebrae, via an aponeurosis called the thoracolumbar fascia. This extends across the space between the costal and iliac attachments;
  - on the half or two thirds of the iliac crest anterior to the medial lip, and the one third lateral to the inguinal ligament.

Fig. 2.92 Psoas major, method of approach – step 1

MA: The subject is supine. The practitioner's thumb and index finger mark the anterior superior iliac spine (thumb) and navel (index finger).

ATTACHMENTS

- Iliopsoas is composed of two muscles, psoas major and iliacus, which unite at their distal insertion.
- Psoas major arises:
  - from the lateral surface of vertebral bodies T12–L5, via fibrous arches;
  - from the adjacent intervertebral discs;
  - from the inferior border of the transverse processes.
- Iliacus arises:
  - from the medial lip of the iliac crest;
  - from the iliac fossa, base of the sacrum, and sacroiliac joint.
- These two muscles have a common insertion into the lesser trochanter of the femur.

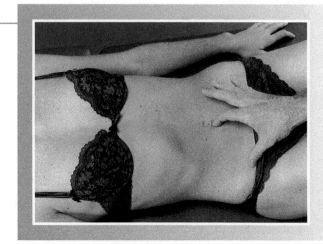

Fig. 2.93 Psoas major, method of approach – step 2

MA: Imagine a hypothetical line running between the practitioner's thumb and index finger, as shown in the figure above (Fig. 2.92). Take the middle of this line, placing your index finger broadly against the lateral border of the rectus abdominis (1).

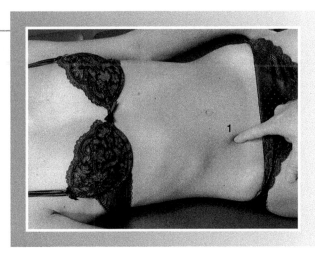

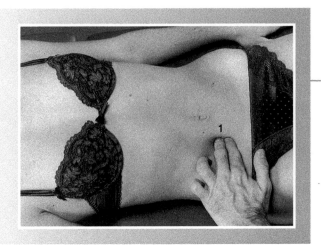

Fig. 2.94 Psoas major, method of approach – step 3

MA: Once you have located the positions described in steps 1 and 2 above (Figs. 2.92 and 2.93), you can palpate this muscle by gently penetrating down through the abdominal wall at the lateral border of rectus abdominis (1). You will detect a fairly significant muscle body beneath your fingers. (It becomes easier to feel if you ask the subject to flex her thigh actively toward the pelvis.)

NERVES AND BLOOD VESSELS

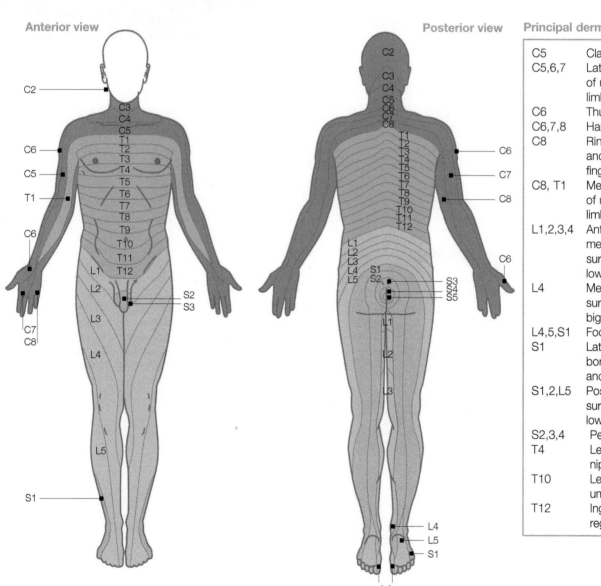

Anterior view

Posterior view

Principal dermatomes:

C5	Clavicles
C5,6,7	Lateral parts of upper limbs
C6	Thumb
C6,7,8	Hand
C8	Ring finger and little finger
C8, T1	Medial parts of upper limbs
L1,2,3,4	Anterior and medial surfaces of lower limbs
L4	Medial surface of big toe
L4,5,S1	Foot
S1	Lateral border of foot and little toe
S1,2,L5	Posterolateral surfaces of lower limbs
S2,3,4	Perineum
T4	Level of nipple
T10	Level of umbilicus
T12	Inguinal region

THE PRINCIPAL BLOOD VESSELS

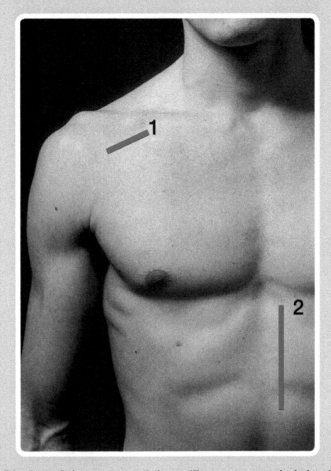

Fig. 2.95 Display of the course of the axillary artery and abdominal aorta
1. Axillary artery
2. Abdominal aorta

The notable structures that can be detected by palpation are:
- Axillary artery (Fig. 2.96)
- Abdominal aorta (Fig. 2.97).

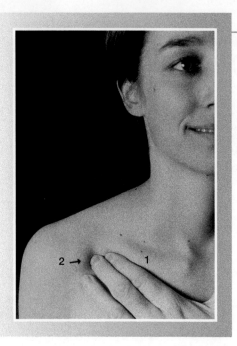

Fig. 2.96 Axillary artery

MA: Place the flat of one hand on the anterior surface of pectoralis major. Here, the practitioner's index finger is resting on the inferior border of the clavicle (1); the ends of his fingers press up against the medial surface of the coracoid process (2) (see Chapter 3). You will feel the pulse beneath your fingers.

Fig. 2.97 Abdominal aorta

MA: This is the continuation of the thoracic aorta, after it has passed through the diaphragm. It passes anteriorly and to the left of the vertebral column before dividing at the level of disc L4–L5 to form its two terminal branches. To take the pulse of this artery, ask the subject to lie supine with her knees bent so as to relax the abdominal tension. Stand to her right side, and place three fingers together just above the navel, one finger's breadth to the left of the linea alba (1). Take great care when penetrating the abdominals.

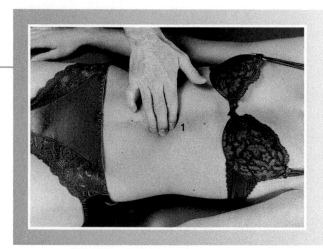

3
The shoulder

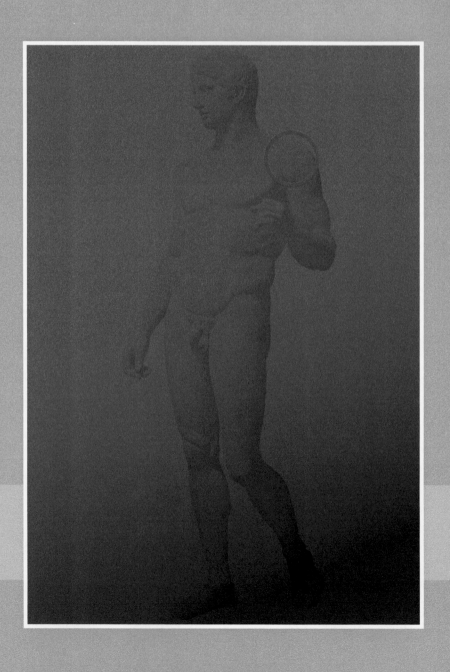

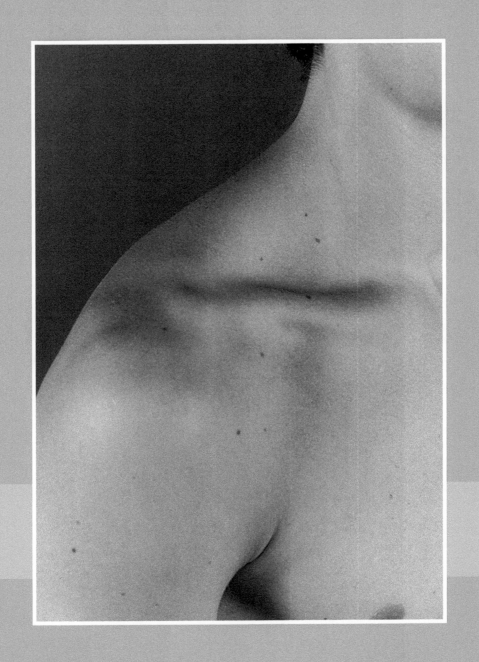

OSTEOLOGY

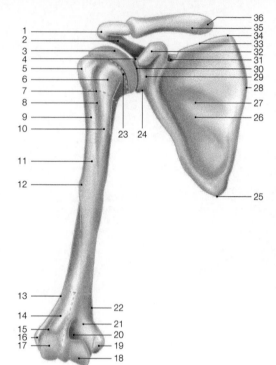

The scapula and humerus (anterior view)

1. Acromial angle
2. Acromion
3. Head of humerus
4. Supraglenoid tubercle
5. Greater tubercle
6. Lesser tubercle
7. Surgical neck
8. Intertubercular sulcus
9. Crest of greater tubercle
10. Crest of lesser tubercle
11. Humerus
12. Deltoid tuberosity
13. Lateral supraepicondylar ridge
14. Lateral condyle
15. Radial fossa
16. Lateral epicondyle
17. Capitulum
18. Trochlea

19. Medial epicondyle
20. Coronoid fossa
21. Medial condyle
22. Medial supraepicondylar ridge
23. Anatomical neck
24. Infraglenoid fossa
25. Inferior angle
26. Scapula
27. Subscapular fossa
28. Medial border
29. Neck
30. Glenoid cavity of scapula
31. Suprascapular notch
32. Coracoid process
33. Superior border
34. Superior angle
35. Clavicle
36. Sternal facet

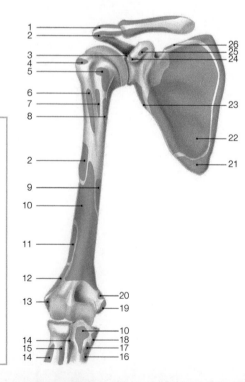

Muscle attachments

1. Trapezius
2. Deltoid
3. Biceps brachii (long head)
4. Supraspinatus
5. Subscapularis
6. Pectoralis major
7. Latissimus dorsi
8. Teres major
9. Coracobrachialis
10. Brachialis
11. Brachioradialis
12. Extensor carpi radialis longus
13. Common extensor tendon
14. Supinator

15. Biceps brachii
16. Flexor pollicis longus
17. Pronator teres
18. Flexor digitorum superficialis
19. Common flexor tendon
20. Pronator teres
21. Serratus anterior
22. Subscapularis
23. Triceps brachii
24. Coracobrachialis and biceps brachii (short head)
25. Pectoralis minor
26. Omohyoid

The scapula and humerus (posterior view)

1. Superior angle
2. Superior border
3. Suprascapular notch
4. Supraspinous fossa
5. Spine
6. Infraspinous fossa
7. Medial border
8. Inferior angle
9. Lateral border
10. Scapula
11. Groove for circumflex scapular vessels
12. Neck
13. Infraglenoid tubercle
14. Medial supraepicondylar ridge
15. Medial epicondyle
16. Trochlea
17. Lateral epicondyle
18. Olecranon fossa
19. Lateral supraepicondylar ridge
20. Humerus
21. Deltoid tuberosity
22. Radial groove
23. Surgical neck
24. Anatomical neck
25. Head of humerus
26. Greater tubercle
27. Notch uniting the supraspinous and infraspinous fossae
28. Coracoid process
29. Acromial angle
30. Acromion
31. Clavicle

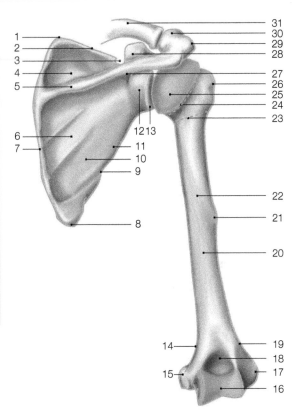

Muscle attachments

1. Levator scapulae
2. Supraspinatus
3. Trapezius
4. Rhomboid minor
5. Infraspinatus
6. Rhomboid major
7. Teres major
8. Latissimus dorsi
9. Teres minor
10. Triceps brachii (long head)
11. Common flexor tendon
12. Triceps brachii
13. Anconeus
14. Common extensor tendon
15. Triceps brachii (medial head)
16. Brachialis
17. Deltoid
18. Triceps brachii (lateral head)

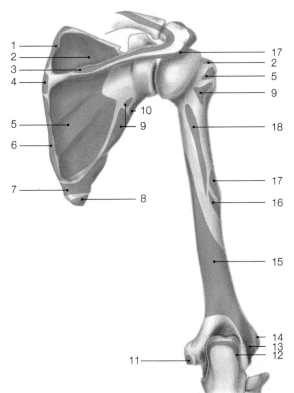

Clavicle
Superior surface

Inferior surface

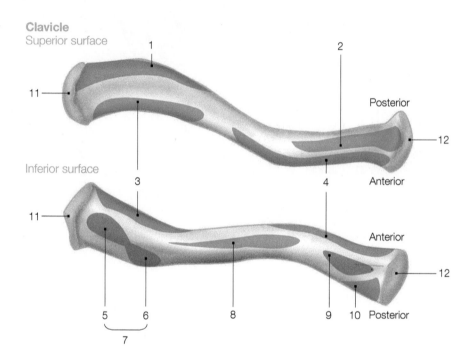

1. Trapezius
2. Sternocleidomastoid
3. Deltoid
4. Pectoralis major
5. Trapezoid ligament
6. Conoid ligament
7. Coracoclavicular ligament
8. Subclavius
9. Costoclavicular ligament
10. Sternocleidohyoid
11. Acromial end
12. Sternal end

The shoulder joint (glenohumeral or scapulohumeral joint): anterior view

1. Capsule of acromioclavicular joint
2. Acromion
3. Coracoacromial ligament
4. Tendon of supraspinatus
5. Coracohumeral ligament
6a. Greater tubercle of humerus
6b. Lesser tubercle of humerus
7. Transverse humeral ligament
8. Intertubercular synovial sheath
9. Subscapularis tendon
10. Biceps brachii tendon (long head)
11. Capsular ligaments
12. Clavicle
13. Trapezoid ligament
14. Conoid ligament
      13 + 14 = Coracoclavicular ligament
15. Superior transverse scapular ligament
16. Suprascapular notch
17. Coracoid process
18. Communication of subtendinous bursa of subscapularis
19. Position of subtendinous bursa of subscapularis (*dotted line*)

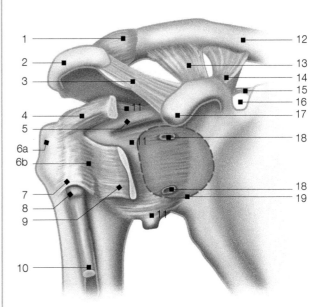

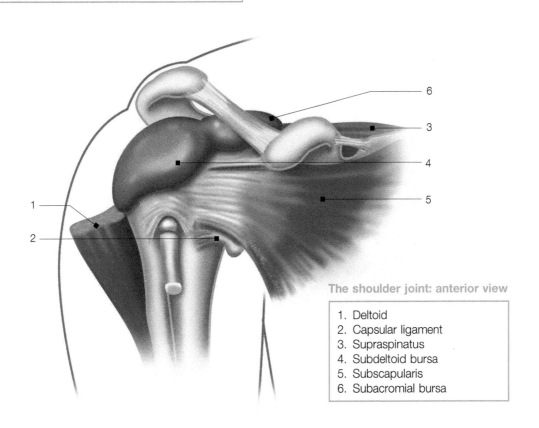

The shoulder joint: anterior view

1. Deltoid
2. Capsular ligament
3. Supraspinatus
4. Subdeltoid bursa
5. Subscapularis
6. Subacromial bursa

THE CLAVICLE

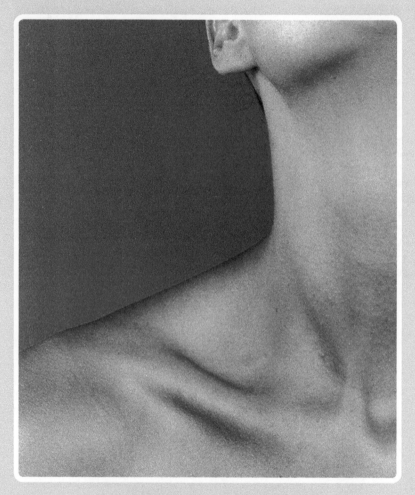

Fig. 3.2 Overall view of the clavicle

The notable structures that can be detected by palpation are:
- The anterolateral concavity (Fig. 3.3)
- The posterolateral convexity (Fig. 3.4)
- The anteromedial convexity (Fig. 3.5)
- The posteromedial concavity (Fig. 3.6)
- The sternal end (Fig. 3.7)
- The acromial end (Fig. 3.8).

Fig. 3.3 The anterolateral concavity of the clavicle

MA: The clavicle is a long bone shaped like an italic letter *"S."* It runs in a transverse direction between the scapula and sternum, and forms a key part of the pectoral girdle. The structure provides attachment to the clavicular (anterior) fibers of the deltoid.

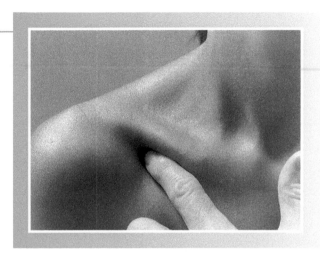

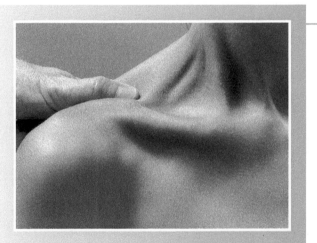

Fig. 3.4 The posterolateral convexity of the clavicle

MA: This part of the clavicle is part of the posterior border. It is convex, with a rough surface that provides attachment to the clavicular fibers of the trapezius. This attachment covers the lateral two thirds of the posterior border.

Fig. 3.5 The anteromedial convexity of the clavicle

MA: This convexity occupies the medial two thirds of the anterior border and provides attachment to the pectoralis major.

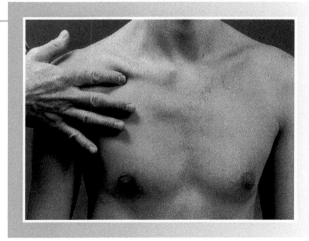

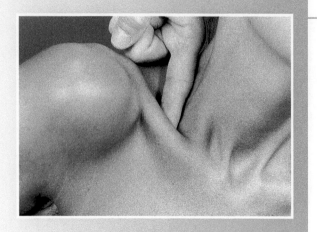

Fig. 3.6 The posteromedial concavity of the clavicle

MA: This concavity occupies the medial two thirds of the posterior border of the clavicle.

CLINICAL NOTE

Fracture of the clavicle

This is one of the commonest fractures in sports.

The skin may be raised by one of the fractured ends, creating a highly indicative "bump"; palpation or pressure produces exquisite point tenderness. Seen early, the precise type of displacement can clearly be identified by palpation: if the fractured medial part of the clavicle is prominent, this indicates anterior displacement; if it forms a depression, it indicates posterior displacement. Posterior displacement is a medical emergency, because of the risk that it may compress vascular and neural structures supplying the arm.

Fig. 3.7 The sternal end of the clavicle

MA: This extremity of the clavicle broadens into a shape resembling a saddle. It articulates with the sternum and first costal cartilage.

Note: These three structures constitute the sternoclavicular joint.

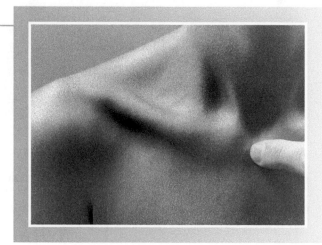

CLINICAL NOTE

Sternoclavicular dislocation

This condition is rare, because it involves violent trauma (e.g., road traffic accident, or certain kinds of sports such as rugby). The dislocation may be anterior or posterior.

Fig. 3.8 The acromial end of the clavicle

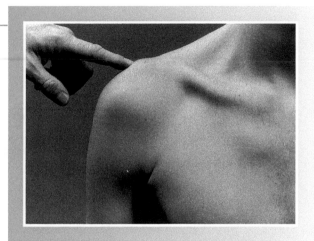

MA: The acromial end is flattened from top to bottom, and articulates with the acromion by means of a downward, outward, and anterior-facing oval articular surface.

Note: These two structures, the acromion and the acromial end of the clavicle, constitute the acromioclavicular joint.

CLINICAL NOTE

Acromioclavicular sprain and dislocation

These are common in sports. The main causes are direct impact on the body of the shoulder, or violent traction of the upper limb. Diagnosis needs to distinguish between three stages:

- Stage I: Simple straining of the capsule. The line of the joint is tender to pressure.

- Stage II: Rupture of the acromioclavicular ligament and overstretching of other ligaments (trapezoid, conoid, and medial coracoclavicular). The acromioclavicular line is tender to pressure. Palpation can also detect displacement of the lateral end of the clavicle.

- Stage III: The lateral (acromial) end of the clavicle is drawn upward by the muscles of the neck, and can be depressed by applying pressure (the "piano key" sign).

The two techniques used here are:

- Palpation, applying pressure to examine for tenderness or the piano key sign of stage III.

- Palpation, mobilizing to examine for "drawer" movement in the sagittal direction.

THE SCAPULA

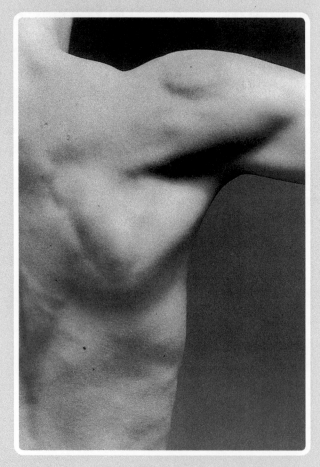

Fig. 3.9 Overall view of the scapula

The notable structures that can be detected by palpation are:

- Scapula (Fig. 3.10)
- Costal (anterior) surface of scapula (Figs. 3.11 and 3.12)
- Spine of the scapula and acromion (its lateral extension) (Figs. 3.13 and 3.14)
- Acromial angle (Fig. 3.15)
- Posteroinferior border of acromion medial to the acromial angle (Fig. 3.16)
- Lateral border of acromion (Fig. 3.17)
- Tip of acromion (Fig. 3.18)
- Medial border of acromion (Fig. 3.19)
- Spine of scapula (Fig. 3.20)
- Medial extremity of scapular spine (Fig. 3.21)
- Tubercle of the scapular spine (Fig. 3.22)
- Supraspinous fossa (Fig. 3.23)
- Infraspinous fossa (Fig. 3.24)
- Medial (vertebral) border of scapula (Fig. 3.25)
- Lateral border of scapula (Fig. 3.26)
- Neck of scapula (Fig. 3.27)
- Coracoid process (Fig. 3.28)
- Superior border of scapula (Fig. 3.29)
- Inferior angle of scapula (Fig. 3.30)
- Superior angle of scapula (Figs. 3.31 and 3.32)
- Superior angle and anterior surface of scapula (Fig. 3.33)
- Cranial border of scapula (Fig. 3.34).

Fig. 3.10 Scapula, global approach

MA: The scapula is a flat bone that lies on the posterior surface of the thoracic cage between the second and seventh ribs. It articulates with the clavicle and the humerus.

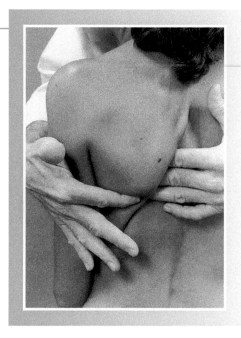

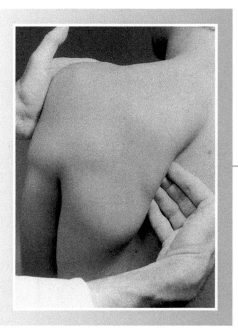

Fig. 3.11 Costal (anterior) surface of the scapula, vertebral approach

MA: The figure alongside shows how this approach from the vertebral direction brings the practitioner's contact to the attachments of serratus anterior muscle, which lie along the medial border of the bone.

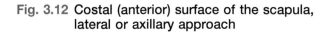

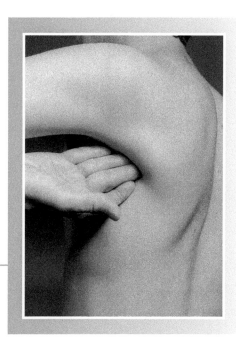

Fig. 3.12 Costal (anterior) surface of the scapula, lateral or axillary approach

MA: Using this approach, the practitioner's contact is directed toward subscapularis. This muscle attaches to the anterior surface of the scapula.

Note: There is a ridge along the lateral (axillary) border, linking the neck of the scapula and the inferior angle. It is called the pillar of the scapula.

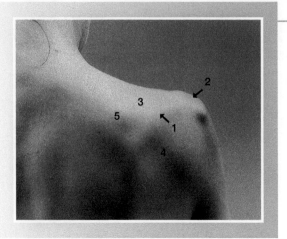

Fig. 3.13 Display of the spine of the scapula and acromion

MA: The spine of the scapula (1) is a triangular structure with a medial crest. It lies perpendicularly to the surface of the scapula, crossing it at the point where the superior quarter joins the inferior three quarters of the bone. So the anterior border of the scapular spine is, in effect, implanted in the posterior surface of the scapula, separating it into two parts. These are the supraspinous fossa (3) and infraspinous fossa (4). The lateral and posterior borders of the scapular spine broaden laterally to form the acromion (2).

Note: The superior angle of the scapula (5) (see also Fig. 3.31) can also be seen here.

Fig. 3.14 Spine of the scapula and acromion

MA: The figure alongside shows the lateral extremity of the scapular spine, between the practitioner's two index fingers. It broadens laterally to form the structure called the acromion. This is quadrangular, and flattened in the opposite direction to the scapular spine, at right angles to it. It has a superior and an inferior surface, a medial border, a lateral border, tip, and acromial angle.

Note: The superior surface seems to have been created by enlargement of the posterior border of the scapular spine. The inferior surface seems to be the result of enlargement of the lateral border of the scapular spine.

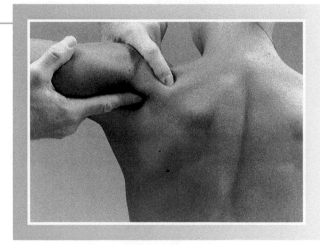

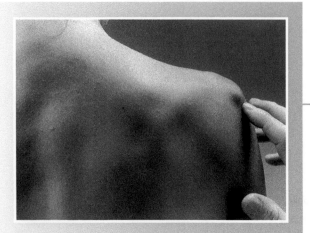

Fig. 3.15 The acromial angle

MA: This is an anatomical reference point, marking the change in direction of the posteroinferior border of the acromion. It provides attachment to deltoid.

Fig. 3.16 Posteroinferior border of the acromion medial to the acromial angle

MA: The practitioner's index finger in the figure alongside indicates this border. It provides attachment to deltoid.

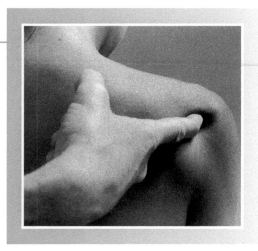

Fig. 3.17 Lateral border of the acromion

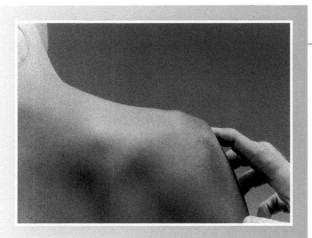

MA: In this figure, the practitioner's index finger indicates this structure. It provides attachment to deltoid.

> **CLINICAL NOTE**
>
> **Fracture of the acromion** is extremely rare. This type of fracture is most often associated with **anteromedial dislocation** of the **humeral head.** In those circumstances it should therefore be considered. Palpation examines for tenderness to pressure on the various points of the acromion. Avoid any action of deltoid and any contact between the acromion and the greater tubercle (which occurs when the arm is raised beyond 90° abduction).

Fig. 3.18 Tip of the acromion

MA: Indicated here by the practitioner's index finger, this lies just lateral and anterior to the acromial end of the clavicle. It provides attachment to the deltoid. The acromial angle (1) can also be seen in this figure.

> **CLINICAL NOTE**
>
> **Subacromial bursitis**
>
> Examine by palpation, looking for tenderness to pressure in the deltoid region. The patient will often indicate the location of the pain. Passive and active circumduction beyond 90° is painful. Everyday actions such as hair combing or putting on a garment, which involve raising the arm above the shoulder – let alone the head – are painful. These movements cause pressure to the subacromial bursa between the humeral head and the acromion.

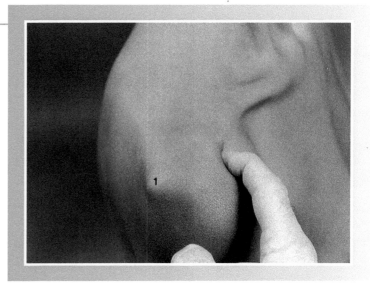

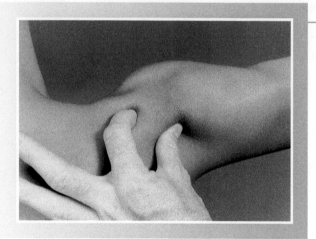

Fig. 3.19 Medial border of the acromion

MA: A superiorly and medially facing, oval articular surface occupies two thirds of this border. It articulates with the acromial end of the clavicle. In this figure, the practitioner's index finger rests on the location of this structure. His thumb is in contact with the posteroinferior border of the acromion.

Fig. 3.20 Spine of the scapula

MA: This is a triangular bony structure, set in the posterior surface of the scapula and lying transversely across it where the superior quarter joins the inferior three quarters of the scapula.

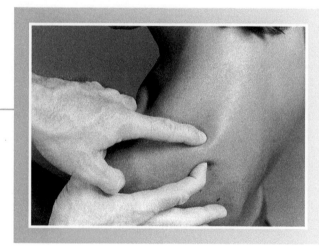

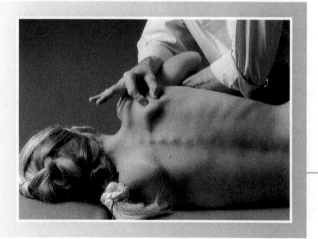

Fig. 3.21 Medial extremity of the scapular spine

MA: The medial extremity of the scapular spine expands into a triangular area which can be seen clearly in this figure beneath the practitioner's thumb-and-finger contact. It ends at the medial border of the scapula.

Fig. 3.22 Tubercle of the scapular spine

MA: Along the posterior border of the scapular spine, just beneath the skin, the middle part enlarges to form a prominence[1] that you can feel as a bulge beneath your fingers. This provides attachment to trapezius (1).

[1]The name "deltoid tubercle" is sometimes used.

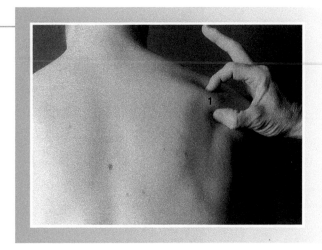

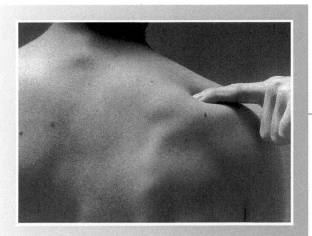

Fig. 3.23 Supraspinous fossa

MA: This lies on the posterior surface of the scapula, above the scapular spine, and provides attachment to supraspinatus.

Fig. 3.24 Infraspinous fossa

MA: This lies on the posterior surface of the scapula, below the scapular spine, and provides attachment to infraspinatus.

> **CLINICAL NOTE**
> **Fracture of the infraspinous fossa** is possible. Tenderness to pressure together with a history consistent with such an injury (e.g., the patient falling on the stairs and landing on her back) should lead you to suspect it.

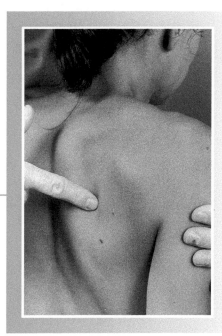

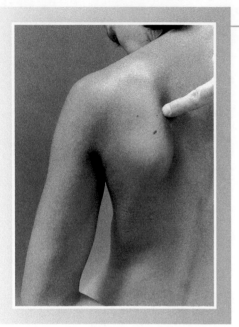

Fig. 3.25 Medial (vertebral) border of the scapula

MA: This is the longest of the three borders of the scapula. It has an obtuse angle, the tip of which corresponds to the medial extremity of the scapular spine. Above this angle is the insertion of levator scapulae. Below the angle are the insertions of rhomboid minor and rhomboid major.

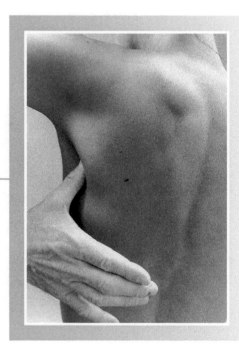

Fig. 3.26 Lateral border of the scapula

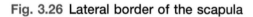

MA: The lateral border broadens at its upper end, below the glenoid cavity, creating a tubercle, the infraglenoid tubercle. This provides attachment to the long head of triceps brachii.

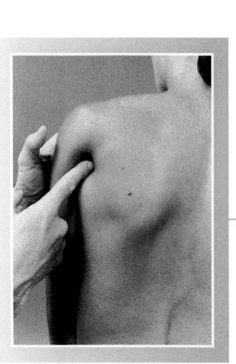

Fig. 3.27 Neck of scapula

MA: The neck of the scapula, which supports the glenoid cavity, forms part of the lateral angle of the scapula, along with the glenoid cavity and the coracoid process. There is a groove on the posterior surface of the neck which links the supraspinous and infraspinous fossae, laterally, to the spine of the scapula.

> **CLINICAL NOTE**
>
> **Fracture of the scapula** is possible. Examine by application of pressure, to find if this evokes or exacerbates pain.

Fig. 3.28 Coracoid process

MA: This process can be found just medial to the head of the humerus and inferior to the clavicle, as shown in this figure. It is shaped like a semiflexed finger. The tip and medial border are accessible to palpation.

MUSCLE ATTACHMENTS

This bony structure provides the insertion of pectoralis minor (indicated here by the horizontal part of the practitioner's partly flexed finger), the origin of coracobrachialis, and the origin of the short head of biceps brachii (both at the tip of the coracoid process).

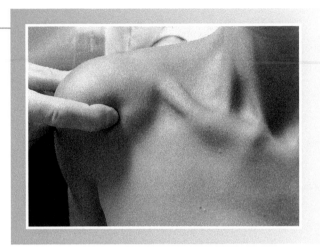

> **CLINICAL NOTE**
>
> **Fracture of the coracoid process** alone is extremely rare. Examine for exquisite pain in response to pressure. Certain movements are to be avoided: flexion of the forearm on the arm, and flexion of the shoulder, especially if accompanied by adduction and respiration using the upper ribs. In practice this means avoiding any action involving any of the three muscles mentioned under Figure 3.28 as having an attachment on the coracoid process, whether the muscle contracts or stretches. Also avoid anything that brings the coracoid process into contact with the lesser tubercle, which happens in adduction and medial rotation.

Fig. 3.29 Superior border of the scapula

MA: This short, thin, sharp border terminates laterally in the suprascapular notch, which provides passage to the suprascapular nerve.

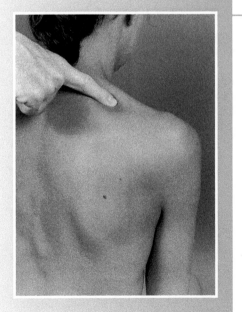

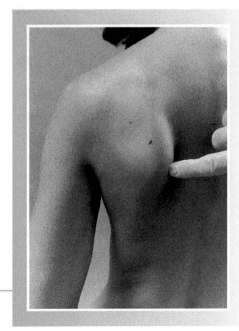

Fig. 3.30 Inferior angle of the scapula

MA: The inferior angle is thick, rough, and rounded in shape, and lies at the junction of the medial (vertebral) and lateral (axillary) borders.

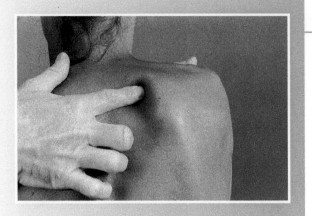

Fig. 3.31 Superior angle of the scapula, dorsal (posterior) approach

MA: The subject is seated. Take hold of her shoulder with one hand, pushing it backward and upward so that the medial (vertebral) border of the scapula becomes prominent. The superior angle is indicated here by the practitioner's index finger.

Fig. 3.32 Superior angle of the scapula, anterior approach

MA: The subject is seated. Ask her to move her arm posteriorly, in such a way that the scapula glides superiorly and anteriorly over the thoracic cage. Another approach is to carry out this movement passively. It causes the superior angle to protrude beneath your fingers, in the muscle mass of trapezius (1). Levator scapulae is indicated by (2). Although she is seated in the adjacent figure, this method of approach can also be used with the subject lying on the contralateral side.

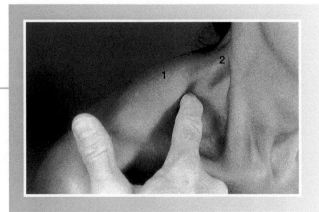

Fig. 3.33 Superior angle and anterior surface of the scapula (facing the supraspinous fossa)

MA: The subject lies on the contralateral side, with his arm straight and medially rotated, and the back of his hand against his back. Take hold of the inferior angle of the scapula with one hand and push it in the cranial direction. Use the index finger of your other hand to palpate the superior (superomedial) angle or the anterior surface of the scapula.

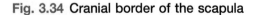

Fig. 3.34 Cranial border of the scapula

MA: The subject lies on the contralateral side. His arm should be straight and medially rotated, and the back of his hand against his back. Take hold of the inferior angle of the scapula with one hand and push it in the cranial direction. Palpate the cranial border of the scapula with your other hand.

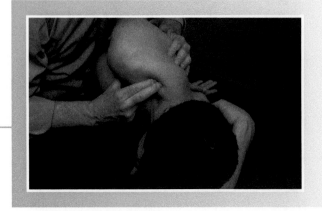

THE SUPERIOR EXTREMITY OF THE HUMERUS

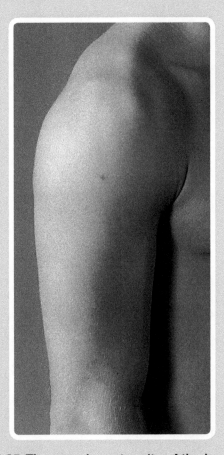

Fig. 3.35 The superior extremity of the humerus

The notable structures that can be detected by palpation are:

- **Humerus:**
  - Global contact for the head of the humerus (Fig. 3.36)
- **The five structures belonging to the humerus:**
  - Lesser tubercle (Figs. 3.37 and 3.38)
  - Intertubercular sulcus (bicipital groove) (Figs. 3.37 and 3.38)
  - Greater tubercle (Figs. 3.37 and 3.38)
  - Crest of greater tubercle (Fig. 3.39)
  - Crest of lesser tubercle (Fig. 3.40).

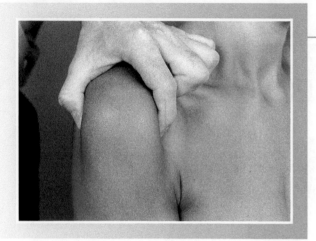

Fig. 3.36 Humerus: global contact for the head of the humerus

MA: The figure here shows a global contact straddling the lateral end of the clavicle and the acromion to take hold of the head of the humerus. Ask the subject to rotate his shoulder alternately in the lateral and medial direction. His elbow can be held at an angle of 90°. You will feel the head of the humerus rotating beneath your fingers.

Note: Begin from the position in which the subject's shoulder is medially rotated. You will then clearly detect the greater and lesser tubercles (see also Figs. 3.37 and 3.38) as they pass beneath your fingers. You will also be able to detect the intertubercular sulcus (see also Figs. 3.37 and 3.38) between the two tubercles.

CLINICAL NOTE

Scapulohumeral dislocation

This is very common in sports. Dislocation may be anterior, posterior, superior, or inferior; anterior dislocation is the most frequently encountered. In this case the humeral head may be:

- anterior to the glenoid cavity;
- inferior to the coracoid process;
- medial to the coracoid process;
- inferior to the clavicle.

Complications:

Always bear in mind the possibility that the dislocation may be accompanied by fracture, either intra-articular (humeral head; glenoid cavity) or extra-articular (lesser tubercle; surgical neck). Likewise, there may be accompanying damage to tendons (tendinopathies or rupture of the rotator cuff) or neurovascular structures (circumflex nerve; axillary artery and/or vein). The cause is usually either indirect mechanical force (e.g., falling onto the hand) or a direct blow to the shoulder (e.g., rugby or judo). Dislocation can recur, caused by some simple movement such as brushing the hair. Palpation shows very clearly that the head of the humerus is out of place.

Fig. 3.37 Global approach to three structures belonging to the humerus: lesser tubercle, intertubercular sulcus, and greater tubercle

MA: The subject is seated. His arm rests against his body, his elbow is bent at an angle of 90°, and his hand is supinated. Use a broad contact with the pads of several fingers, positioned on pectoralis major and the clavicular part of deltoid. With your other hand, draw the subject's arm into lateral rotation. In this position, you will feel the coracoid process beneath your fingers. Just lateral to this you can feel the lesser tubercle. If you ease the subject's arm into medial rotation, you will sense laterally, and in this order, the intertubercular sulcus and the greater tubercle beneath your fingers.

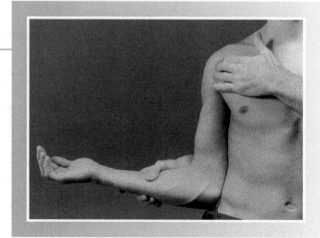

CLINICAL NOTE

Tenderness to pressure on palpation should give rise to suspicion of **fracture of the greater or lesser tubercle.**

Fig. 3.38 Another global approach to three structures belonging to the humerus

MA: The subject is seated, with her shoulder abducted at 90°, and elbow flexed at an angle of 90°. The practitioner should stand behind her. Place one hand on the deltopectoral groove, using a broad contact with several fingers together. With your other hand, take hold of the subject's elbow; using rapid but low-amplitude, alternating movements, rotate her shoulder laterally and medially. The dense structure you detect beneath your fingers in the more medial position is the lesser tubercle, and the more lateral one is the greater tubercle. The depression between these two structures is the intertubercular sulcus (bicipital groove).

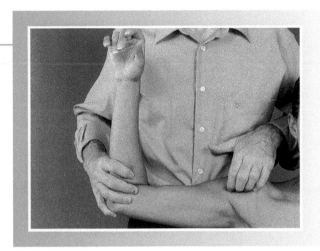

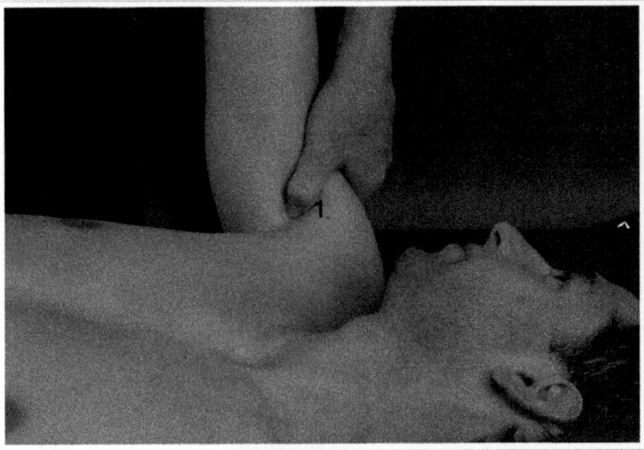

Fig. 3.39 Crest of the greater tubercle

MA: The crest of the greater tubercle can be palpated inferior to the tendon of pectoralis major (1), whose insertion is on this tubercle.

> **CLINICAL NOTE**
>
> There is a possible **fracture site** here, at the **surgical neck:** the most frequent fracture of the humerus. This should be considered where there is a history involving a fall onto the point of the shoulder. In younger subjects, this might be a fall from a horse; in the elderly, a fall downstairs, for example. When examining for this, begin with palpation, looking for increased tenderness to pressure. Bear in mind the possibility of damage to the circumflex nerve.

Fig. 3.40 Crest of the lesser tubercle

MA: This is located medial to the greater tubercle. In some subjects, it helps to separate the long and short heads of biceps brachii. Care is needed on approaching this structure, because the main nerves supplying the arm run nearby, in a fairly limited space.

Teres major and latissimus dorsi (medially) both have their insertion here.

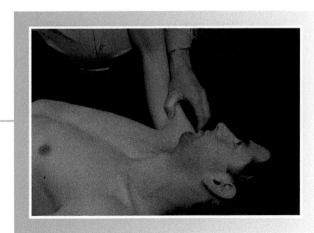

MYOLOGY

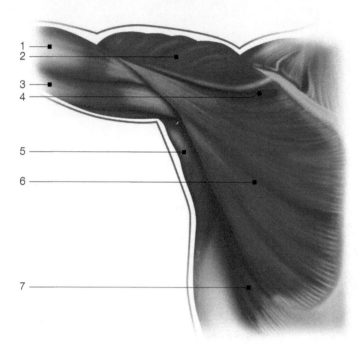

The anterior muscle group: superficial layer (pectoralis major)

1. Long head of biceps brachii
2. Deltoid
3. Short head of biceps brachii
4. Deltopectoral triangle
5. Latissimus dorsi
6. Pectoralis major
7. Pectoralis major (abdominal part)

Anterior muscle group: deep layer (subclavius and pectoralis minor; attachments of pectoralis major)

1. Deltoid
2. Pectoralis minor
3. Coracobrachialis
4. Tendon of pectoralis major
5. Long head of biceps brachii
6. Short head of biceps brachii
7. Serratus anterior
8. Pectoralis major (clavicular part)
9. Subclavius
10. Pectoralis major
11. First costal head
12. Second costal head
13. Third costal head
14. Fourth costal head
15. Fifth costal head

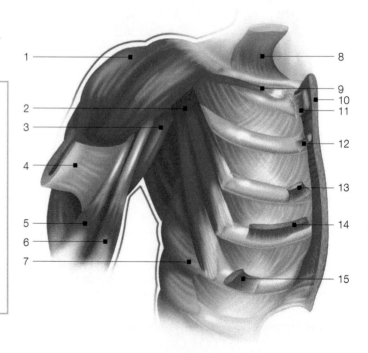

Supraspinatus, infraspinatus, teres minor, and teres major

1. Supraspinatus
2. Medial axillary space
3. Teres minor
4. Infraspinatus
5. Rhomboid major
6. Deltoid (cut and reflected)
7. Lateral axillary space
8. Lateral head of triceps brachii
9. Long head of triceps brachii
10. Teres major
11. Latissimus dorsi
12. Clavicle
13. Trapezius

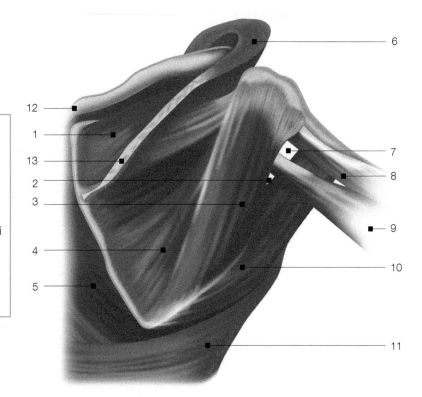

Subscapularis

1. Coracobrachialis
2. Pectoralis minor
3. Lateral axillary space
4. Deltoid
5. Pectoralis major
6. Long head of biceps brachii
7. Subclavius
8. Subscapularis
9. Long head of triceps brachii
10. Medial axillary space
11. Teres major
12. Latissimus dorsi

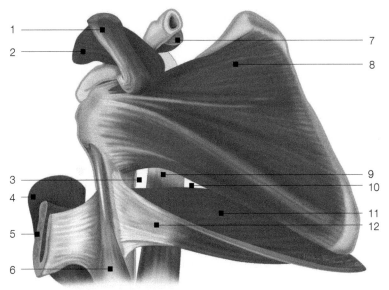

THE ANTERIOR MUSCLE GROUP

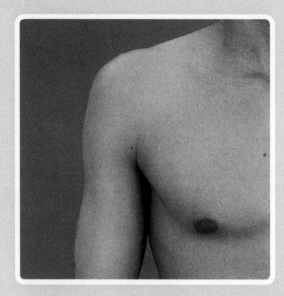

Fig. 3.41 The shoulder: anterior muscle group

The notable structures that can be detected by palpation are:

- **Superficial layer:**
  - **Pectoralis major:**
    - General view (Fig 3.42)
    - Clavicular head (Fig. 3.43)
    - Sterno-chondro-costal head (Fig. 3.44)
    - Manubrial head (Fig. 3.45)
    - Abdominal head (Fig. 3.46)
- **Deep layer:**
  - **Subclavius** (Fig. 3.47)
  - **Pectoralis minor:**
    - Presentation of pectoralis minor (Fig. 3.48)
    - Coracoid attachment of pectoralis minor (Fig. 3.49).

ACTIONS

- Pectoralis major:
  - When the fixed end is on the thorax, this muscle adducts the arm and rotates it medially.
    - The clavicular head raises the arm and adducts it toward the contralateral shoulder.
    - The sterno-chondro-costal head adducts the arm horizontally.
  - The abdominal part lowers and adducts the arm toward the contralateral hip.
  - When the fixed end is on the humerus, it is an accessory inspiratory muscle and assists in raising the trunk.
- Subclavius:
  - When the fixed end is caudal: it draws the clavicle downward.
  - When the fixed end is cranial: It serves as an accessory inspiratory muscle.
- Pectoralis minor:
  - When the fixed end is caudal: it draws the coracoid process superiorly and anteriorly.
  - When the fixed end is cranial: it serves as an accessory inspiratory muscle.

INNERVATIONS

- Pectoralis major: lateral and medial pectoral nerves (C6–C7–C8)
- Subclavius: ramus of the superior trunk of the brachial plexus (C5–C6)
- Pectoralis minor: medial pectoral nerve (C7–C8–T1)

Fig. 3.42 Pectoralis major: Display of the different heads

Note: Not all four heads of pectoralis major are present in every case; this depends on the morphology of the subject. The manubrial and sternal heads will not always be found.

1. Clavicular head
2. Manubrial head
3. Sternal head
4. Abdominal head

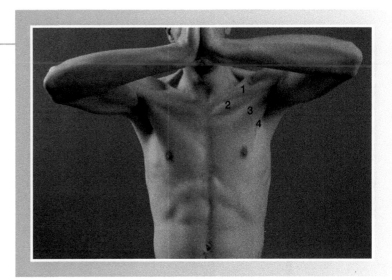

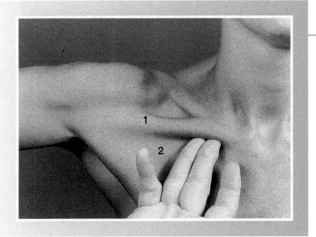

Fig. 3.43 Clavicular head of pectoralis major

MA: Abduct the subject's arm to an angle of 90°, with his elbow also bent at 90° so that his forearm points upward. Ask him to adduct his arm horizontally as you offer resistance to the medial part of the arm. Using your two fingers together, place your contact underneath the subject's clavicle, looking for a groove between the clavicular head (1) and the sterno-chondro-costal head (2).

ATTACHMENTS

- The clavicular head of pectoralis major arises from the medial two thirds of the anterior border of the clavicle.
- Insertion: see Figure 3.46.

Fig. 3.44 Sterno-chondro-costal head of pectoralis major (1)

MA: Abduct the subject's arm to an angle of 90°, and provide resistance to the horizontal adduction of his arm. The sterno-chondro-costal head (1) will appear under the groove that separates it from the clavicular head (2) (see Fig. 3.43).

ATTACHMENTS

- The sterno-chondro-costal head of pectoralis major arises:
  - from the anterior surface of the sternal manubrium;
  - from the body of the sternum;
  - from the costal cartilages of the second to sixth ribs;
  - from the costal (bony) part in the case of the fifth and sixth ribs.
- Insertion: see Figure 3.46.

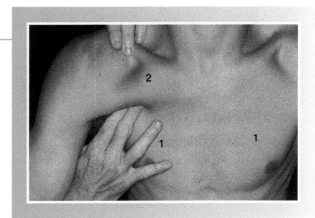

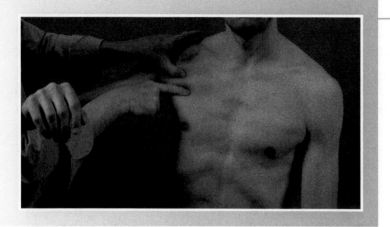

Fig. 3.45 Manubrial head of pectoralis major

MA: Here, the practitioner's left thumb and right index finger surround the manubrial head.

Note: This head is not always individually present.

Fig. 3.46 Abdominal head of pectoralis major

MA: Resist the adduction of the subject's arm with one hand (not visible on photograph). Ease the index finger of the other hand between the sterno-chondro-costal (3) and abdominal (4) heads of the pectoralis major.

ATTACHMENTS

- The abdominal part of pectoralis major arises from the rectus sheath.
- The three or four parts of pectoralis major (clavicular, manubrial, sterno-chondro-costal, and abdominal) terminate in a tendon inserting into the crest of the greater tubercle of the humerus, lateral to the latissimus dorsi. These are separated by a bursa.

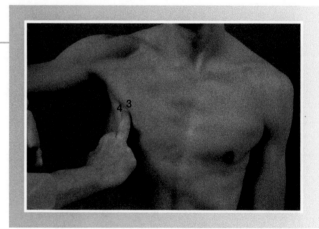

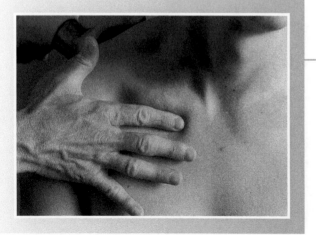

Fig. 3.47 Subclavius

MA: The general location of this muscle is indicated here by the practitioner's fingers. The muscle is not easy to detect by palpation.

Note: This muscle functions as an active ligament of the sternocostoclavicular joint and forms a key element in the various movements of the clavicle.

ATTACHMENTS

- The origin of subclavius is tendinous, and located on the first costal cartilage of the first rib.
- Its insertion is into the middle part of the inferior surface of the clavicle.

Fig. 3.48 Pectoralis minor

MA: The subject is seated or supine. Support the arm concerned by cradling his forearm in one hand. His elbow should be bent at 90° and resting on your forearm. Use this supporting hold to ease the subject's shoulder upward and medially so as to slacken pectoralis major as much as possible. Then, using the pads of the fingers of your other hand and stabilized by the thumb, in the contact shown in the adjacent figure, slide your fingers under pectoralis major to try to locate a fairly significant cord of muscle. This is pectoralis minor. It is very easy to detect, even in the relaxed state, but can be made more prominent by calling on the actions of the muscle. To do this, you can either ask the subject to take short, repeated in-breaths, to mobilize the third, fourth, and fifth ribs to which the muscle is attached (in this case the fixed end is on the coracoid process), or, as illustrated here, you can ask him to move his shoulder forward. Pectoralis minor is then responsible for performing this action, as the fixed end of the muscle is costal and its insertion is into the coracoid process of the scapula.

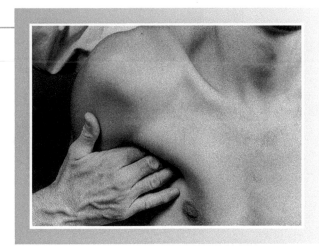

ATTACHMENTS

- Pectoralis minor has a tendinous origin on the third, fourth, and fifth ribs.
- It inserts into the medial border of the horizontal portion of the coracoid process.

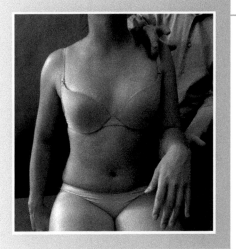

Fig. 3.49 Coracoid attachment of pectoralis minor

MA: The subject is seated, with her arm against the side of her thorax and elbow flexed. Stand behind her and take hold of her arm with one hand. Place the middle finger of your other hand anterior to the coracoid process, and ask the subject to move her shoulder forward. You will be able to palpate pectoralis minor through pectoralis major, inferior to the coracoid process.

THE MEDIAL MUSCLE GROUP

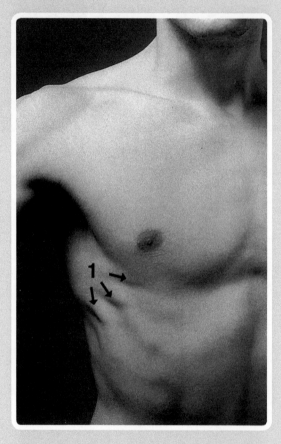

**Fig. 3.50 Anterolateral view of the trunk:
the medial muscle group of the shoulder**

1. Serratus anterior

This comprises just one muscle, serratus anterior. (Figs 3.51 and 3.52)

ACTIONS

Serratus anterior abducts the scapula in relation to the vertebral column, i.e., it moves it laterally across the thorax, at the same time moving it anteriorly.

INNERVATION

- Serratus anterior: Long thoracic nerve (C5–C6)

Fig. 3.51 Serratus anterior – palpation on the ribs

MA: The subject should be either seated or standing. Ask him to take short, repeated in-breaths so as to make the muscular digitations (1) attached to the ribs appear in between latissimus dorsi (2) posteriorly and pectoralis major (3) anteriorly.

ATTACHMENTS

• Serratus anterior arises from the lateral surfaces of the first ten ribs, by means of muscular digitations.
• It is inserted into the superomedial and inferior angles of the scapula and the medial border of the scapula between these two angles.

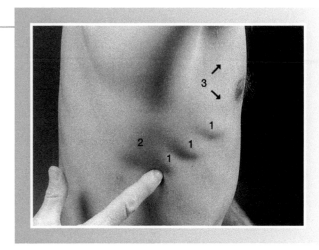

Fig. 3.52 Serratus anterior – another approach

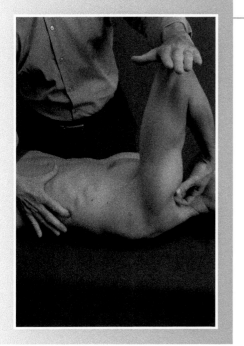

MA: The subject lies supine, with his arm flexed at 90° and elbow bent to the maximum extent, as shown. Place one hand on the subject's elbow and ask him to push his elbow upward toward the ceiling, so as to abduct the scapula. With your other hand, palpate the digitations of serratus anterior at their origins on the lateral surface of the ribs.

CLINICAL NOTE

If testing of serratus anterior reveals any deficit, this may indicate a problem affecting the **long thoracic nerve.** It is possible to palpate this nerve in subjects who are sufficiently thin. In others, follow the course of the nerve, examining for tenderness to palpation.

THE POSTERIOR MUSCLE GROUP

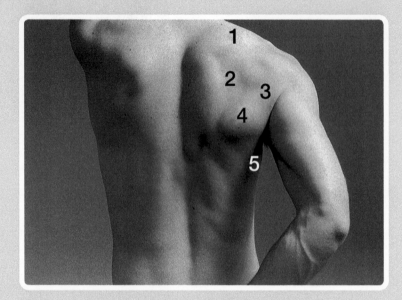

Fig. 3.53 The posterior muscle group

1. Supraspinatus
2. Infraspinatus
3. Teres minor
4. Teres major
5. Latissimus dorsi

Note: The position of subscapularis cannot be seen in this figure. (It lies on the anterior surface of the scapula.)

The notable structures that can be detected by palpation are:

- Subscapularis (Figs. 3.54–3.57)
- Supraspinatus (Figs. 3.58–3.60)
- Humeral insertion of supraspinatus (Fig. 3.61)
- Infraspinatus (Figs. 3.62 and 3.63)
- Teres minor (Figs. 3.64 and 3.65)
- Humeral insertions of infraspinatus and teres minor muscles (Fig. 3.66)
- Teres major (Figs. 3.67–3.69)
- Latissimus dorsi (Figs. 3.70 and 3.71).

ACTIONS

- Supraspinatus:
  - Abducts the arm.
  - Functions as an active ligament of the glenohumeral joint (opposes downward dislocation of the head of the humerus).
- Infraspinatus and teres minor:
  - Rotate the arm laterally.
  - Supinate the forearm, assisting when this function is required to be performed forcefully.
  - Assist in holding the head of the humerus inside the glenoid cavity.
- Teres major:
  - When the fixed end is on the scapula: provides retropulsion, adduction, and medial rotation of the arm.
  - When the fixed end is on the humerus: draws the angle of the scapula forward and laterally.
- Latissimus dorsi:
  - When the fixed end is on the pelvis:
    - The superior fibers provide retropulsion, adduction, and medial rotation of the arm.
    - The lateral and inferior fibers ipsilaterally incline the trunk and lower the shoulder.
    - The two latissimus dorsi muscles working together extend the vertebral column.
  - When the fixed end is on the humerus: ipsilateral closure of the costovertebral space.
- Subscapularis:
  - Rotates the arm medially, with a slight adduction component.
  - When pronation of the forearm is to be performed forcefully, subscapularis assists this function.

INNERVATIONS

- Subscapularis: subscapular nerve (C5–C6)
- Supraspinatus: suprascapular nerve (C5–C6)
- Infraspinatus: suprascapular nerve (C5–C6)
- Teres minor: axillary nerve (C5–C6)
- Teres major: subscapular nerve (C5–C6)
- Latissimus dorsi: thoracodorsal nerve (C6–C7–C8)

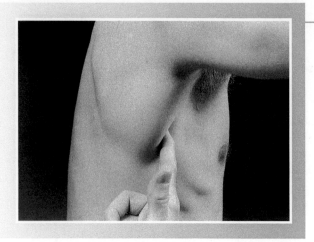

Fig. 3.54 Subscapularis

MA: To gain access to this muscle it is necessary to draw the scapula away from the thoracic cage, and slide your contact over the anterior surface of the scapula between latissimus dorsi laterally and pectoralis major medially and anteriorly.

ATTACHMENTS

- Subscapularis arises from the anterior surface of the scapula:
  - by means of tendinous fibers on the crests;
  - by means of muscle fibers between the crests.
- The muscle fibers cross the anterior surface of the glenohumeral joint, adhering to the capsule.
- The muscle inserts into the lesser tubercle of the humerus.

Note: The neurovascular bundles of the axilla traverse the anterior surface of this muscle. The muscle forms part of what has traditionally been called the rotator cuff.

Fig. 3.55 Subscapularis, lateral approach to the anterior surface of the muscle body

MA: The subject lies on the contralateral side, resting his head on one hand and placing the other against the edge of the table, as shown. Stand behind the subject, and place the palm of one hand against the dorsal surface of the subject's scapula. Abduct the scapula, swinging it laterally so as to overlap the side of the thoracic cage. Ask the subject to press onto the edge of the table, putting his weight on it. This causes medial rotation of the shoulder, which is the action of the subscapularis. You will then be able to palpate the contracted muscle with your other hand.

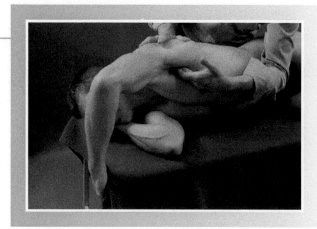

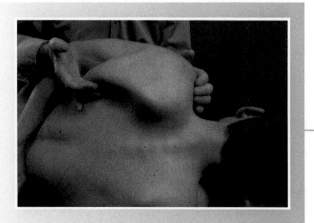

Fig. 3.56 Subscapularis, medial approach

MA: The subject lies on the contralateral side, with his arm medially rotated and the back of his hand resting on his sacrum or lumbar region. The practitioner is shown using his left hand to push the scapula medially, posteriorly, and inferiorly. His right hand palpates the medial part of the subscapularis, through serratus anterior.

Fig. 3.57 Subscapularis, humeral insertion

MA: The subject is seated. The practitioner stands behind him. Take hold of the subject's flexed elbow with one hand, and laterally rotate his arm. Use your other hand to palpate the lesser tubercle, the point of attachment of subscapularis, as the muscle separates from the coracoid process during the lateral rotation.

> **CLINICAL NOTE**
> There is tenderness to pressure on palpation of the lesser tubercle if the **tendon of subscapularis** is affected. This structure also forms part of the rotator cuff. When the muscle is tested, the finding is deficit and/or pain. (Oppose medial rotation of glenohumeral joint.)

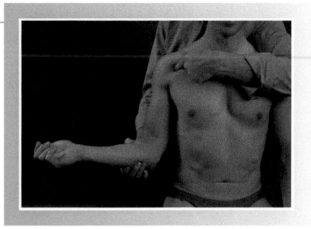

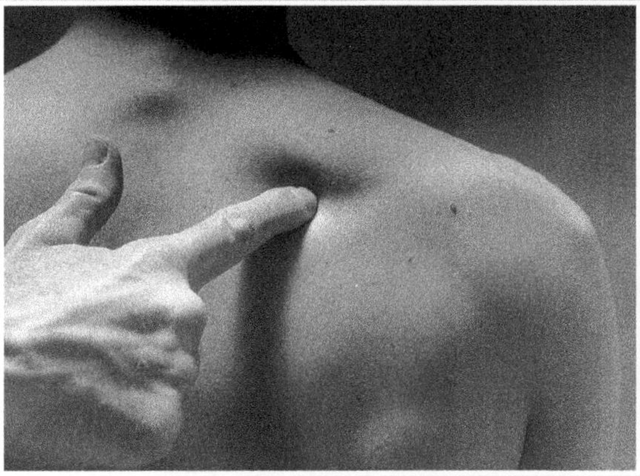

Fig. 3.58 Supraspinatus

MA: Above the spine of the scapula, supraspinatus can only be palpated through trapezius, in the supraspinous fossa. Abduction of the arm makes it possible to detect the muscle beneath your fingers, because this motion brings it into action to stabilize the shoulder.

ATTACHMENTS

- Supraspinatus arises from the medial two thirds of the supraspinous fossa and the deep surface of the supraspinous fascia.
- It crosses the superior part of the glenohumeral joint, adhering to the joint capsule there.
- It is inserted into the superior facet of the greater tubercle of the humerus.

Note: This muscle forms part of what has traditionally been called the rotator cuff.

> **CLINICAL NOTE**
> Testing of this muscle may reveal deficit if there is entrapment of the suprascapular nerve (tunnel syndrome), which involves compression of the nerve as it passes through the suprascapular notch.

Fig. 3.59 Supraspinatus, another approach

MA: The subject lies on his left side, with his right arm resting along the right side of his chest. Use your left hand at the subject's elbow to resist isometric abduction of his right arm. Use your right thumb to palpate the contraction of supraspinatus above the spine of the scapula.

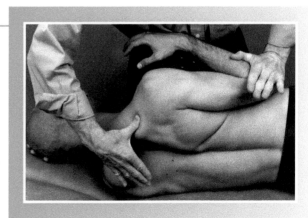

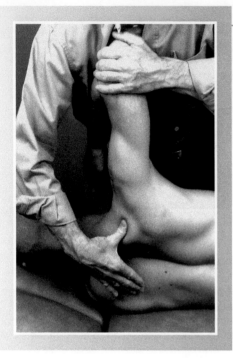

Fig. 3.60 Supraspinatus, another approach

MA: The subject lies on his left side, with his shoulder and elbow both flexed at 90°, and his right forearm flat against the right side of the practitioner's chest. Use your left hand at the subject's elbow to resist isometric abduction of his right arm. As you do so, palpate the contraction of supraspinatus, above the spine of the scapula, with your right thumb.

Fig. 3.61 Humeral insertion of supraspinatus

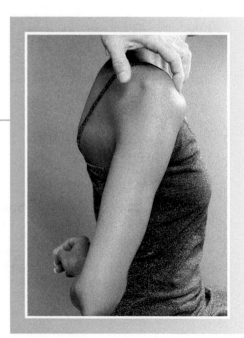

MA: Position the subject's arm as shown here. Her shoulder is medially rotated and pulled back, with the dorsal surface of her hand and the posterior surface of her forearm against her back. This tendinous insertion attaches to the superior facet of the greater tubercle of the humerus, which can be palpated anterior to the top of the acromion.

Note: This muscle contributes to the acromioclavicular arch and forms part of what has traditionally been called the rotator cuff.

> **CLINICAL NOTE**
>
> **Tendinitis** here produces tenderness to pressure or exacerbation of pain on palpation. Testing (abduction of the shoulder against resistance) may reveal deficit and/or evoke pain.

Fig. 3.62 Infraspinatus

MA: The subject is seated. The practitioner should support the subject's arm (shoulder abducted at 90°, elbow flexed at 90°). From this starting position, ask him to rotate his shoulder laterally, as shown in the adjacent figure. (This means that he brings the posterior surface of his forearm upward and backward.) The contraction can be detected in the infraspinous fossa of the scapula, where this muscle arises (1).

ATTACHMENTS

- The origin of infraspinatus is muscular, arising from the medial three fourths of the infraspinous fossa and the deep surface of the infraspinous fascia.
- The muscle fibers adhere to the capsule, crossing the posterosuperior part of the glenohumeral joint.
- The muscle inserts into the middle facet of the posterior surface of the greater tubercle of the humerus.

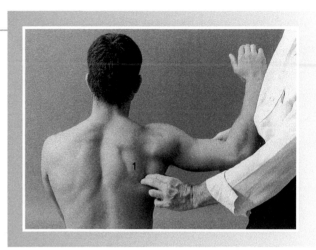

> ### CLINICAL NOTE
>
> Testing of infraspinatus may reveal deficit if the **suprascapular nerve** is affected. A possible cause is entrapment of the suprascapular nerve, which can be compressed as it passes through the suprascapular notch or spinoglenoid notch.

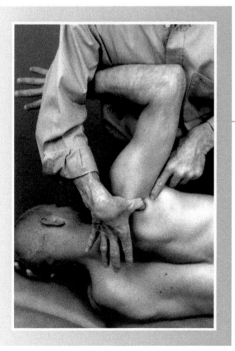

Fig. 3.63 Infraspinatus, another approach

MA: The subject lies on his left side, with shoulder flexed at 90°, elbow at 90°, and with his right forearm lying against the right half of the practitioner's chest. Ask the subject to rotate his shoulder laterally, and use the medial surface of your arm to offer isometric resistance.

This will leave both your hands free to take hold of the most lateral part of the body of infraspinatus between your right thumb and left index finger. This is near the point where infraspinatus attaches to the middle facet of the greater tubercle of the humerus.

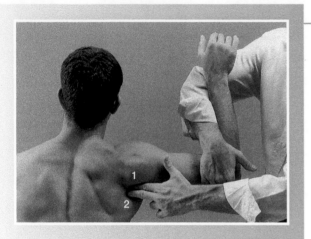

Fig. 3.64 Teres minor

MA: The subject is seated, shoulder abducted at 90°, elbow flexed at 90°. Grasp the subject's arm with a supporting hold. The anterior surface of the subject's forearm should be pronated, resting on your arm. Use a two-finger contact with the pads of the fingers of your other hand on the lateral border of the scapula, between the spinal (posterior) part of the deltoid (1) cranially and teres major (2) caudally. Ask the subject to rotate his shoulder laterally (i.e., to move his hand and forearm backward) repeatedly. This will cause the muscle to contract beneath your fingers.

ATTACHMENTS

- The origin of teres minor (which is muscular) is in the infraspinous fossa, along the superior half of the lateral border of the scapula.
- It is inserted by means of a tendon into the inferior facet of the greater tubercle of the humerus.

Fig. 3.65 Teres minor, palpation of the relaxed muscle

MA: The subject lies on the contralateral side. The practitioner stands facing him. Grasp his elbow with one hand and guide the arm to a 90° angle of abduction. With your other hand, palpate teres minor – caudal to the spinal part of deltoid (1) – by rolling it beneath your fingers against the lateral border of the scapula.

Note: Teres minor is inconstant. When present, it lies covered by the muscle mass of teres major.

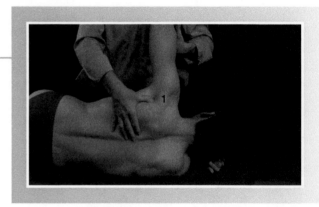

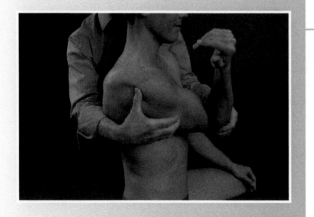

Fig. 3.66 Humeral insertions of infraspinatus and teres minor

MA: The subject is seated. Take hold of his elbow with one hand and guide the arm concerned into a position of flexion, adduction, and lateral rotation. The three elements of this movement cause the greater tubercle of the humerus to shift posteriorly and separate from the acromion. This enables you to palpate the insertions of infraspinatus and teres minor on the humerus. The bony landmark on the spine of the scapula is the acromial angle.

Note: These two muscles form part of what has traditionally been called the rotator cuff.

> **CLINICAL NOTE**
>
> Tenderness to pressure, or an increase in existing pain, on palpation is a sign of **tendinitis.** To test, ask the patient to rotate his shoulder laterally against resistance. This may be painful and/or reveal deficit. These two muscles are normally both affected together. Their humeral insertions are very close to each other, and the action of both is to rotate the shoulder laterally.

Fig. 3.67 Teres major (1)

MA: The subject should be lying prone or placed in a sitting position, with the back of his hand and posterior surface of the relevant forearm resting on the sacrum. Offer resistance to the medial surface of his arm, and resist retropulsion of the arm. Teres major (here indicated by the practitioner's index finger) creates a raised prominence that is usually clearly marked.

ATTACHMENTS

- The origin of teres major (which is muscular) is in the infraspinous fossa, along the inferior half of the lateral border of the scapula.
- It inserts by means of a broad tendon into the crest of the lesser tubercle of the humerus, posterior to latissimus dorsi. A synovial bursa separates these.

Note: The attachment of this muscle is to the inferior third of the lateral quarter of the infraspinous fossa.

> **CLINICAL NOTE**
> This muscle is also part of the rotator cuff. Any disorder at the humeral insertion may cause or exacerbate tenderness to pressure here. Testing of the muscle may also produce pain and/or reveal deficit.

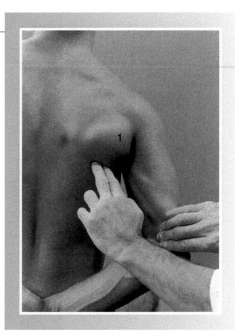

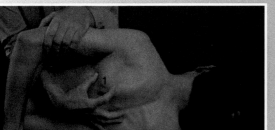

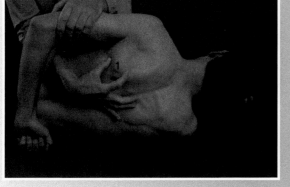

Fig. 3.68 Teres major, another approach

MA: The subject should lie on the contralateral side. The practitioner stands facing him. Guide the subject's arm into retropulsion and medial rotation, using one hand on the medial surface of his arm to offer resistance to this movement. With your other hand, palpate the body of the muscle (1) that appears at the postero-infero-lateral part of the scapula.

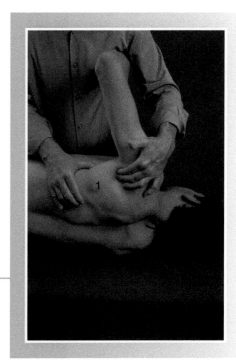

Fig. 3.69 Teres major, another approach

MA: The subject lies on the contralateral side and the practitioner stands facing him. Abduct the subject's arm to an angle of 90°, and let his hand rest flat against the side of your chest. Ask him to rotate his shoulder medially, which presses the subject's hand against your chest. The round mass of teres major (1) then appears at the postero-infero-lateral part of the scapula.

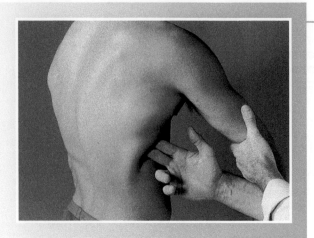

Fig. 3.70 Latissimus dorsi

MA: Resist the adduction of the subject's arm by placing resistance at the medial surface of his arm. This causes the muscle to become prominent on the posterolateral part of the thorax.

Fig. 3.71 Latissimus dorsi, another approach

MA: The subject is supine. Place the four fingers of your right hand on the inferior part of his shoulder, and ask him to bend his trunk to the right while you resist this action. Palpate latissimus dorsi with your left hand.

Note: In the adjacent figure, the practitioner has begun by asking the subject to place his forearm flat against the practitioner's chest, as a way of disengaging the latissimus dorsi.

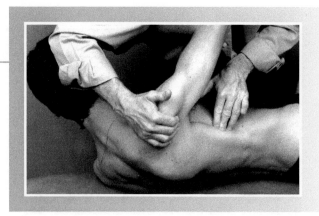

THE LATERAL MUSCLE GROUP

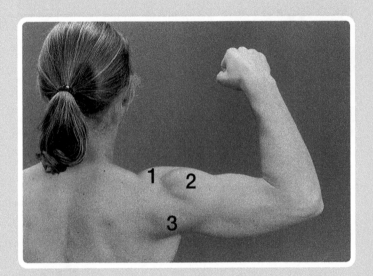

Fig. 3.72 Posterior view of the shoulder region
1. Clavicular (anterior) part of the deltoid
2. Acromial (middle) part of the deltoid
3. Spinal (posterior) part of the deltoid

This group consists of a single muscle, deltoid, which lies on the lateral part of the shoulder.

The notable structures that can be detected by palpation are:
- Spinal (posterior) part of deltoid (Fig. 3.73)
- Acromial (middle) part of deltoid (Fig. 3.74)
- Clavicular (anterior) part of deltoid (Fig. 3.75).

ACTIONS

- The clavicular part of deltoid participates in the following actions:
  - Antepulsion (drawing forward) of the arm
  - Direct abduction, together with the acromial part of deltoid
  - Horizontal anterior adduction, together with the clavicular head of pectoralis major.
- The acromial part of deltoid is responsible for abduction of the arm, together with supraspinatus.
- The spinal part of deltoid is responsible for:
  - Posterior horizontal abduction of the arm
  - Retropulsion of the arm, together with teres major and latissimus dorsi muscles. (Its role in this movement is, however, a specific one; the spinal part of deltoid operates in a neutral position or in abduction, while the other two muscles perform this motion in adduction.)

INNERVATION

- Deltoid: axillary nerve (C5–C6)

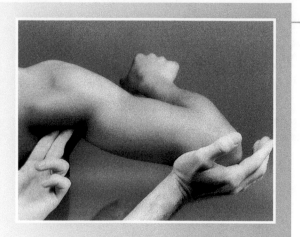

Fig. 3.73 Spinal part of the deltoid

MA: The subject's shoulder is abducted at 90°, with elbow flexed. Place resistance, as shown here, against the posterior, inferior part of the arm just above the elbow. Ask the subject to draw his arm backward and horizontally. You will feel or see the body of the muscle on the posterior part of his shoulder. Here it is indicated by the two-finger contact of the practitioner's other hand.

ATTACHMENTS OF THE THREE PORTIONS OF DELTOID

- Deltoid arises:
  – by means of a tendinous attachment: on the anterior border and superior surface of the acromial end of the clavicle, and on the lower border of the spine of the scapula;
  – by means of a muscular attachment: on the lateral border of the acromion.
- Deltoid inserts via a tendon into the deltoid tuberosity of the humerus.

Note: The subdeltoid bursa lies between the acromial part of deltoid and the greater tubercle.

Fig. 3.74 Acromial part of deltoid

MA: The subject should adopt the same position as in the previous figure (Fig. 3.73). In the adjacent figure, the practitioner's two thumbs indicate the limits of the acromial part (1), which lies between the clavicular part (2) and the spinal part (3). Ask the subject to abduct his arm, while you resist this movement.

Note: Deltoid covers the glenohumeral joint, and is separated from it by the subdeltoid bursa.

> **CLINICAL NOTE**
>
> When the **subdeltoid bursa** is affected, there is tenderness to pressure on palpating the muscle body of deltoid. Active circumduction is painful. Testing is by abduction of the shoulder against resistance, and may reveal deficit and/or cause pain. Testing of each of the muscles of the rotator cuff causes neither.

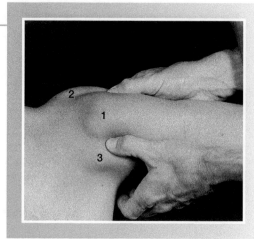

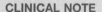

Fig. 3.75 Clavicular part of deltoid

MA: The subject's shoulder is again at 90° abduction, with elbow flexed. In the adjacent figure, the practitioner's thumb and index finger indicate the limits of the clavicular part. Ask the subject to draw his shoulder forward horizontally while you resist this movement.

> **CLINICAL NOTE**
>
> (All three parts of the muscle.) If testing reveals deficit and there is pain at the point of the shoulder, consider the possibility of a problem affecting the **circumflex nerve,** such as nerve entrapment (tunnel syndrome), involving compression of the nerve in the lateral axillary space.

4
The arm

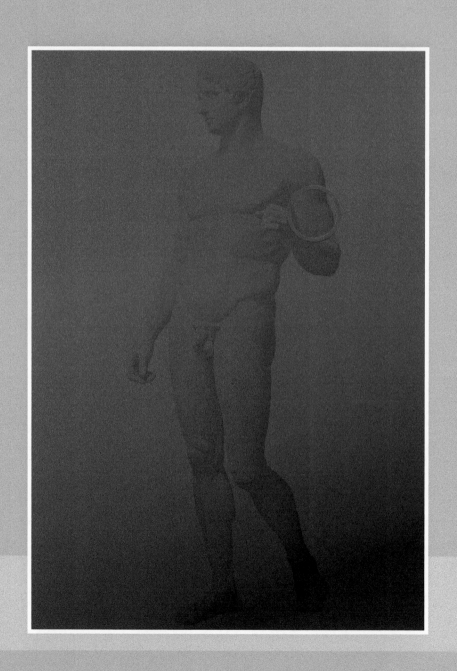

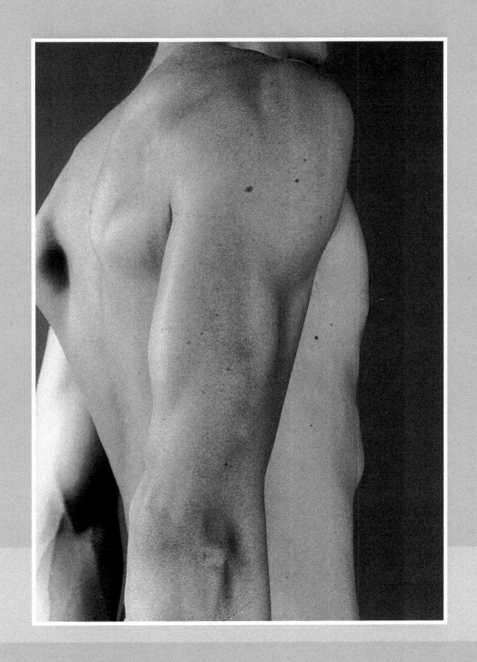

MYOLOGY

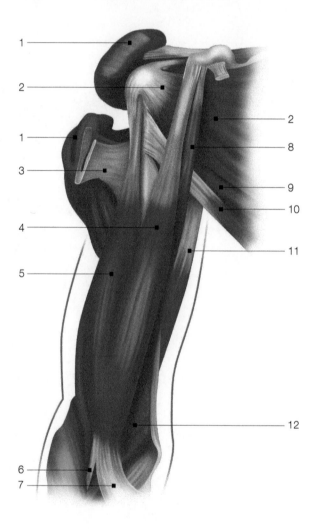

Anterior muscle group: superficial layer (biceps brachii)

1. Deltoid
2. Subscapularis
3. Pectoralis major
4. Short head of biceps brachii
5. Long head of biceps brachii
6. Tendon of biceps brachii
7. Aponeurosis of biceps brachii
8. Coracobrachialis
9. Teres major
10. Latissimus dorsi
11. Triceps brachii
12. Brachialis

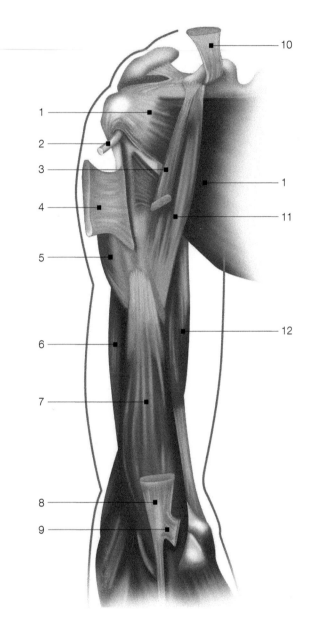

Anterior muscle group: deep layer (coracobrachialis and brachialis)

1. Subscapularis	7. Brachialis
2. Tendon of biceps brachii (long head)	8. Biceps brachii
3. Short head of biceps brachii	9. Aponeurosis of biceps brachii
4. Pectoralis major	10. Pectoralis minor
5. Deltoid	11. Coracobrachialis
6. Lateral head of triceps brachii	12. Long head of triceps brachii

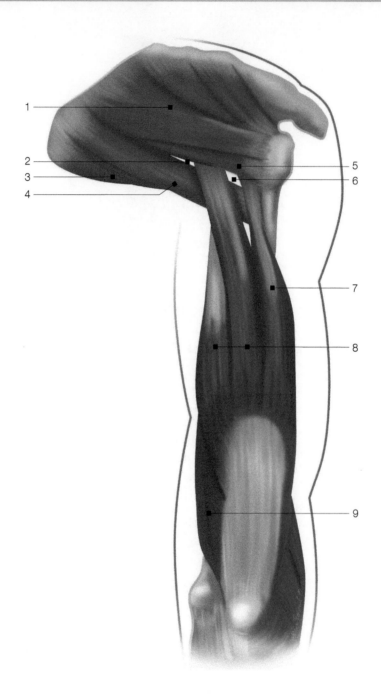

1
2
3
4
5
6
7
8
9

Posterior muscle group of the arm: triceps brachii

1. Infraspinatus
2. Medial axillary space
3. Latissimus dorsi
4. Teres major
5. Teres minor

6. Lateral axillary space
7. Lateral head of triceps brachii
8. Long head of triceps brachii
9. Medial head of triceps brachii

THE ANTERIOR MUSCLE GROUP

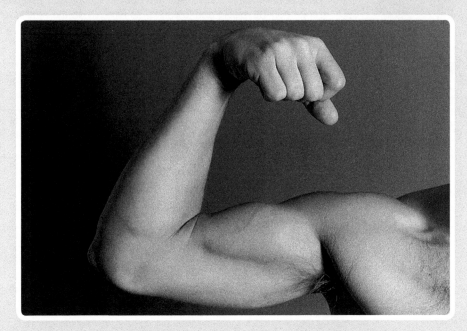

Fig. 4.2 The anterior region of the arm

This group consists of three muscles: biceps brachii, coracobrachialis, and brachialis. These muscles overlie each other, arranged in two layers: a superficial and a deep layer.

The notable structures that can be detected by palpation are:

- Superficial layer:
  - Body of the long head of biceps brachii (Fig. 4.3)
  - Body of the short head of biceps brachii (Figs. 4.4 and 4.5)
  - Tendon of biceps brachii (Fig. 4.6)
  - Bicipital aponeurosis (Fig. 4.7)
- Deep layer:
  - Body of coracobrachialis (Fig. 4.8)
  - Brachialis (Figs. 4.9–4.12).

ACTIONS

- Biceps brachii:
  - Flexes and supinates the forearm upon the arm.
  - Helps to retain the head of the humerus in the glenoid cavity.
- Coracobrachialis flexes and slightly adducts the arm.
- Brachialis flexes the forearm on the arm. (Forearm pronated.)

INNERVATIONS

- Biceps brachii: musculocutaneous nerve (C5–C6)
- Coracobrachialis: musculocutaneous nerve (C5–C6)
- Brachialis: musculocutaneous nerve (C5–C6)

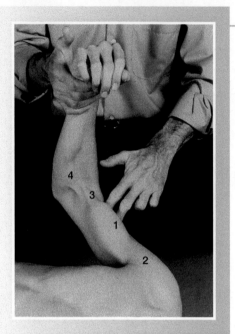

1. Body of biceps
2. Proximal tendon of the long head of biceps
3. Distal tendon of biceps
4. Bicipital aponeurosis

Fig. 4.3 Body of the long head of biceps brachii

MA: As shown in this figure, the long head can easily be palpated on the anterior surface of the arm, from the elbow region to the point where the muscle disappears behind deltoid. Ask the subject to contract and relax the muscle repeatedly by raising and lowering his forearm on the arm several times, with the forearm supinated. This makes it easier to see the body of the muscle.

ATTACHMENTS

Biceps brachii is made up of two parts, the long and short heads.

- The long head arises from the supraglenoid tubercle of the scapula, and the glenoid labrum.
- The short head arises from the apex of the coracoid process of the scapula.
- These two portions of the muscle rejoin and are inserted into the posterior surface of the radial tuberosity. The aponeurosis that radiates out from biceps (Fig. 4.7) leaves the medial tendon level with the elbow and disappears into the antebrachial fascia.

> **CLINICAL NOTE**
>
> **The following problems can affect the tendon of the long head:**
>
> - Tendinopathy: Examination looks for tenderness to palpation in the bicipital groove, and for pain in the palm-up test. (See Glossary.)
>
> - Rupture: On palpation, the body of the long head feels flaccid and appears to have sunk to the middle of the arm.
>
> - Displacement (total or partial) medial to the crest of the lesser tubercle. The patient reports having heard a click, and palpation finds pain at the bicipital groove.

Fig. 4.4 Body of the short head of biceps brachii

MA: In order to distinguish between the short (1) and long head (2) of the muscle, use one of your hands to offer slight resistance as the subject flexes his supinated forearm on the arm. Then place two or three fingers of your other hand flat on the proximal third of anterior surface of the subject's arm, with your palm resting on pectoralis major, as shown. Moving downward toward the subject's elbow and easing medially, seek a groove separating the two bodies of the long and short heads of biceps brachii. This is best done by asking the subject to flex his elbow, so as to contract and relax the muscle, a few times in succession.

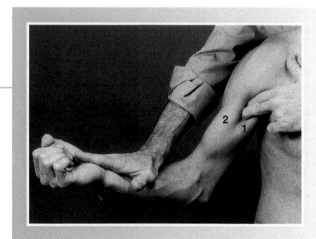

Fig. 4.5 Short head of biceps brachii

MA: Place the subject's forearm so that it rests between your arm and your thoracic cage, and hold it there. Both your hands need to be free to perform this investigation. In this illustration, the practitioner has isolated the short head (1) of biceps brachii, separating it from the long head (2) and from coracobrachialis (3). His right thumb is resting on coracobrachialis.

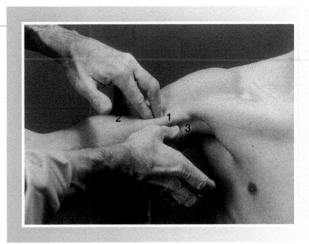

Fig. 4.6 Distal tendon of biceps brachii

MA: This tendon is very strong and can easily be palpated in the fold of the elbow. If you do need to make the tendon more prominent, ask the subject to flex his supinated forearm, and resist this action.

Note: The attachment of this tendon is to the posterior part of the radial tuberosity.

> **CLINICAL NOTE**
>
> **Problems affecting the distal tendon** are rare. There are two possibilities:
>
> - Tendinopathy: There is tenderness to palpation at the distal insertion of the tendon. Flexion of the elbow and supination against resistance cause pain, as does stretching of the muscle.
>
> - Distal rupture: Treatment requires surgery. Complications are stiffness on extension and wasting of the muscle. Bear in mind the possibility that complex regional pain syndrome could develop.

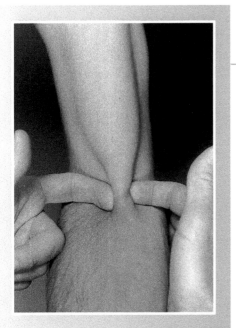

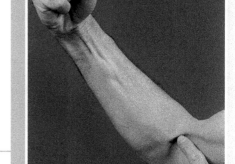

Fig. 4.7 Aponeurosis of biceps brachii

MA: Begin by asking the subject to flex his supinated forearm upon the arm. Place your index finger on the medial part of his elbow, against the tendon of biceps brachii. You can then detect where the aponeurosis leaves the medial border and anterior surface of this tendon to disappear into the aponeurosis of the medial epicondylar muscles (forearm flexors).

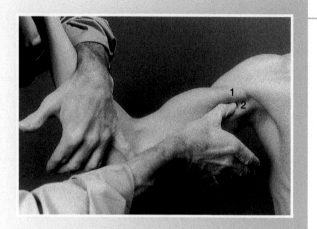

Fig. 4.8 Body of coracobrachialis

MA: Place a contact using the pad of your thumb on the medial surface of the subject's upper arm behind the short head (1) of biceps brachii (Fig. 4.5). To help you locate coracobrachialis, first ask the subject to flex his elbow, then to flex and adduct his shoulder, as shown in this figure, while you resist these movements by placing your other hand against the anterior surface of his forearm. This will throw biceps into full contraction and make it easier for you to distinguish biceps from coracobrachialis, which you are seeking. You will sense a muscular cord (2) tensing beneath your fingers.

ATTACHMENTS

- Coracobrachialis arises via a tendon, fused with that of the short portion of biceps, from the medial side of the apex of the coracoid process of the scapula.
- Its insertion is into the middle third of the medial surface of the humerus.

Note: This muscle runs from the coracoid process to the medial surface of the upper arm.

Fig. 4.9 Body of brachialis in the inferior third of the upper arm

MA: Place a global contact, between thumbs and fingers, on the lateral and medial parts of the upper arm, behind and to either side of biceps brachii (1). Ask the subject to pronate his forearm and then flex his elbow against resistance.

ATTACHMENTS

- Brachialis arises via muscle fibers:
  - from the inferior half of the medial and lateral surfaces of the humerus;
  - from the medial and lateral intermuscular septa.
- It is inserted into the medial part of the tuberosity of the ulna.

Note: This muscle runs from the humerus to the tuberosity of the ulna.

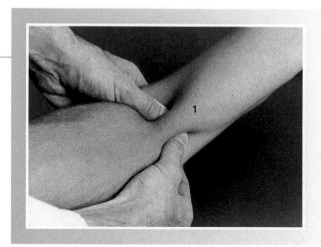

Fig. 4.10 Brachialis at the arm, another approach – step 1

MA: It is possible to roll the body of the muscle beneath your fingers against the lateral border of the humerus. To do this, abduct the subject's arm at 90° and position it so that biceps is pulled downward by gravity. This makes it easier to separate out brachialis. The subject's elbow should also be bent at 90° so as to relax biceps and brachialis muscles. Ease biceps brachii (1) aside with your fingers and take hold of as much as possible of the body of brachialis.

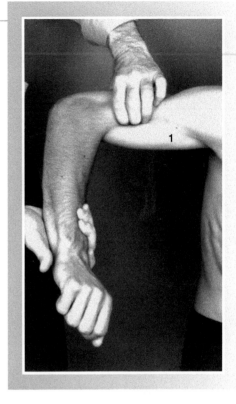

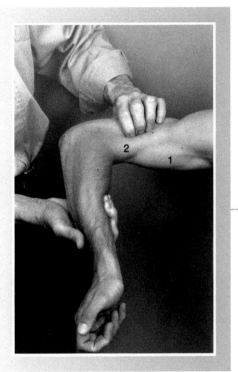

Fig. 4.11 Brachialis at the arm, another approach – step 2

MA: With the subject's shoulder and elbow still positioned as described above (Fig. 4.10), roll your fingers onto brachialis (2), working backward from anterior until you locate the muscle on the lateral border of the humerus. You will find it quite separate from biceps (1), which normally covers it (particularly the anterior part), leaving the lateral and medial parts free.

Fig. 4.12 Brachialis at the arm, other method of approach

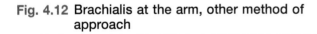

MA: Another way to separate brachialis from biceps is to ease back biceps medially. This enables you to take hold of it between the thumb of your right hand and the index, middle, and ring fingers of your left hand (as shown in the adjacent figure).

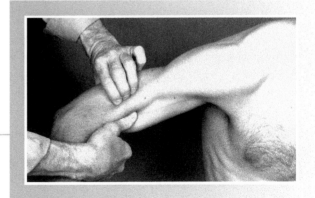

CLINICAL NOTE

If testing reveals any deficit of this muscle, or other muscles of the anterior compartment of the arm (biceps brachii, coracobrachialis), a **neurogenic cause** should be considered. Entrapment of the musculocutaneous nerve where it passes through the body of coracobrachialis is one possibility. Examine by palpating this muscle, looking for the place that causes pain to be exacerbated.

THE POSTERIOR MUSCLE GROUP

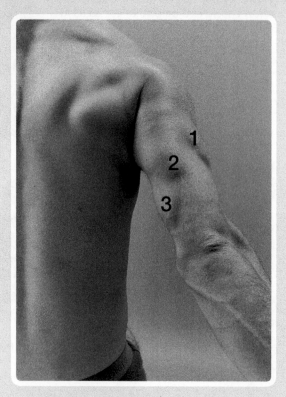

Fig. 4.13 The posterior region of the arm
1. Lateral head of triceps brachii
2. Long head of triceps brachii
3. Medial head (deep head) of triceps brachii

This muscle group consists of just one muscle, triceps brachii.
  The notable structures that can be detected by palpation are:

- Proximal tendon of the long head of triceps brachii (Figs. 4.14 and 4.15)
- Body of the long head of triceps brachii (Fig. 4.16)
- Lateral head of triceps brachii (Fig. 4.17)
- Medial head (deep head) of triceps brachii (Figs. 4.18 and 4.19)
- Distal tendon of the long head of triceps brachii (Fig. 4.20).

ACTIONS

- The long head of triceps brachii extends the forearm on the arm, acting together with anconeus. (The force of the medial and lateral heads when performing this action is greater than that of the long head.)
- The long head is involved in retropulsion of the arm, and maintains the head of the humerus in the glenoid cavity (for example, during extension of the arm together with extension of the elbow).

INNERVATIONS

- Triceps brachii: radial nerve (C6–C7–C8)

Fig. 4.14 Proximal tendon of the long head of triceps brachii

MA: The subject is seated. The practitioner should stand beside the subject, on the side of the arm to be examined. Position the subject's arm as shown in the adjacent figure, with his shoulder abducted at 90° and elbow flexed at 90°. Place your contact on the posterior part of the subject's shoulder using the pad of one or two fingers of your palpating hand as shown, in contact with the spinal part of deltoid and lateral to teres minor (see Chapter 3). Ask the subject to extend his forearm on the arm, while you resist this action by placing your other hand on the distal end of his forearm. You will detect the tendon beneath your fingers, on the posterior surface of the subject's shoulder.

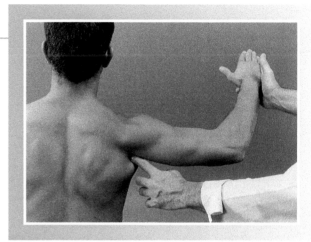

ATTACHMENTS

Triceps brachii consists of three heads: the lateral, medial, and long heads.

- The long head arises from the infraglenoid tubercle and glenoid labrum, by means of a tendon.
- The lateral head arises via tendinous fibers:
  - from the lateral part of the posterior surface of the humerus, proximal to the radial groove;
  - from the lateral intermuscular septum of the arm.
- The medial head arises via fleshy fibers:
  - from the medial intermuscular septum of the arm;
  - from the posterior surface of the shaft of the humerus, distal to the radial groove.

The three heads converge toward the middle of the posterior surface, on a tendon that is flattened from front to back.

- The fibers of the long head terminate on the superficial part of this tendon.
- The fibers of the lateral head terminate on the deep part and the lateral border of this tendon.
- The fibers of the medial head terminate on the deep part and the medial border of this tendon.

The muscle is inserted:

- by means of a tendon into the posterior part of the superior surface of the olecranon of the ulna;
- by means of fleshy fibers from the lateral and medial heads, into the lateral and medial surfaces of the olecranon of the ulna.

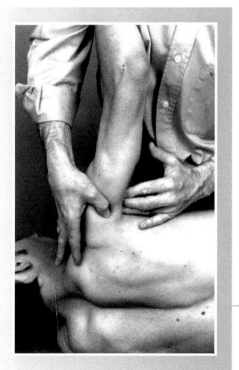

Fig. 4.15 Proximal tendon of the long head of triceps brachii, another approach

MA: The subject lies on his left side, with his right arm abducted at 90° and forearm resting inside the pit of the practitioner's right arm. Ask the subject to extend his forearm upon the arm. This action enables you to sense the contraction at the tendon and to take hold of the tendon between your fingers.

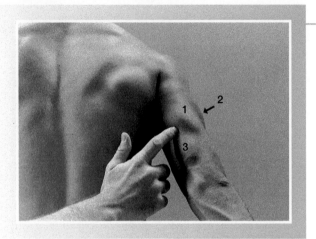

Fig. 4.16 Body of the long head of triceps brachii

MA: The long head (1) of triceps brachii should not be confused with the lateral head (2), which lies anterior and laterally to it, or with the medial head (3), which is distal to the long head and more medially situated. Ask the subject to extend his forearm on the arm against resistance in order to make the body of the long head more prominent, or to enable you to palpate it when it is contracted.

Fig. 4.17 Lateral head of triceps brachii (1)

MA: The lateral head is situated on the lateral surface of the arm, lateral and anterior to the long head (2) of triceps brachii. Extension of the subject's forearm on the arm against resistance will help to display it.

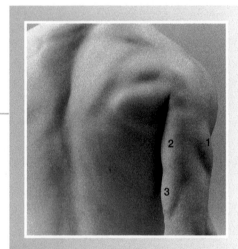

1. Lateral head of triceps brachii
2. Long head of triceps brachii
3. Medial head of triceps brachii

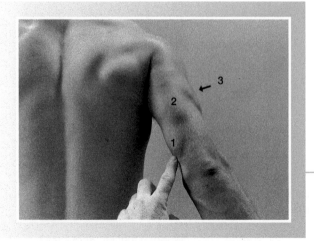

Fig. 4.18 Medial head of triceps brachii, posterior view

MA: Ask the subject to extend and flex his forearm repeatedly on the arm against resistance, in order to help you display the medial head (1). It is situated at the distal prolongation of the long head, and is medial to it.

1. Medial head of triceps brachii
2. Long head of triceps brachii
3. Lateral head of triceps brachii

Fig. 4.19 Medial head of triceps brachii, medial view

MA: In the adjacent figure, the body of the medial head (1) can be seen on the medial part of the arm, medial and posterior to biceps brachii (2) and proximal to the medial epicondyle (3). Ask the subject to extend his forearm on the arm against resistance to assist you in displaying and detecting it.

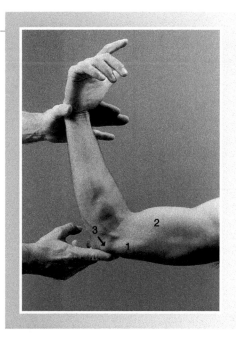

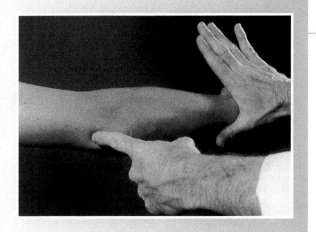

Fig. 4.20 Distal tendon of triceps brachii

MA: The distal tendon is generally flattened from front to back, although it is sometimes found as a full, cylindrical cord that can be perceived on the posterior surface of the elbow, just before its insertion into the superior surface of the olecranon. Ask the subject to extend his forearm on the arm against resistance to help you detect it.

CLINICAL NOTE

Tendinopathy

To investigate this, apply palpation to look for tenderness to pressure at one or more points on the elbow. Isometric testing can be done by opposing extension of the elbow, to find whether this evokes pain.

NERVES AND BLOOD VESSELS

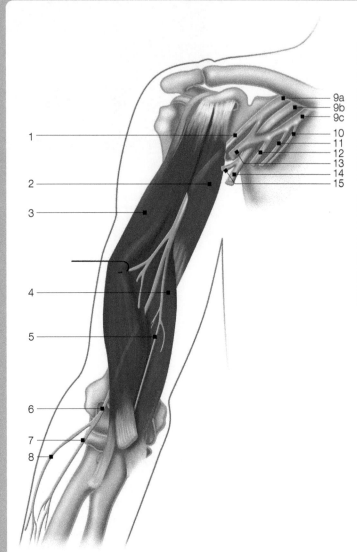

Musculocutaneous nerve (anterior view) and muscles innervated by musculocutaneous nerve

1. Musculocutaneous nerve (C5, C6, C7)
2. Coracobrachialis
3. Biceps brachii
4. Brachialis
5. Articular branch
6. Lateral cutaneous nerve of forearm
7. Anterior division
8. Posterior division
9a. Lateral cord of brachial plexus
9b. Posterior cord of brachial plexus
9c. Medial cord of brachial plexus
10. Medial cutaneous nerve of arm
11. Medial cutaneous nerve of forearm
12. Ulnar nerve
13. Median nerve
14. Radial nerve
15. Axillary nerve

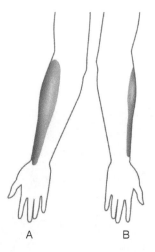

Cutaneous innervation by lateral cutaneous nerve of forearm

A. Anterior (palmar) view
B. Posterior (dorsal) view

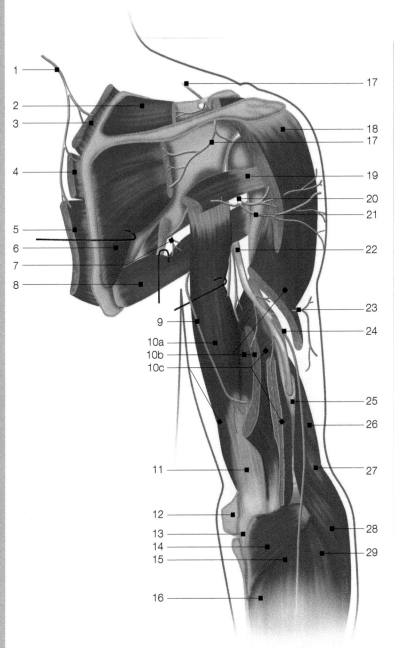

1. Dorsal scapular nerve (C5)
2. Supraspinatus
3. Levator scapulae (innervated by rami of C3 and C4)
4. Rhomboid minor
5. Rhomboid major
6. Infraspinatus
7. Inferior subscapular nerve (C5, C6)
8. Teres major
9. Posterior cutaneous nerve of arm (branch of radial nerve in axillary fossa)
10abc. Triceps brachii, (a) long head, (b) lateral head, (c) medial head
11. Tendon of triceps brachii
12. Medial epicondyle
13. Olecranon
14. Anconeus
15. Extensor digitorum
16. Extensor carpi ulnaris
17. Suprascapular nerve (C5, C6)
18. Deltoid
19. Teres minor
20. Axillary nerve (C5, C6)
21. Superior lateral cutaneous nerve of arm
22. Radial nerve (C5–C8)
23. Inferior lateral cutaneous nerve of arm
24. Posterior cutaneous nerve of forearm
25. Lateral intermuscular septum
26. Brachialis (lateral part; the rest of the muscle is innervated by the musculocutaneous nerve)
27. Brachioradialis
28. Extensor carpi radialis longus
29. Extensor carpi radialis brevis

THE PRINCIPAL NERVES AND BLOOD VESSELS

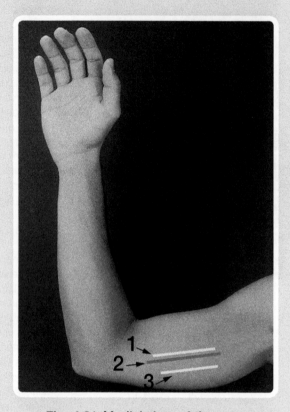

Fig. 4.21 Medial view of the arm

1. Median nerve
2. Brachial artery
3. Ulnar nerve

The notable structures that can be detected by palpation are:
- Brachial artery (Fig. 4.22)
- Median nerve and distal part of the brachial artery (Fig. 4.23)
- Ulnar nerve in the distal part of the arm (Fig. 4.24)
- Radial nerve at the posterior surface of the arm (Figs. 4.25 and 4.26).

Fig. 4.22 Brachial artery (proximal part)

MA: Begin by locating coracobrachialis. Flexion and abduction of the subject's shoulder (as shown here) will help you to do this. Place a broad contact – with the pads of two or more fingers – behind the body of the muscle. You will be able to detect the pulse of the brachial artery.

Note: Take great care when taking the pulse, as the median nerve passes close to the brachial artery.

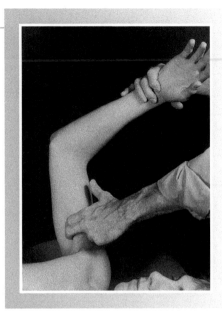

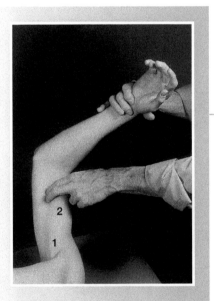

Fig. 4.23 Median nerve and brachial artery (distal part)

MA: Begin by locating the body of coracobrachialis (1) by flexion and abduction of the subject's shoulder. Place a broad contact – with the pads of two or more fingers – behind the body of this muscle, and draw the whole arm into a position of horizontal abduction. The subject's forearm may be flexed and pronated. You can follow the entire course of the nerve along the anteromedial surface of the arm to the fold of the elbow, easing aside biceps brachii (2) laterally to roll the nerve beneath your fingers. It is also possible to follow the brachial artery along the course of the median nerve, on the medial part of the arm. The pulse of this artery can be felt beneath your fingers as far as the fold of the elbow.

Note: Care should be taken when taking the pulse of the brachial artery, as the medial nerve passes close to the brachial artery. (Exceptionally, the nerve lies behind the artery.)

CLINICAL NOTE

1. **Tunnel syndrome (entrapment of a nerve in a normal tunnel of bone/muscle/aponeurosis)**

   The median nerve can be affected at three points:

   - at the forearm, where the nerve passes between the heads of pronator teres;

   - at the forearm, at the arch of flexor digitorum superficialis;

   - at the wrist, at the carpal tunnel. In this case, the nerve is compressed because the tunnel is reduced in size due to tenosynovitis (through microtrauma in the course of the patient's professional work). Clinically, the patient complains of pain or paresthesia (pins and needles, burning sensation, etc.) at the hand or fingers. The patient may also report clumsiness (tendency to drop objects held in the hand). The thenar eminence is sometimes atrophied.

2. **Trauma**

   Injury to the nerve can occur following a fracture, along the whole of its course, or may result from dislocation of the lunate bone.

3. **Other pathologies**

   The nerve may be the site of neuritis or of a tumor.

   Examination seeks to locate the problem (in addition to the history) by asking the patient to point to the site of the pain or paresthesia, or by giving details of the accident. The examination itself, in the case of post-traumatic pain, involves:

   - Palpation: apply pressure as you palpate the possible sites of nerve entrapment. Pain and/or paresthesia denotes a positive finding. In the case of dislocation of the lunate, if seen early, palpation will detect the bone concerned and the possible sequelae.

   - Stretching the nerve also evokes pain and/or paresthesia in the area of skin concerned.

   - Motricity: muscle testing of the myotome enables you to locate the muscles affected.

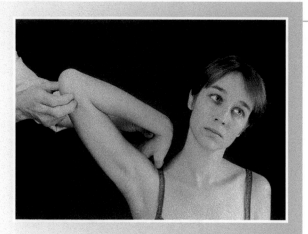

Fig. 4.24 Ulnar nerve in the distal part of the arm

MA: At the point where the superior third of the arm meets the middle third, the nerve takes an inferior, posterior, and medial direction. It passes through the medial intermuscular septum. From here on, until it reaches the groove between the epicondyle and the olecranon, it is in the posterior compartment of the arm, so that you can roll the nerve beneath your fingers at the contact with the medial head of triceps brachii. It is easier to perceive this nerve if the subject's arm is placed in maximum antepulsion, as shown here (it may or may not be abducted). Her elbow should be flexed to the maximum, forearm pronated, and wrist extended. Take care not to allow the subject to remain in this position for too long, because it is a biomechanical situation in which pressure buildup within the nerve is at its greatest. (See Chapter 5.)

CLINICAL NOTE

Compression of the ulnar nerve may occur following fracture of the distal end of the humerus or the medial epicondyle. Two sites of entrapment should be considered:

- The groove for the ulnar nerve: findings are paresthesia at the little finger and ulnar portion of the fourth finger, through microtrauma in professional work, and/or valgus of the ulna. Palpation with the use of pressure may evoke or exacerbate these.

- The ulnar canal (Guyon's canal): paresthesia at the palm of the hand, through microtrauma in professional work or sports, probably due to prolonged pressure at the base of the hypothenar eminence.

Fig. 4.25 Radial nerve (posterior surface of the arm)

MA: Place one hand distal to the deltoid tuberosity of the humerus, on the posterior surface of the arm, at the radial groove. The structure to be investigated can be rolled beneath your fingers, through the muscular mass of triceps brachii.

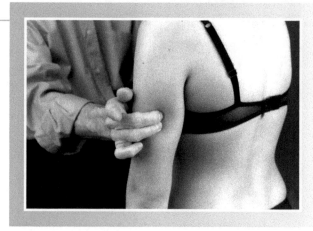

CLINICAL NOTE

Problems affecting the **radial nerve** can occur as complications following dislocation of the head of the humerus or fracture of the surgical neck of the shaft. This nerve, in common with all others, can be the site of a tumor or neuritis. Tunnel syndrome is possible if the nerve is compressed at the arcade of Frohse (supinator arch). Paralysis is only complete (muscle test score 0) if the lesion is in the axilla.

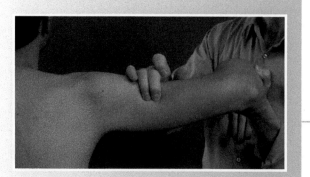

Fig. 4.26 Radial nerve, another approach

MA: Grasp the subject's elbow with one hand. Guide his arm into the position shown here, flexed and abducted at an angle of 90°. Use your other hand to palpate the radial nerve in the depression that forms between deltoid and the lateral head of triceps brachii.

5
The elbow

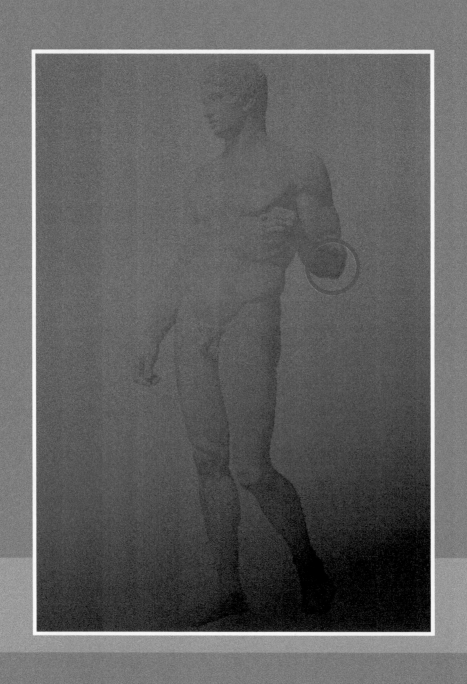

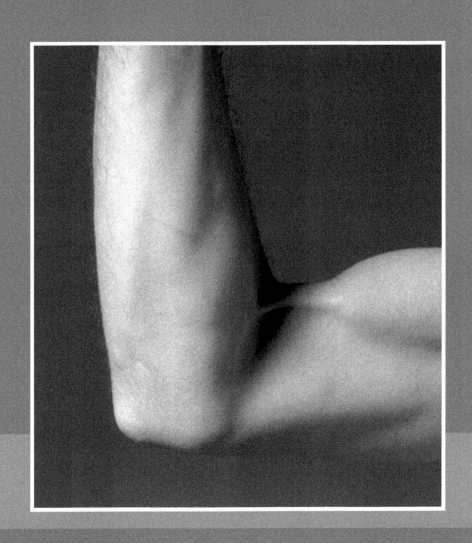

OSTEOLOGY

Anterior view

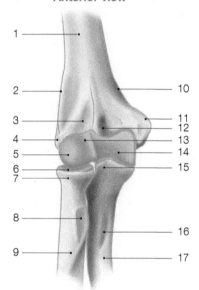

Posterior view

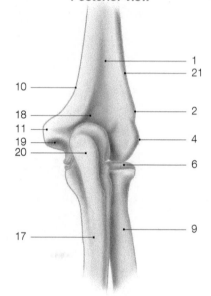

Lateral view

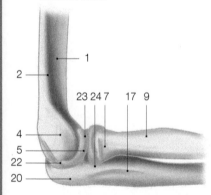

Medial view

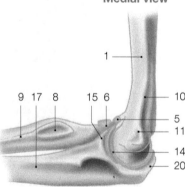

The elbow joint

1. Humerus
2. Lateral supraepicondylar ridge
3. Radial fossa
4. Lateral epicondyle
5. Capitulum of humerus
6. Head of radius
7. Neck of radius
8. Radial tuberosity
9. Radius
10. Medial supraepicondylar ridge
11. Medial epicondyle
12. Coronoid fossa
13. Capitulotrochlear groove
14. Trochlea of humerus
15. Coronoid process
16. Tuberosity of ulna
17. Ulna
18. Olecranon fossa
19. Radial groove
20. Olecranon
21. Lateral border
22. Humeroulnar joint
23. Humeroradial joint
24. Radioulnar joint

THE ELBOW: OVERVIEW

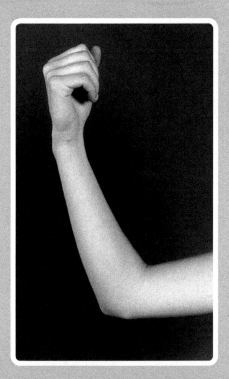

Fig. 5.2 Topographical presentation of the elbow

The notable structures that can be detected by palpation are:

- **Humerus:**
  - Capitulum of the humerus (Figs. 5.3 and 5.20)
  - Lateral epicondyle (Fig. 5.4)
  - Lateral supraepicondylar ridge (Fig. 5.5)
  - Olecranon fossa (Fig. 5.6)
  - Medial epicondyle (Figs. 5.7 and 5.8)
  - Medial supraepicondylar ridge (Fig. 5.9)
  - Groove for the ulnar nerve (Fig. 5.10)
  - Trochlea of humerus (Fig. 5.21)
- **Radius:**
  - Head of the radius (Fig. 5.11)
  - Neck of the radius (Fig. 5.12)
  - Radial tuberosity (Fig. 5.13)
- **Ulna:**
  - Display of the olecranon at the elbow (Fig. 5.14)
  - Superior surface of the olecranon (Fig. 5.15)
  - Medial surface of the olecranon (Fig. 5.16)
  - Lateral surface of the olecranon (Fig. 5.17)
  - Posterior border of the shaft (body) of the ulna (Fig. 5.18)
  - Coronoid process of the ulna (Fig. 5.19).

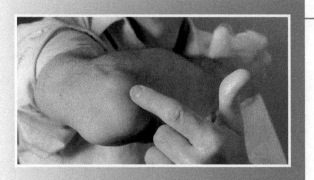

Fig. 5.3 Capitulum of the humerus, posterior surface

MA: This lies at the distal and lateral extremity of the humerus, and articulates with the articular facet of the radius. In order for you to palpate the full extent of the capitulum, the subject's elbow needs to be fully flexed. This muscular action will also reveal the posterior and inferior parts of this structure. The capitulum will appear smooth beneath your fingers.

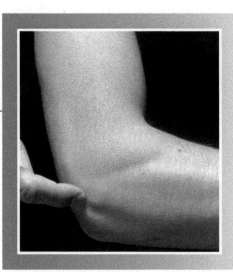

Fig. 5.4 Lateral epicondyle

MA: This structure is proximal and lateral to the capitulum, and distal to the distal extremity of the lateral supraepicondylar ridge. You can feel its rough surface beneath your fingers. It gives attachment to the lateral epicondylar muscles (forearm extensors) and the radial collateral ligament.

Note: The lateral epicondylar muscles (also called the forearm extensors) are a muscle group consisting of the following: anconeus, extensor carpi radialis brevis, extensor digitorum, extensor digiti minimi, extensor carpi ulnaris, and supinator. The attachment of anconeus is by means of its own tendon on the posterior surface of the lateral epicondyle of the humerus. The origin of the other muscles is by means of a common tendon.

CLINICAL NOTE

Four types of pathology can occur at the lateral epicondyle, either in isolation or superimposed:

1. **Epicondylitis:** This is the most frequently seen. It consists of tendinopathy of the epicondylar muscles; those most commonly affected are extensor carpi radialis brevis, extensor digitorum, and, to a lesser extent, supinator. Two others can (very rarely) be involved: extensor digiti minimi and extensor carpi ulnaris. Three methods of investigation are used in diagnosis:
   - palpation by applying pressure;
   - isometric testing of each of the muscles concerned;
   - stretching of these muscles.

   Each of these tests replicates or exacerbates the pain.
2. **Arthropathy of the humeroradial joint:** These are the articular/abarticular structures concerned.
3. **Compression of the posterior branch of the radial nerve.**
4. **Cervicobrachial neuralgia:** The source of the pathology lies at C5–C6 or C6–C7. (See Chapter 1.)

Fig. 5.5 Lateral supraepicondylar ridge

MA: This can be sensed as a marked, sharp ridge beneath your fingers. It is directly accessible beneath the skin, proximal to the lateral epicondyle (Fig. 5.4), and is considerably more marked than the medial supraepicondylar ridge.

Note: The proximal continuation of this ridge runs along the lateral border of the humerus (this can be sensed clearly beneath your fingers) as far as the (lateral) deltoid tuberosity.

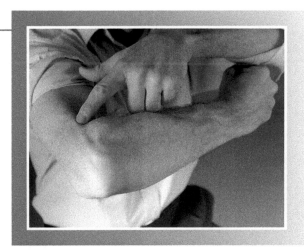

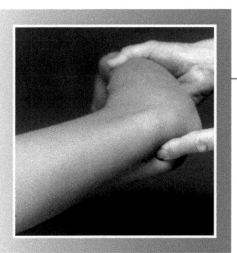

Fig. 5.6 Olecranon fossa

MA: This lies at the distal extremity of the posterior surface of the humerus. The fossa receives the proximal extremity of the olecranon when the forearm is extended on the arm. The approach is easier if the subject's elbow is flexed at an angle of 130°–140°, so as to relax the tendon of triceps brachii. Using a contact with the pads of two fingers, supported against the capitulum of the humerus, direct your contact posteriorly, easing the tendon of triceps brachii aside medially. The fossa will appear beneath your fingers, proximal to the olecranon.

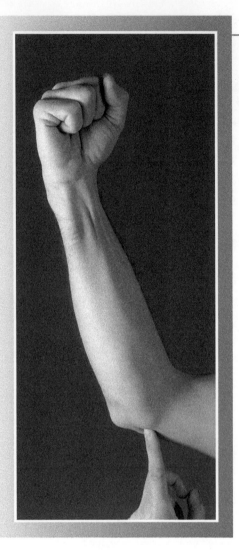

Fig. 5.7 Medial epicondyle

MA: This structure is proximal and medial to the trochlea of the humerus, at the distal extremity of the medial border of the shaft of the bone.

ATTACHMENTS

- The anterior surface and tip of the medial epicondyle provide attachment to the medial epicondylar muscles (forearm flexors), i.e., pronator teres, flexor carpi radialis, palmaris longus, flexor carpi ulnaris, and flexor digitorum superficialis.
- The posterior surface of the medial epicondyle is smooth, traversed by a vertical groove through which the ulnar nerve passes.
- The inferior border provides attachment to the ulnar collateral ligament of the elbow joint.

> **CLINICAL NOTE**
>
> **Medial collateral ligament sprain**
>
> On palpation, there is tenderness to pressure or exacerbation of pain at the medial epicondyle. Valgus stress is applied to test the ligament; it is positive if it reawakens the pain.

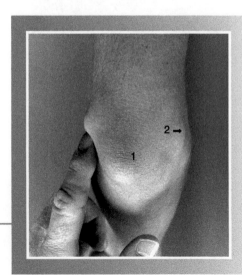

Fig. 5.8 Posterior view of the medial epicondyle

MA: This figure shows the position of the medial epicondyle, indicated by the practitioner's index finger, relative to the olecranon (1) and the lateral epicondyle (2).

Fig. 5.9 Medial supraepicondylar ridge

MA: This ridge is much less marked than the lateral supraepicondylar ridge. It can be found above the medial epicondyle, and is felt beneath your fingers as a blunt ridge which is easy to access.

Note: This ridge approximately follows the medial border of the humerus.

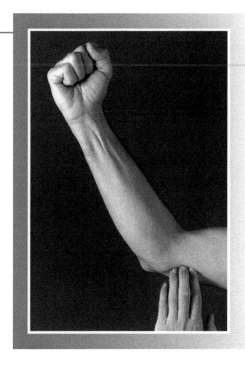

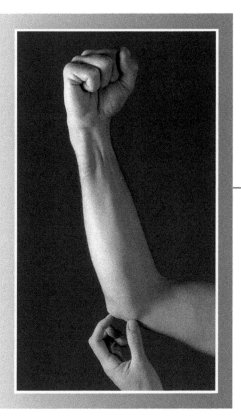

Fig. 5.10 Groove for the ulnar nerve

MA: This is a vertical groove crossing the posterior surface of the medial epicondyle. In this figure, the practitioner's thumb and finger contact indicates the extent of the groove. The practitioner's thumb rests medially, on the medial epicondyle, while the index finger is on the olecranon.

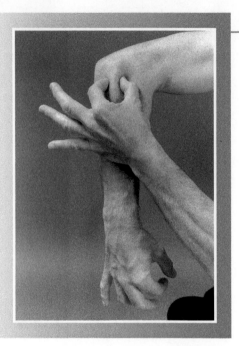

Fig. 5.11 Head of the radius

MA: Position your thumb and index finger at the capitulum of the humerus, with the subject's elbow flexed at 90°. Then slide the contact distally, maintaining your contact with the skin. You will sense the joint cavity between the humerus and radius beneath your fingers. You can then take hold of the head of the radius between thumb and index finger. (If you are in any doubt, you can identify the head of the radius by asking the subject to pronate and supinate his forearm, so that the head of the radius turns beneath your fingers.)

CLINICAL NOTE

Fracture of the head of the radius is possible. On palpation, pressure causes exquisite pain. Pronation and supination are particularly painful. The elbow can be flexed fairly normally, but it cannot be fully extended.

Fig. 5.12 Neck of the radius

MA: Take as your starting point the thumb and index finger contact on the head of the radius, as described above (Fig. 5.11). Descend roughly one finger's breadth distally, where you will detect a narrowing. This is the structure you are looking for.

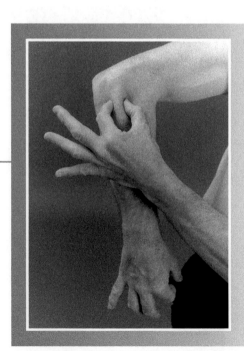

Fig. 5.13 Radial tuberosity

MA: Place your thumb in the base of the lateral groove of the fold of the elbow, as shown here (see Note below). Position your thumb against the distal, lateral extremity of the tendon of biceps brachii, and you will make contact with the bony structure of the radial tuberosity. Note that supination of the forearm brings the radial tuberosity toward your contact, and pronation moves it away.

Note: The lateral groove of the fold of the elbow runs obliquely inferiorly and medially. It is formed by the lateral part of biceps brachii medially and anteriorly, laterally by brachioradialis, and posteriorly by brachialis. The radial tuberosity is an ovoid structure situated on the anteromedial part of the bone, at the junction of the neck and shaft of the radius. On its posterior surface, it provides attachment to the tendon of biceps brachii.

Care should be taken when palpating this structure, because there is a synovial bursa between the tendon and the anterior part of the tuberosity.

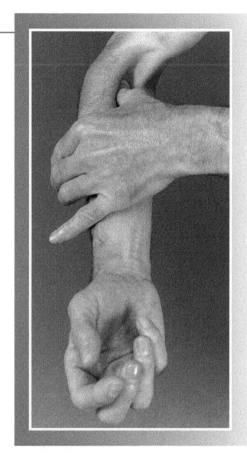

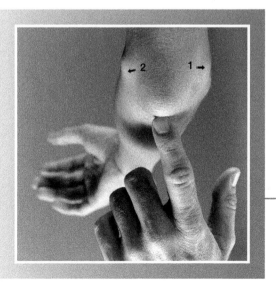

Fig. 5.14 Display of the olecranon at the elbow

MA: This is the posterior vertical process of the proximal extremity of the ulna. In the adjacent figure, the practitioner's index finger shows the topographical location of the olecranon relative to the lateral epicondyle (1) and medial epicondyle (2). These three bony structures are among the most important making up the elbow joint.

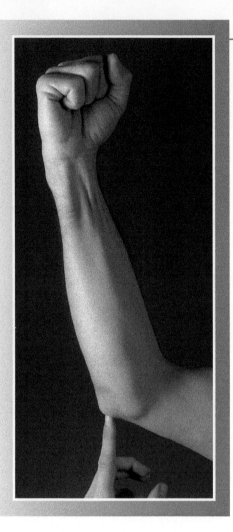

Fig. 5.15 Superior surface of the olecranon

MA: This lies immediately beneath the skin and so presents no difficulties of access, as the adjacent figure demonstrates. A beaklike process extends forward; this rests in the olecranon fossa of the humerus when the forearm is extended at the elbow.

Note: The posterior part gives attachment to the tendon of triceps brachii.

Fig. 5.16 Medial surface of the olecranon

MA: This surface (indicated by the practitioner's index finger) is important because it gives insertion to the posterior part of the ulnar collateral ligament of the elbow joint and to flexor carpi ulnaris.

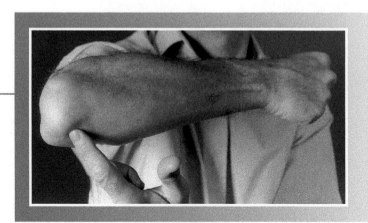

Fig. 5.17 Lateral surface of the olecranon

MA: The posterior part of the radial collateral ligament of the elbow joint has its attachment here. So too does anconeus.

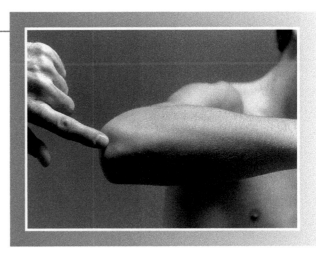

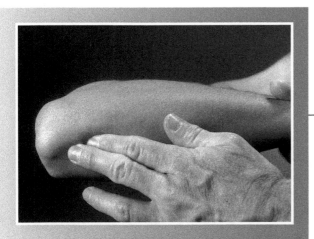

Fig. 5.18 Posterior border of the shaft of the ulna

MA: This bony structure is the distal extension of the posterior surface of the olecranon. Examination presents no difficulties.

Fig. 5.19 Coronoid process of the ulna

MA: The subject's elbow should be slightly flexed. Place one hand on the posterior surface of the elbow, at the olecranon (Fig. 5.14), and the other on the medial border of the proximal extremity of the ulna. Position your thumb medial to the distal tendon of biceps brachii. Grasp the posterior border of the ulna with your other fingers. The practitioner's thumb can be seen here opposite the coronoid process, a bony structure which can only be accessed indirectly, through the mass of muscle: in this case, the anterior group of the muscles of the forearm.

Note: The coronoid process is one of the two processes of the superior extremity of the ulna; the other is the olecranon (Fig. 5.14). These two bony structures unite to form a hook-shaped articular cavity, the trochlear notch of the ulna.

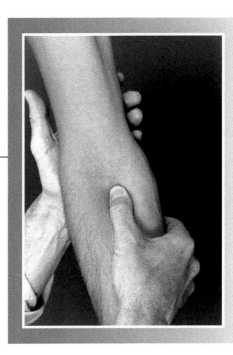

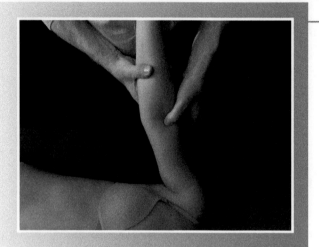

Fig. 5.20 Capitulum of the humerus, anterior surface

MA: The subject's elbow is extended. With the index finger of your palpating hand, the left, seek the posterior part of the joint space between the humerus and radius. Then place your left thumb above the fold of the elbow, in the lateral bicipital groove between the lateral epicondyle and the tendon of the biceps. You will sense the smooth articular surface of the capitulum beneath your left thumb.

Note: It is easier to detect this structure if the elbow is hyperextended.

Fig. 5.21 Trochlea of the humerus

MA: The subject's elbow is extended. With your palpating hand, seek the medial epicondyle of the humerus. Use your thumb to help you position this hand between the epicondyle and the tendon of the biceps, in the medial bicipital groove. You will sense the smooth articular surface of the trochlea beneath your fingers.

Note: It is easier to detect this structure if the elbow is hyperextended.

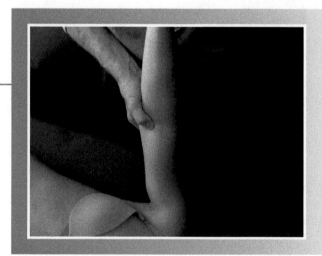

NERVES AND BLOOD VESSELS

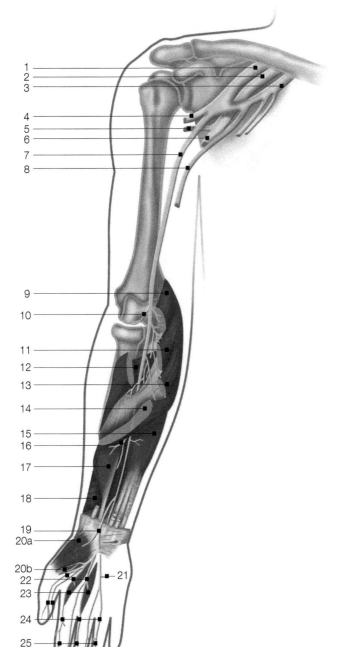

Median nerve (anterior view) and muscles innervated by the median nerve

1. Lateral cord of brachial plexus
2. Posterior cord of brachial plexus
3. Medial cord of brachial plexus
4. Musculocutaneous nerve
5. Axillary nerve
6. Radial nerve
7. Median nerve (C6, C7, C8, T1)
8. Ulnar nerve
9. Pronator teres (humeral head)
10. Articular branch
11. Flexor carpi radialis
12. Pronator teres (ulnar head)
13. Palmaris longus
14. Flexor digitorum superficialis
15. Flexor digitorum profundus
16. Anterior interosseous nerve
17. Flexor pollicis longus
18. Pronator quadratus
19. Palmar branch of median nerve
20. Thenar muscles:
20a. Abductor pollicis brevis
20b. Superficial head of flexor pollicis brevis
21. Anastomosis uniting branch of median nerve and ulnar nerve
22. Common palmar digital nerves
23. First and second lumbricals
24. Proper palmar digital nerves
25. Dorsal branches

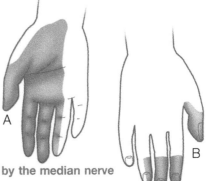

Cutaneous innervation by the median nerve
Palmar view (A) and dorsal view (B)

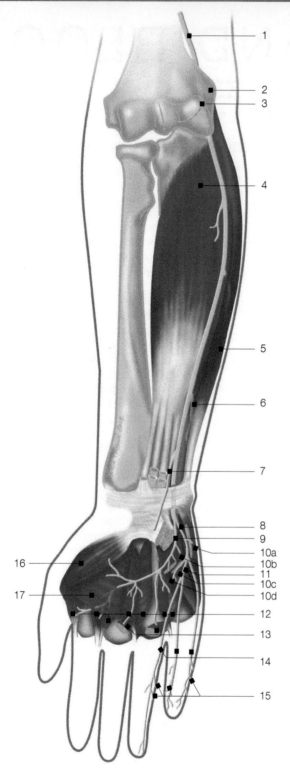

Ulnar nerve

1. Ulnar nerve (C8, T1)
2. Medial epicondyle
3. Articular branch (behind condyle)
4. Flexor digitorum profundus (medial part)
5. Flexor carpi ulnaris
6. Dorsal branch of ulnar nerve
7. Palmar branch
8. Superficial branch
9. Deep branch
10. Hypothenar muscles:
10a. Palmaris brevis
10b. Abductor digiti minimi
10c. Flexor digiti minimi brevis
10d. Opponens digiti minimi
11. Common palmar digital nerve
12. Palmar and dorsal interossei
13. Third and fourth lumbricals
14. Proper palmar digital nerves
15. Dorsal branches
16. Flexor pollicis brevis
17. Adductor pollicis

Cutaneous innervation by the ulnar nerve

Palmar view (A) and dorsal view (B)

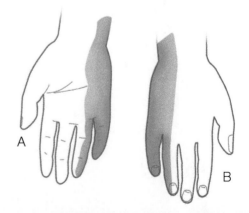

THE PRINCIPAL NERVES AND BLOOD VESSELS

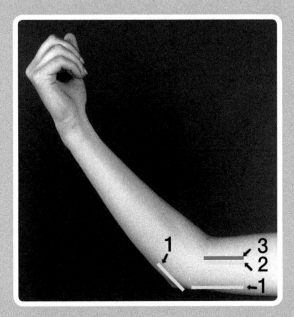

Fig. 5.22 Display of the course of the main nerves and blood vessels of the medial part of the elbow

1. Ulnar nerve
2. Median nerve
3. Brachial artery

Note: The nerves can be palpated by one of the following means: scratching the location with your fingernail; rolling it beneath the pads of your fingers; or displaying them by inducing a state of tension in them (according to region).

The notable structures that can be detected by palpation are:

- Ulnar nerve in the groove for the ulnar nerve (Fig. 5.23)
- Ulnar nerve in the proximal part of the forearm (Fig. 5.24)
- Median nerve in the medial bicipital groove (Fig. 5.25)
- Radial nerve (Figs. 5.26 and 5.27)
- Musculocutaneous nerve (Fig. 5.26)
- Brachial artery at the medial bicipital groove (Fig. 5.28).

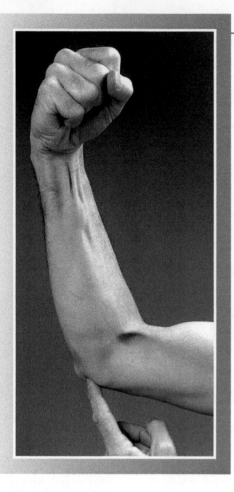

Fig. 5.23 Ulnar nerve in the groove for the ulnar nerve

MA: Examination presents no difficulty. Simply place your index finger in the groove for the ulnar nerve to contact the structure concerned. The nerve can be sensed beneath your fingers as a full, cylindrical cord. Great care is needed in the approach to the nerve. It lies in the groove for the ulnar nerve and then enters beneath the arch that unites the humeral head and ulnar head of the flexor carpi ulnaris muscle.

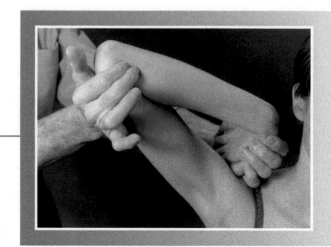

Fig. 5.24 Ulnar nerve in the proximal part of the forearm

MA: Beyond the groove for the ulnar nerve, it is still possible to palpate the ulnar nerve in the proximal part of the forearm. To do this, ease the subject's arm into flexion with her forearm pronated and hand extended. The nerve can be palpated in the "antebrachial" extension of the groove for the ulnar nerve of the medial epicondyle. It can be felt beneath your fingers as a full, cylindrical cord in the proximal third of the forearm.

Fig. 5.25 Median nerve in the medial bicipital groove

MA: To palpate this nerve, use the pad of two fingertips, medial to the tendon of biceps brachii. It is fairly simple to locate it in this position, as shown in the photograph. You will sense a full, cylindrical cord that can be rolled beneath the pads of your index and middle fingers. This is the median nerve.

Note: The brachial artery lies lateral to the median nerve.

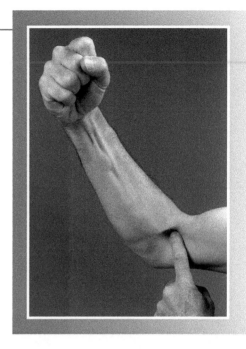

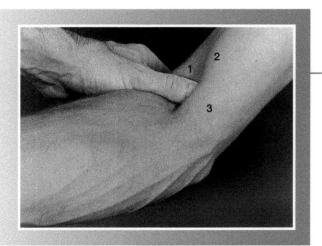

Fig. 5.26 Radial nerve and musculocutaneous nerve

MA: The musculocutaneous nerve is the one that lies closest to the tendon of biceps. It continues as the lateral cutaneous nerve of the forearm, which in turn divides into an anterior and a posterior branch. It is more superficial than the radial nerve, which lies deeper and more laterally in the lateral bicipital groove.

These two nerves are accessible to palpation, either by rolling them under the pads of your fingers, or by scratching with the nail of your thumb or index finger.

1. Brachioradialis
2. Biceps brachii
3. Tendon of biceps

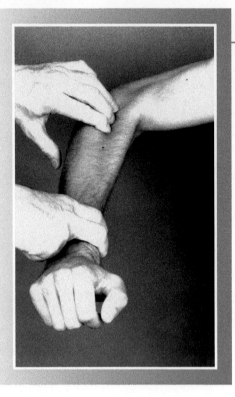

Fig. 5.27 Radial nerve at the neck of the radius and posterior surface of the forearm

MA: The motor deep branch of this nerve can be palpated at the neck of the radius; it can also be palpated more distally, on the posterior surface of the forearm. To do this, you should first locate the bodies of two muscles, extensor carpi radialis brevis and extensor digitorum. Place a broad contact in between these two muscles, and roll the radial nerve beneath the pads of your fingers, easing extensor digitorum aside medially as you do so.

Fig. 5.28 Brachial artery at the medial bicipital groove

MA: Place a two-finger contact in the fold of the elbow, medial and posterior to the tendon of biceps brachii (1). Here you can clearly detect the pulse of the brachial artery. Note that the median nerve lies medially to it.

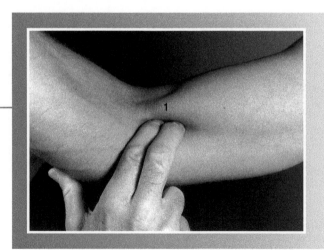

6
The forearm

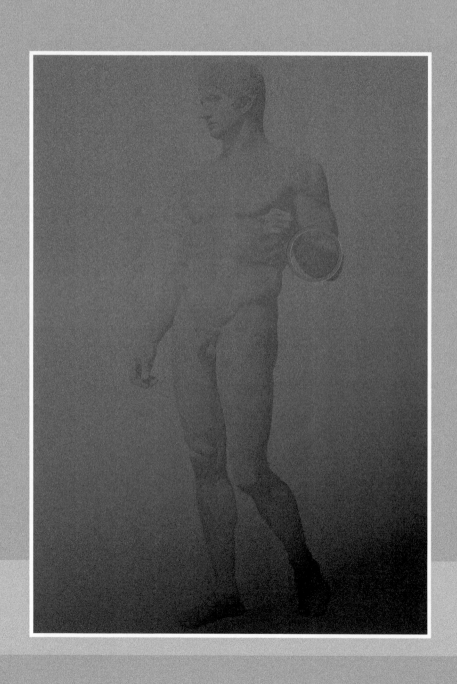

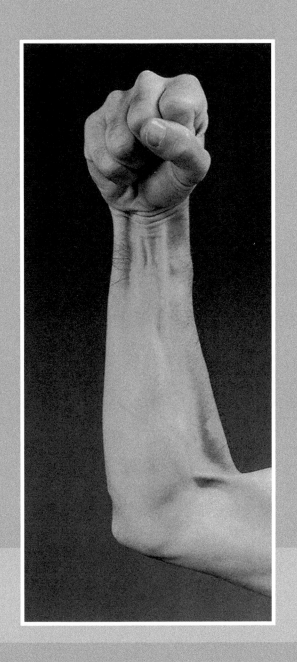

MYOLOGY

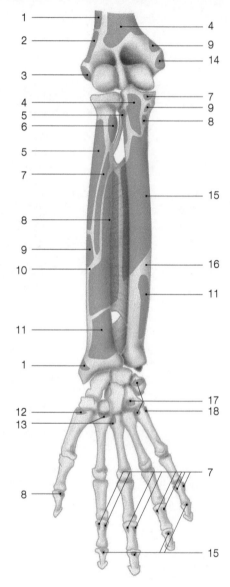

Muscles of the forearm (anterior view)

1. Brachioradialis	7. Flexor digitorum superficialis	13. Flexor carpi radialis
2. Extensor carpi radialis longus	8. Flexor pollicis longus	14. Common flexor tendon
3. Common extensor tendon	9. Pronator teres	15. Flexor digitorum profundus
4. Brachialis	10. Radius	16. Ulna
5. Supinator	11. Pronator quadratus	17. Flexor carpi ulnaris
6. Biceps brachii	12. Abductor pollicis longus	18. Extensor carpi ulnaris

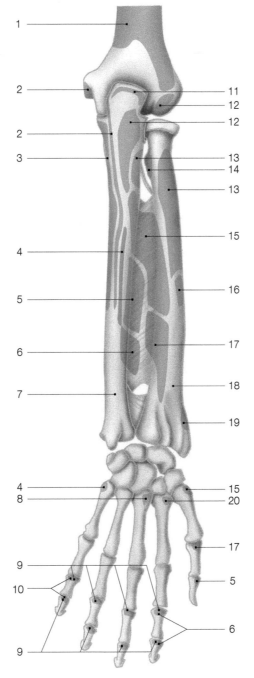

Muscles of the forearm (posterior view)

1. Triceps brachii	8. Extensor carpi radialis brevis	14. Biceps brachii
2. Flexor carpi ulnaris	9. Extensor digitorum	15. Abductor pollicis longus
3. Flexor digitorum profundus	10. Extensor digiti minimi	16. Pronator teres
4. Extensor carpi ulnaris	11. Tendon of triceps brachii	17. Extensor pollicis brevis
5. Extensor pollicis longus	12. Anconeus	18. Radius
6. Extensor indicis	13. Supinator	19. Brachioradialis
7. Ulna		20. Extensor carpi radialis longus

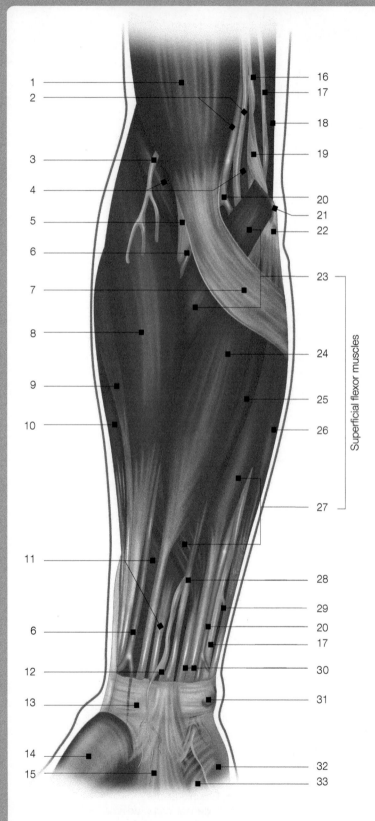

1
2
3
4
5
6
7
8
9
10
11
6
12
13
14
15

16
17
18
19
20
21
22
23
24
25
26
27
28
29
20
17
30
31
32
33

Superficial flexor muscles

Muscles of the forearm (superficial layer): anterior view

1. Biceps brachii
2. Median nerve and brachial artery
3. Lateral cutaneous nerve of forearm
4. Brachialis
5. Tendon of biceps brachii
6. Radial artery
7. Bicipital aponeurosis
8. Brachioradialis
9. Extensor carpi radialis longus
10. Extensor carpi radialis brevis
11. Flexor pollicis longus muscle and tendon
12. Median nerve
13. Transverse fibers of palmar aponeurosis (palmar carpal ligament)
14. Thenar muscles
15. Palmar aponeurosis
16. Medial cutaneous nerve of forearm
17. Ulnar nerve
18. Triceps brachii
19. Medial intermuscular septum
20. Ulnar artery
21. Medial epicondyle of humerus
22. Common flexor tendon
23. Pronator teres
24. Flexor carpi radialis
25. Palmaris longus
26. Flexor carpi ulnaris
27. Flexor digitorum superficialis
28. Tendon of palmaris longus
29. Dorsal branch of ulnar nerve
30. Tendons of flexor digitorum superficialis
31. Pisiform
32. Palmar branch of median nerve
33. Hypothenar muscles

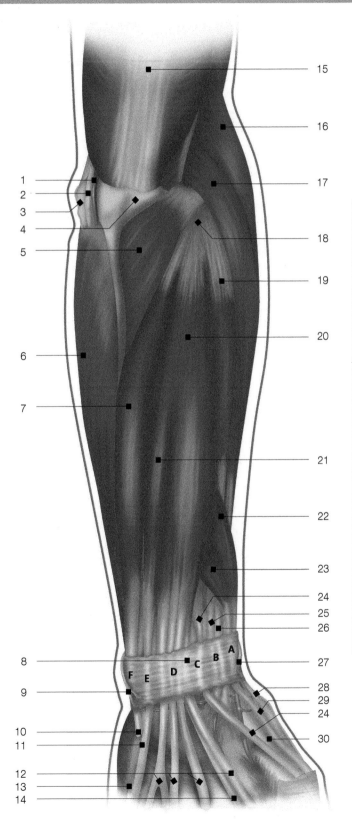

15
16
17
18
19
20
21
22
23
24
25
26
27
28
29
24
30

1
2
3
4
5
6
7
8
9
10
11
12
13
14

B A
C
F E D

Muscles of the forearm (superficial layer): posterior view)

1. Superior ulnar collateral artery
2. Ulnar nerve
3. Medial epicondyle of humerus
4. Olecranon
5. Anconeus
6. Flexor carpi ulnaris
7. Extensor carpi ulnaris
8. Extensor retinaculum (compartments A–F)
9. Dorsal branch of ulnar nerve
10. Tendon of extensor carpi ulnaris
11. Tendon of extensor digiti minimi
12. Tendons of extensor digitorum
13. Fifth metacarpal
14. Tendon of extensor indicis
15. Triceps brachii
16. Brachioradialis
17. Extensor carpi radialis longus
18. Common extensor tendon
19. Extensor carpi radialis brevis
20. Extensor digitorum
21. Extensor digiti minimi
22. Abductor pollicis longus
23. Extensor pollicis brevis
24. Tendon of extensor pollicis longus
25. Tendon of extensor carpi radialis brevis
26. Tendon of extensor carpi radialis longus
27. Superficial branch of radial nerve
28. Tendon of abductor pollicis longus
29. Tendon of extensor pollicis brevis
30. Anatomic snuffbox

THE LATERAL MUSCLE GROUP

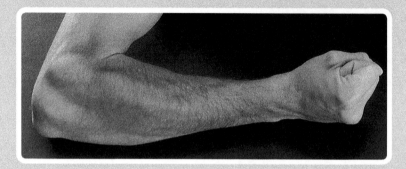

Fig. 6.2 View of the lateral muscle group

This group consists of four muscles, arranged in two layers.

The notable structures that can be detected by palpation are:

- **Superficial layer.** There are three muscles in this layer. Working across medially, these are:
  - Brachioradialis (Figs. 6.3–6.5)
  - Extensor carpi radialis longus (Figs. 6.6–6.12, and 6.17)
  - Extensor carpi radialis brevis (Figs. 6.13–6.17)
- **Deep layer.** This consists of a single muscle, supinator (Fig. 6.18).

ACTIONS

- Brachioradialis flexes the forearm on the arm in the neutral position (neither pronated nor supinated).
- Extensor carpi radialis longus extends and abducts the wrist (inclines it radially).
- Extensor carpi radialis brevis extends the wrist. It also helps to incline the wrist radially when it is semipronated.
- Supinator (together with biceps) helps to supinate the forearm on the arm (assisted, where the impulse to supinate the forearm is strong, by the adductors and lateral rotator muscles of the shoulder, which work together to bring about this action).

INNERVATIONS

- Brachioradialis: radial nerve (C5–C6)
- Extensor carpi radialis longus: radial nerve (C5–C6–C7)
- Extensor carpi radialis brevis: radial nerve (C5–C6–C7)
- Supinator: Radial nerve (C5–C6–C7)

Fig. 6.3 Proximal part of brachioradialis

MA: With the subject's arm in a neutral position, neither pronated nor supinated, apply resistance on the inferior third of the radius, and ask him to flex his forearm on the arm. You will sense the contraction on the distal part of the lateral border of the humerus.

ATTACHMENTS

- Brachioradialis arises:
  - on the inferior third of the lateral border of the humerus, by means of tendinous fibers;
  - on the lateral intermuscular septum of the arm, by means of fleshy fibers.
- It is inserted into the lateral surface of the base of the radial styloid process.

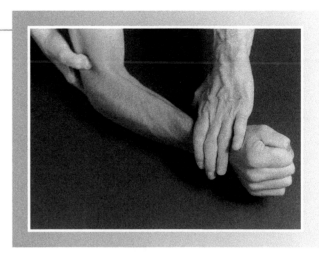

Fig. 6.4 Body of brachioradialis

MA: Apply the same resistance and request the same action as that described above. The body of the muscle becomes prominent, appearing clearly as indicated by the practitioner's index finger in the adjacent figure.

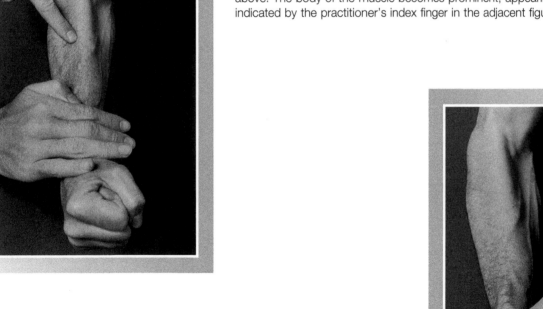

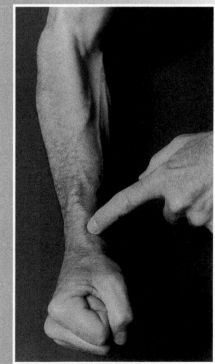

Fig. 6.5 Insertion of brachioradialis

MA: The muscle is inserted into the base of the radial styloid process, by means of a flat tendon. This attachment is indicated here by the practitioner's index finger.

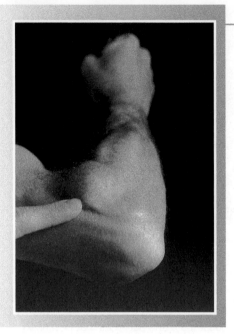

Fig. 6.6 Origin of extensor carpi radialis longus

MA: The subject's elbow should be flexed. Ask him to extend his wrist and incline it radially. You will see the muscle contract on the lateral border of the humerus, approximately three finger-breadths distal to the attachment of brachioradialis.

ATTACHMENTS

- Extensor carpi radialis longus arises on the lateral supraepicondylar ridge and the lateral intermuscular septum of the arm.
- It is inserted into the lateral tuberosity of the base of the second metacarpal.

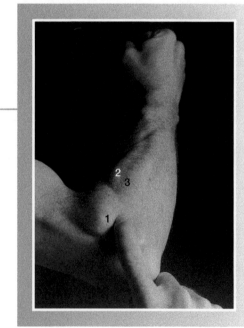

Fig. 6.7 Body of extensor carpi radialis longus at the elbow

MA: In many subjects, the body of this muscle appears clearly on the lateral surface of the elbow if you ask them to extend their wrist and incline it in the radial direction. In other subjects, you may find that the contraction of the muscle appears on the lateral surface of the elbow, lateral to the proximal part of brachioradialis (Fig. 6.3) (level with the fold of the elbow).

1. Body of extensor carpi radialis longus
2. Extensor carpi radialis brevis
3. Extensor digitorum

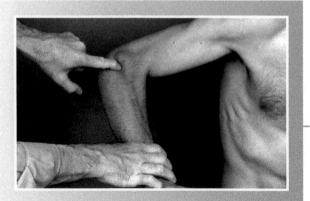

Fig. 6.8 Extensor carpi radialis longus at the forearm

MA: The adjacent figure shows the body of this muscle from another angle. It becomes visible when contracted, and tends to appear as a short, fairly voluminous muscle in males (depending on profession and type or degree of physical activity) and is more elongated in females.

Fig. 6.9 Tendon of extensor carpi radialis longus

MA: In the middle third of the forearm, the body of the muscle gives way to a tendon, located on the anterolateral part of the body of extensor carpi radialis brevis. The two tendons can be distinguished in the more distal region by using a broad two-finger contact and "rolling" the tendons on the shaft of the radius.

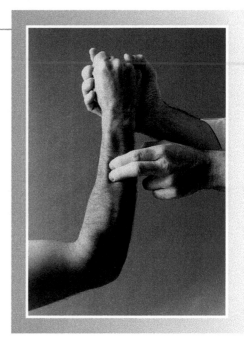

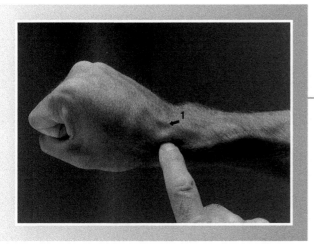

Fig. 6.10 Displaying the tendon of extensor carpi radialis longus at the wrist

MA: This tendon is inserted into the lateral part of the dorsal surface of the base of the second metacarpal, and becomes clearly visible in some subjects (as in the adjacent figure, indicated by the practitioner's index finger), lateral to the tendon of extensor carpi radialis brevis (1), if you ask the subject to clench his fist.

Fig. 6.11 Distal palpation of the tendon of extensor carpi radialis longus, another approach – step 1

MA: A triangle with a proximal apex (1) and distal base can clearly be seen in the adjacent figure. The two tendons belonging to extensor carpi radialis longus and extensor carpi radialis brevis can be palpated in this angle. The triangle has a distal base (the first commissure); its ulnar side is formed by the tendon of extensor digitorum going to the index (second) finger (2) and its radial side by the tendon of extensor pollicis longus (3).

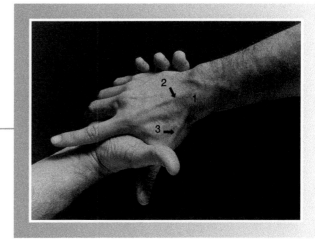

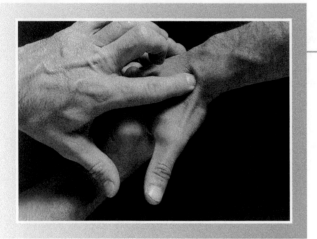

Fig. 6.12 Distal palpation of the tendon of extensor carpi radialis longus, another approach – step 2

MA: Contact the ulnar border of the tendon of extensor pollicis longus with one finger and ease the tendon aside radially, feeling for the tendon of extensor carpi radialis longus.

Fig. 6.13 Extensor carpi radialis brevis in the forearm

MA: This figure shows the body of extensor carpi radialis brevis, from another angle. It is indicated by the practitioner's index finger. You can also see the course of the muscle and how it relates to other muscles of the forearm.

ATTACHMENTS

- Extensor carpi radialis brevis arises on the anterior surface of the lateral epicondyle of the humerus (via the common tendon of the epicondylar muscles – the forearm extensors).
- It is inserted into the dorsal and lateral base of the third metacarpal.

> **CLINICAL NOTE**
>
> **Lateral epicondylitis**
>
> This muscle is the one most frequently involved in lateral epicondylitis. Ask the patient to extend his wrist against resistance applied at the dorsal surface of the head of the third metacarpal. (Isometric testing of extensor carpi radialis brevis.) Diagnosis can be confirmed or ruled out by palpation: tenderness to pressure may be evoked or exacerbated.
>
> Care should be taken: palpation of this muscle can be very painful, because the radial nerve runs deep to it.

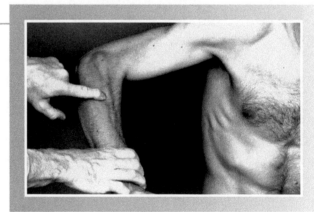

1. Extensor carpi radialis longus
2. Brachioradialis
3. Extensor digitorum

Fig. 6.14 Topographical relations of extensor carpi radialis brevis

MA: The body of this muscle is indicated here by the practitioner's index finger; it is situated radially to extensor digitorum (1). At this level it runs along the tendon of extensor carpi radialis longus (2) (not visible in this photograph), which lies laterally to it. Brachioradialis (3) is also situated lateral to it.

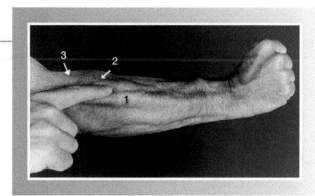

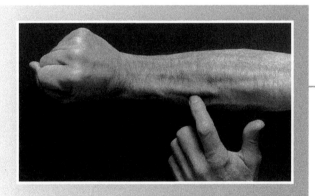

Fig. 6.15 Extensor carpi radialis brevis in the inferior third of the forearm

MA: At this level the tendon (indicated by the practitioner's index finger), along with that of extensor carpi radialis longus, passes anterior to abductor pollicis longus. More distally they also pass anterior to extensor pollicis brevis.

Fig. 6.16 Insertion of extensor carpi radialis brevis

MA: This tendon can be seen in the adjacent figure, indicated by the practitioner's index finger. It is situated medially to the tendon of extensor carpi radialis longus (1).

Note: The tendon of this muscle inserts into the dorsal aspect of the base of the third metacarpal.

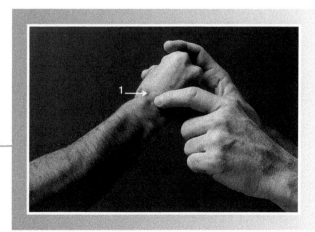

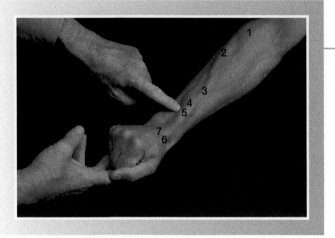

Fig. 6.17 Relations of extensor carpi radialis longus and brevis with the other muscles of the forearm, another view

MA: Extensor carpi radialis longus and brevis run to a point midway down the forearm, where they give way to tendons that can be seen in some subjects, but can in any case easily be palpated. These then pass underneath the body of abductor pollicis longus and extensor pollicis brevis. Distally, extensor carpi radialis longus (ECRL) inserts into the posterolateral tuberosity of the base of the second metacarpal, and extensor carpi radialis brevis (ECRB) into that of the third metacarpal.

1. Extensor carpi radialis longus
2. Extensor carpi radialis brevis
3. Tendons of ECRL and ECRB
4. Abductor pollicis longus
5. Extensor pollicis brevis
6. Insertion of ECRL into base of second metacarpal
7. Insertion of ECRB into base of third metacarpal

Fig. 6.18 Supinator

MA: The subject's elbow should be flexed and almost completely supinated. (This muscle is the only one that is effective when the arm is almost fully supinated.) Using your index and middle fingers, place your contact distal to the head of the radius, opposite the neck of the radius, where some fibers of supinator are attached (on the anterior, posterior, and lateral surfaces). Wedge your index and middle fingers against the inferior edge of the head of the radius, and ask the subject to supinate her forearm actively, using repeated, short, rapid movements, to enable you to sense the contraction of the muscle fibers beneath your fingers.

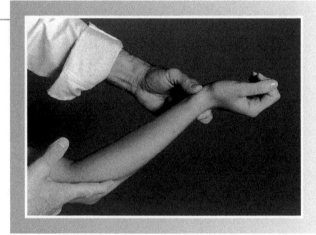

ATTACHMENTS

Supinator has two heads, one superficial and one deep.

• Origins. Taking the muscle as a whole, it arises:
  – from the inferior part of the lateral epicondyle of the humerus;
  – from the middle portion of the radial collateral ligament;
  – from the supinator ridge of the ulna;
  – from the supinator fossa of the ulna.
• Insertions:
  – into the superior part of the oblique line of the anterior border of the radius (superficial portion);
  – into the anterior, lateral, and posterior surfaces of the neck of the radius (deep portion).

CLINICAL NOTE

Supinator is sometimes also involved in epicondylitis, though much more rarely than extensor carpi radialis brevis and extensor digitorum. Isometric testing should be done by resisting supination of the forearm on the arm while the elbow is either completely flexed or almost completely extended. The reason for this is to avoid any participation by the biceps. Examine by palpation, looking for tenderness to pressure at the **lateral epicondyle,** or level with the neck of the radius.

THE POSTERIOR MUSCLE GROUP

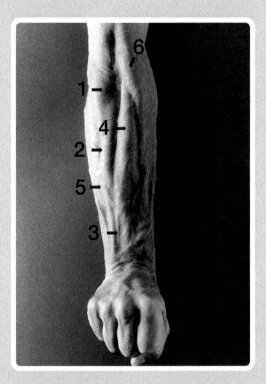

Fig. 6.19 Posterior view of the forearm

1. Anconeus
2. Extensor carpi ulnaris
3. Extensor digiti minimi
4. Extensor digitorum
5. Flexor carpi ulnaris
6. Extensor carpi radialis longus

This group consists of eight muscles, arranged as follows:

- Superficial layer. Working across medially, the muscles of this layer are extensor digitorum, extensor digiti minimi, extensor carpi ulnaris, anconeus.
- Deep layer. Working downward from superior to inferior, the muscles of this layer are abductor pollicis longus, extensor pollicis brevis, extensor pollicis longus, extensor indicis.

The notable structures that can be detected by palpation are:

- Extensor digitorum (Figs. 6.20–6.23):
  - Tendons on the back of the hand (Figs. 6.24 and 6.26)
  - Insertions at the phalanges (Fig. 6.25)
  - Tendon to the second finger and extension of aponeurosis (Figs. 6.27, 6.28, and 6.33)
- Extensor indicis (Figs. 6.26 and 6.27)
- Extensor digiti minimi:
  - Origin (Fig. 6.29)

- Body of muscle (Fig. 6.30)
- Tendon (Figs. 6.31–6.33)
- Extensor carpi ulnaris (Figs. 6.34–6.36)
- Anconeus (Fig. 6.37)
- Abductor pollicis longus:
    - Body of muscle (Figs. 6.38, 6.39, and 6.42)
    - Tendon (Fig. 6.40)
- Extensor pollicis brevis:
    - Body of muscle (Fig. 6.41 and 6.42)
    - Tendon at the wrist (Fig. 6.43)
    - Insertion (Fig. 6.44)
- Extensor pollicis longus (Figs. 6.45–6.47).

ACTIONS

- Anconeus extends the forearm on the arm.
- Extensor carpi ulnaris extends and adducts the wrist (inclines it to the ulnar side).
- Extensor digitorum:
    - extends the three phalanges of the last four fingers; the action is much more marked for the extension of the proximal (first) phalanx;
    - works together with extensor indicis and extensor digiti minimi in the extension of the index and little fingers;
    - works together with the lumbricals and the dorsal and palmar interossei in the extension of the middle and distal phalanges;
    - assists in the extension of the wrist on the forearm.
- Extensor indicis and extensor digiti minimi also assist in the extension of the wrist.
- Abductor pollicis longus:
    - draws the first metacarpal anteriorly when the thumb is abducted;
    - initiates opposition of the thumb together with the most lateral muscles of the thumb;
    - assists in flexing the wrist.
- Extensor pollicis brevis:
    - extends the proximal phalanx on the first metacarpal, and abducts the first metacarpal. (This is essentially the muscle that abducts the thumb.)
    - assists in the radial inclination of the thumb.
- Extensor pollicis longus:
    - extends the distal phalanx on the proximal one;
    - extends the proximal phalanx on the first metacarpal;
    - then draws the first metacarpal posterior to the plane of metacarpals.

INNERVATIONS

- Extensor digitorum: radial nerve (C6–C7–C8)
- Extensor digiti minimi: radial nerve (C6–C7–C8)
- Extensor carpi ulnaris: radial nerve (C6–C7–C8)
- Anconeus: radial nerve (C6–C7–C8)
- Abductor pollicis longus: radial nerve (C6–C7–C8)
- Extensor pollicis brevis: radial nerve (C6–C7–C8)
- Extensor pollicis longus: radial nerve (C6–C7–C8)
- Extensor indicis: radial nerve (C6–C7–C8)

Fig. 6.20 Extensor digitorum, proximal part

MA: This muscle (1) is situated posteriorly and medially to extensor carpi radialis longus (2). It can be revealed by asking the subject to make a fist and then repeatedly open it and extend his fingers.

Note: Palpation of this muscle with application of pressure can be very painful, because the radial nerve lies deep to it.

ATTACHMENTS

* Origins:
  – From the lateral epicondyle, via the common tendon of origin of the epicondylar muscles (forearm extensors).
* Insertions:
  – At the proximal phalanx, each tendon of extensor digitorum receives the tendinous expansion of the lumbricals and of the interossei on its lateral and medial borders.
  – Each tendon is inserted into the three phalanges as follows:
    - At the metacarpophalangeal joint, each tendon has a fibrous expansion that is inserted into the base of the proximal phalanx.
    - Each tendon then subdivides into three slips at the proximal phalanx: a middle slip is attached to the dorsal surface of the superior extremity of the middle phalanx; two lateral slips unite on the dorsal surface of the middle phalanx, and are inserted into the superior extremity of the dorsal surface of the distal phalanx.

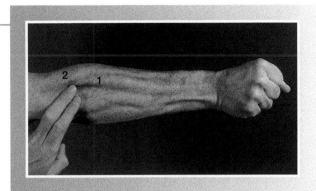

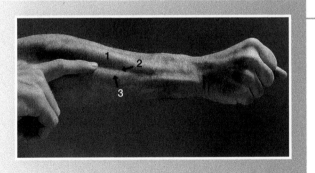

Fig. 6.21 Extensor digitorum on the forearm

MA: This muscle (1) is situated centrally on the posterior surface of the forearm. It runs down behind supinator and the four muscles of the deep layer of the posterior region of the forearm. It is bounded by extensor digiti minimi (2) (not visible on this photograph) medially, and by extensor carpi ulnaris (3). Ask the subject to perform the same muscular action as that described in Figure 6.20.

Note: At this level the body of the muscle is made up of four portions.

Fig. 6.22 Extensor digitorum, distal part

MA: On the distal part of the posterior surface of the forearm, the muscle consists of a group of four tendons, issuing from the four portions of the muscle described in the note to Figure 6.21.

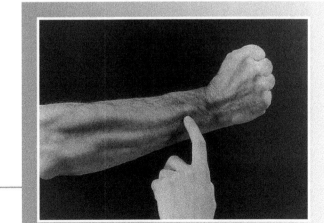

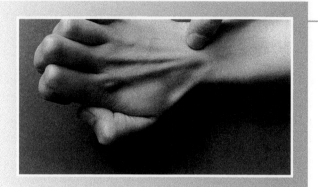

Fig. 6.23 Extensor digitorum at the wrist

MA: At this level the four tendons of extensor digitorum and the tendon of extensor indicis come together and pass through an osteofibrous sheath, part of the extensor retinaculum, which holds them against the posterior surface of the radius before they pass onto the dorsal surface of the hand.

Fig. 6.24 Tendons of extensor digitorum

MA: Extend the subject's hand, applying resistance on the posterior surface of the proximal phalanges, as shown in the adjacent figure. This will make the tendons appear on the back of her hand.

> **CLINICAL NOTE**
>
> This muscle is often involved in **epicondylitis.** Examine by isometric testing of the muscle, placing resistance on the dorsal surface of the head of the proximal phalanges. Pain at the epicondyle suggests that this muscle is affected. The diagnosis can be confirmed or otherwise by palpation of the lateral surface of the elbow, at the epicondyle, looking for tenderness to pressure.

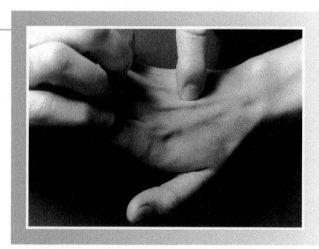

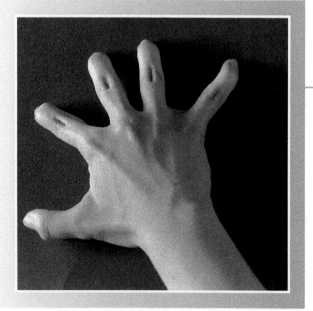

Fig. 6.25 Insertions of extensor digitorum at the phalanges

MA: Each tendon is inserted into the respective base of each of the three phalanges of the four fingers on which the tendons operate.

Note: The photograph in the adjacent figure shows extensor digitorum tendons that are each divided into two at the level of the phalanges. This is an exceptional case, and not the usual rule.

> **CLINICAL NOTE**
>
> **Mallet finger**
>
> This is caused by rupture of the tendon of extensor digitorum at its most distal attachment (on the distal phalanx) following harsh flexion of the distal phalanx on the second. Extension of the distal phalanx on the second (middle phalanx) becomes impossible.

Fig. 6.26 Extensor indicis on the back of the hand

MA: This muscle extends from the ulna to the index finger. On the dorsal surface of the wrist and hand, the tendon of extensor indicis (1) lies by the ulnar border of the tendon of extensor digitorum going to the index finger (2). In most cases it unites with this tendon at the metacarpophalangeal joint.

ATTACHMENTS

• Extensor indicis arises:
  – from the inferior third of the posterior surface of the ulna;
  – from the interosseous membrane of the forearm.
• It is inserted at the metacarpophalangeal joint of the index finger, where it fuses with the tendon of extensor digitorum going to the index finger.

Note: In the figure shown here, the practitioner's index finger points between the two tendons described above.

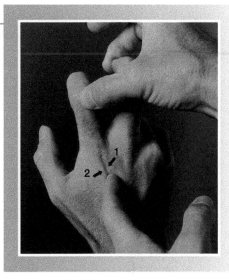

Fig. 6.27 Topographical relations of the tendon of extensor indicis and tendons of extensor digitorum

MA: Ask the subject first of all to flex his metacarpophalangeal joints, and then to extend his second finger (the index). The tendon of extensor digitorum (1) going to the second finger "goes over" the tendon of extensor indicis (indicated here by the practitioner). It is drawn across by an expansion of the aponeurosis (2) which links it to the tendon of extensor digitorum going to the middle finger (3). This has the effect of drawing the tendon of extensor digitorum going to the second finger to the ulnar border of the tendon of extensor indicis.

Note: The italic "S"-shaped tendon (1) seen on the back of the hand when performing the action described here is the tendon of extensor digitorum going to the second finger.

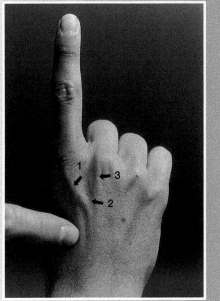

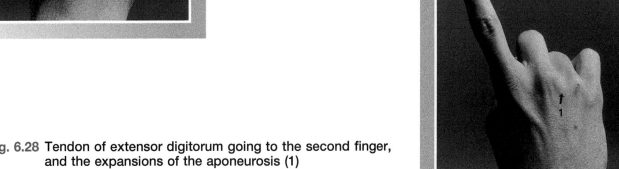

Fig. 6.28 Tendon of extensor digitorum going to the second finger, and the expansions of the aponeurosis (1)

MA: On the back of the hand, the tendons of extensor digitorum are interlinked by fibrous slips (1). These may be transverse or oblique.

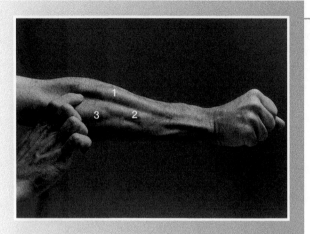

1. Extensor digitorum
2. Extensor carpi ulnaris
3. Anconeus

Fig. 6.29 Extensor digiti minimi: origin

MA: This muscle arises from the lateral epicondyle of the humerus, medial to the origin of extensor digitorum (1).

In the adjacent figure, the practitioner's index finger indicates the location of extensor digiti minimi in the groove between extensor digitorum and extensor carpi ulnaris.

ATTACHMENTS

- Extensor digiti minimi arises:
  - from the lateral epicondyle of the humerus;
  - from the antebrachial fascia.
- Distally, it fuses with the tendon of extensor digitorum going to the fifth finger near the fifth metacarpal (this varies from one individual to another).

Fig. 6.30 Body of extensor digiti minimi

MA: This is a very long, slender muscle situated in the depression between the bodies of extensor digitorum (1) and extensor carpi ulnaris (2). It is indicated here by the practitioner's index finger. To sense the contraction of this muscle, place a broad contact (with the pads of two or three fingers) in the depression described above. Then ask the subject to extend his little finger repeatedly.

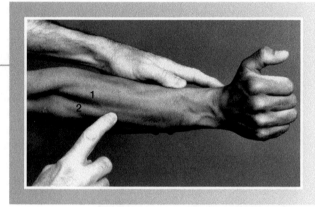

Fig. 6.31 Tendon of extensor digiti minimi

MA: In order to locate this tendon, place your contact (using your index finger, or two or three fingers) medial to the tendon of extensor digitorum (1), and lateral to the tendon of extensor carpi ulnaris (2). You will feel the tendon you are looking for beneath your fingers. This can be facilitated by asking the subject to extend the proximal phalanx of his fifth finger repeatedly while the other two remain flexed.

Note: The tendon passes behind the head of the ulna and wrist joint in a separate sheath.

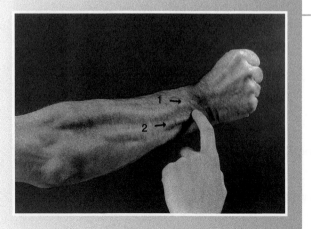

Fig. 6.32 Tendon of extensor digiti minimi on the back of the hand

MA: Occasionally, the tendon of extensor digiti minimi is divided in two, as seen here. This can be displayed by asking the subject to hyperextend the metacarpophalangeal joint of her fifth finger, while you resist this action.

CLINICAL NOTE

This is very seldom involved in epicondylitis. Examine by isometric testing, resisting extension of the proximal phalanx of the fifth finger. The pain is evoked at the **epicondyle.** The diagnosis can be confirmed or otherwise by palpation at the epicondyle, looking for the same tenderness to pressure.

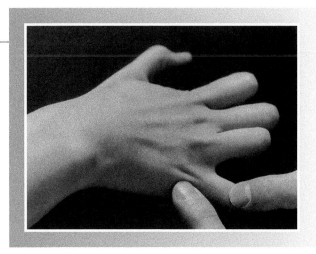

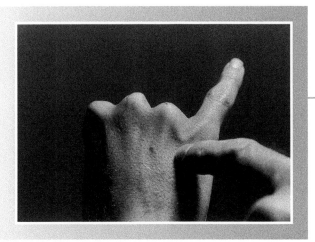

Fig. 6.33 Expansion of the aponeurosis of extensor digitorum on the tendon of extensor digiti minimi

MA: The tendons of extensor digitorum going to the fourth finger and of extensor digiti minimi are normally connected with each other. This connection is indicated here by the practitioner's index finger.

Note: There are similar connections between the tendons of the other fingers.

Fig. 6.34 Origin of extensor carpi ulnaris

MA: The practitioner's index finger in the adjacent figure indicates the proximal part of this muscle (1). Begin by locating extensor digitorum (2). Then position your contact medial to that muscle and ask the subject to extend his wrist repeatedly, inclining it to the ulnar side at the same time. You can then detect extensor carpi ulnaris beneath your fingers. It can help you find the best point of contact if you also locate anconeus (3).

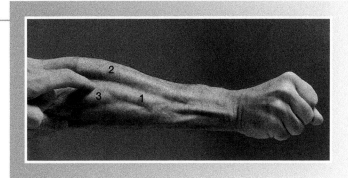

ATTACHMENTS

- Extensor carpi ulnaris arises via the common tendon of the lateral epicondylar muscles:
  - from the lateral epicondyle of the humerus;
  - from the superior two thirds of the lateral side of the posterior border of the ulna;
  - from the deep surface of the antebrachial fascia.
- It is inserted into the posteromedial tuberosity of the base of the fifth metacarpal.

195

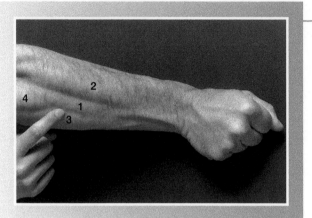

Fig. 6.35 Body of extensor carpi ulnaris

MA: In the adjacent figure, the practitioner's index finger indicates the body of extensor carpi ulnaris (1) between those of extensor digitorum (2) (laterally) and flexor carpi ulnaris (3) (medially). Anconeus (4) lies medially and proximally to it.

Fig. 6.36 Extensor carpi ulnaris: distal part

MA: The tendon of extensor carpi ulnaris (indicated here by the practitioner's index finger) passes behind the distal extremity of the ulna, in an osteofibrous sheath. It is inserted into the medial tuberosity of the fifth metacarpal.

> **CLINICAL NOTE**
>
> This muscle can also be implicated in **epicondylitis,** but extremely rarely. Examine by isometric testing, applying resistance to a movement combining extension of the wrist with inclination to the ulnar side by means of a contact at the ulnar border of the fifth metacarpal. The diagnosis can be confirmed or otherwise by palpation, applying pressure at the lateral epicondyle.

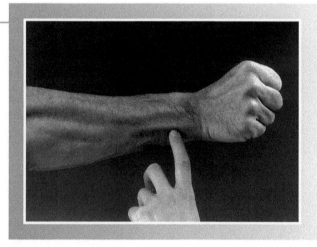

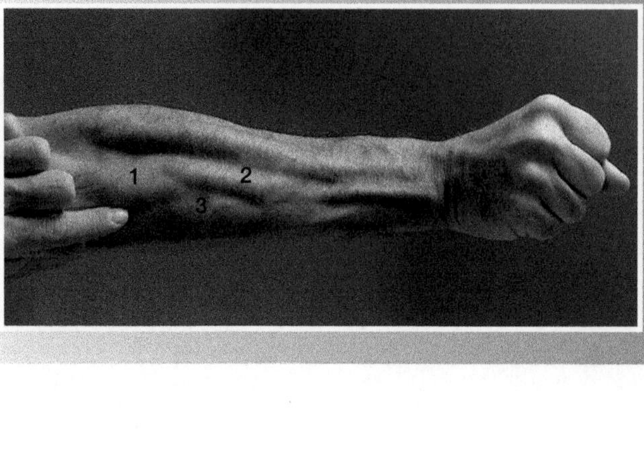

Fig. 6.37 Anconeus (1)

MA: It is easier to palpate this muscle if you begin with a three-finger contact resting against the lateral border of the olecranon. Then, using the same contact, slide your fingers down toward the distal and lateral part of the forearm, maintaining contact with the skin. You will feel the contour of this muscle beneath your fingers. Ask the subject to contract the muscles repeatedly to extend his forearm on the arm. This will make the body of the muscle more prominent.

In the adjacent figure, the practitioner's index finger indicates the anconeus between the bodies of extensor carpi ulnaris (2) (laterally) and flexor carpi ulnaris (3) (medially).

ATTACHMENTS

- Anconeus arises, via a tendon, from the posterior surface of the lateral epicondyle of the humerus.
- It is inserted into the lateral, posterior surface of the olecranon and the superior quarter of the posterior border of the ulna.

Fig. 6.38 Body of abductor pollicis longus

MA: The body of this muscle can be palpated on the posterior surface of the radius. It is shown in the figure alongside, indicated by the practitioner's index finger, at the point where it passes over the lateral surface of the radius. Ask the subject to abduct his thumb repeatedly as shown, extending it away from the other fingers to enable you to detect the contraction of the muscle.

ATTACHMENTS

* Abductor pollicis longus arises:
  – from the posterior surface of the ulna;
  – from the interosseous membrane of the forearm;
  – from the medial part of the posterior surface of the radius.
* It is inserted into the lateral tuberosity of the base of the first metacarpal.

Note: There is an oblique groove (1) separating abductor pollicis longus and extensor pollicis brevis (2).

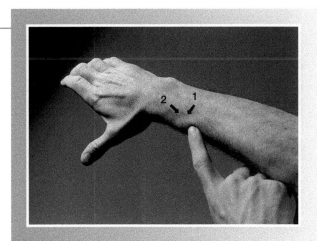

> **CLINICAL NOTE**
>
> **Intersection syndrome**
>
> This condition occurs in the posterolateral part of the distal third of the forearm, at the point where the tendons of extensor carpi radialis longus and brevis cross those of abductor pollicis longus and extensor pollicis brevis.
>
> The syndrome is caused by inflammation of the synovial bursa located here. The bursitis (swelling) is evident on palpation with pressure, which is not only painful but also produces clearly audible crepitus. Isometric testing of the abduction and extension of the thumb reveals deficit and evokes pain.

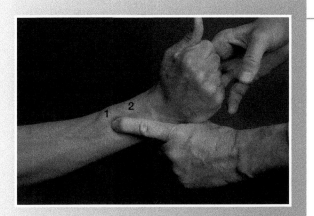

Fig. 6.39 Abductor pollicis longus, another view

MA: The practitioner's index finger is positioned in the groove between extensor pollicis brevis and abductor pollicis longus, easing back the body of abductor pollicis longus proximally.

1. Abductor pollicis longus
2. Extensor pollicis brevis

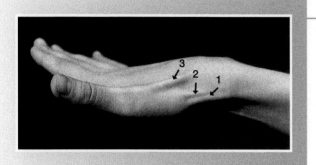

Fig. 6.40 Tendon of abductor pollicis longus

MA: Ask the subject to abduct her thumb as shown, extending it away from the other fingers, to enable you to detect this tendon. It is indicated here by the arrow on the right (1). The tendon is inserted into the lateral tuberosity of the base of the first metacarpal.

Note: It is not always easy to distinguish the tendon of abductor pollicis longus clearly from that of extensor pollicis brevis. The two are often found running closely alongside each other in such a way that they seem to be a single tendon. It helps to remember that the tendon of abductor pollicis longus lies farther anteriorly.

1. Tendon of abductor pollicis longus
2. Tendon of extensor pollicis brevis
3. Tendon of extensor pollicis longus

Fig. 6.41 Body of extensor pollicis brevis

MA: This muscle lies on the posterior surface of the forearm, below abductor pollicis longus. Both turn around the lateral surface of the radius. A point to remember in identifying these two muscles is that extensor pollicis brevis occupies the more distal position. An oblique groove can be palpated between the bodies of the two muscles on the posterolateral part of the radius; extensor pollicis brevis will be found below this groove. Ask the subject to abduct his thumb repeatedly, extending it away from the other fingers, to help you sense the muscle contraction.

ATTACHMENTS

- Extensor pollicis brevis arises:
  – from the medial third of the posterior surface of the radius;
  – from the interosseous membrane of the forearm.
- It is inserted into the dorsal surface of the proximal phalanx of the thumb.

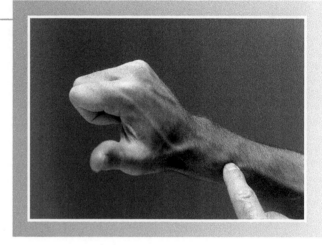

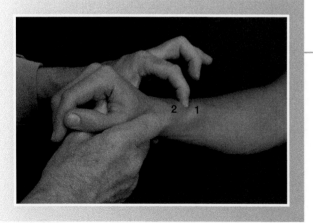

Fig. 6.42 Palpation of abductor pollicis longus and extensor pollicis brevis (relaxed), another view

MA: With one hand, take hold of the subject's hand and guide it into a pronated position. With the index finger of your other hand, seek the groove (depression) between the body of abductor pollicis longus and that of extensor pollicis brevis. Rolling your index finger proximally brings it to rest on abductor pollicis longus, and rolling it distally contacts extensor pollicis brevis.

1. Abductor pollicis longus
2. Extensor pollicis brevis

Fig. 6.43 Tendon of extensor pollicis brevis at the wrist

MA: It is often difficult to distinguish the tendon of this muscle from that of abductor pollicis longus at this level, as the two run closely side by side. To make the tendon apparent at the lateral part of the wrist, ask the subject first to extend all his fingers, and then abduct his thumb away from the other fingers. When trying to identify this tendon, remember that it occupies a dorsal position relative to that of abductor pollicis longus.

Note: This tendon marks the anterolateral extent of the anatomic snuffbox.

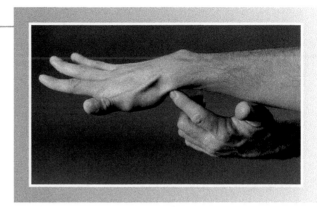

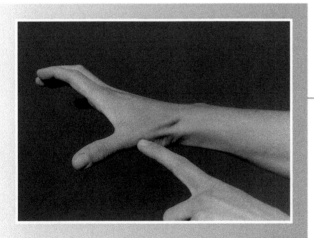

Fig. 6.44 Insertion of extensor pollicis brevis

MA: The tendon indicated here by the practitioner's index finger runs along the dorsal surface of the first metacarpal, and is inserted into the dorsal part of the base of the proximal phalanx.

Fig. 6.45 Extensor pollicis longus on the posterior surface of the radius

MA: Use the pads of two fingers to place a contact on the posterior surface of the radius, medial to the body of extensor pollicis brevis (1). Ask the subject to extend his thumb back beyond the plane of the hand, and you will feel the tendon of extensor pollicis longus becoming taut beneath your fingers.

ATTACHMENTS

- Extensor pollicis longus arises:
  - from the middle third of the posterior surface of the ulna;
  - from the interosseous membrane of the forearm.
- It is inserted into the dorsal surface of the base of the distal phalanx of the thumb.

Note: The body of extensor pollicis longus runs down the posterior surface of the forearm in an oblique lateral and inferior direction; it runs under and closely against extensor pollicis brevis.

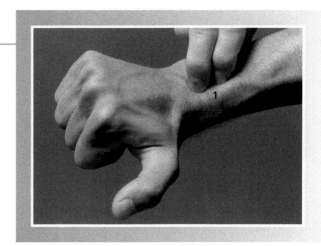

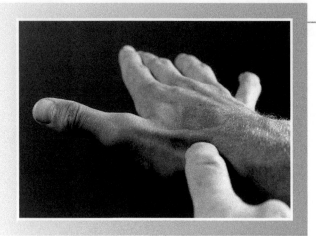

Fig. 6.46 Tendon of extensor pollicis longus at the wrist

MA: This tendon can be made more prominent by asking the subject to perform the same action as that described in Figure 6.45. This tendon marks the posterolateral extent of the anatomic snuffbox at the wrist. The anterolateral boundary of this feature is marked by the tendon of extensor pollicis brevis.

Note: The anatomic snuffbox is a triangular depression which appears on the posterolateral aspect of the wrist when the extensor muscles of the thumb contract. The floor of this depression is formed by the scaphoid bone.

Fig. 6.47 Insertion of extensor pollicis longus

MA: The tendon runs along the dorsal surface of the first metacarpal and proximal phalanx, and is inserted into the dorsal part of the base of the distal phalanx, shown here by the practitioner's index finger.

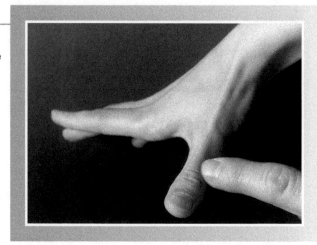

THE ANTERIOR MUSCLE GROUP

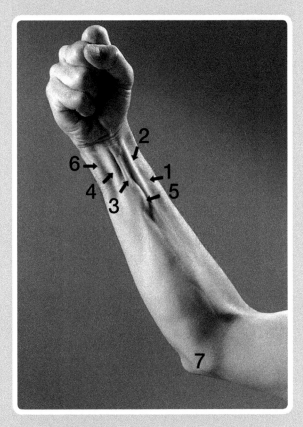

Fig. 6.48 Anterior view of the forearm

1. Flexor pollicis longus
2. Flexor carpi radialis
3. Palmaris longus
   Flexor digitorum superficialis:
4. Tendon to the fourth finger
5. Body of muscle
6. Flexor carpi ulnaris
7. Common tendon of origin of the medial epicondylar muscles (forearm flexors)

This group consists of eight muscles, arranged in four layers as follows:

- The first layer of the anterior compartment consists (working medially) of pronator teres, flexor carpi radialis, palmaris longus, and flexor carpi ulnaris muscles.
- The second layer contains flexor digitorum superficialis.
- The third layer consists of flexor digitorum profundus medially and flexor pollicis longus laterally.
- The fourth layer contains the pronator quadratus.

The notable structures that can be detected by palpation are the medial epicondylar muscles (forearm flexors) (Fig. 6.49) and common tendon of origin (Fig. 6.50).

- Pronator teres (Figs. 6.51 and 6.52)
- Flexor carpi radialis:
  - Body (Fig. 6.53)
  - Tendons (Figs. 6.54 and 6.55)
- Palmaris longus (Figs. 6.56 and 6.57)
- Flexor carpi ulnaris (Figs. 6.58–6.60)
- Flexor digitorum superficialis (Figs. 6.61–6.65)
- Flexor pollicis longus (Figs. 6.66–6.69).

ACTIONS

Flexor pollicis longus:

- Flexes the distal phalanx of the thumb on the proximal one.
- Helps flex the proximal (first) phalanx of the thumb on the first metacarpal.
- Helps oppose the thumb to the other fingers, and in the various grasping actions of the hand.

Flexor digitorum profundus:

- Acts on the last four fingers to:
  - flex the distal (third) phalanges on the middle (second) ones;
  - help flex the middle phalanges on the proximal (first) ones;
  - help flex the proximal phalanges on the metacarpals.
- Helps to flex the wrist.
- Helps oppose the thumb to the other fingers, and in the various grasping actions of the hand.

Flexor digitorum superficialis:

- Acts on the last four fingers to:
  - flex the middle phalanges on the proximal ones;
  - help flex the proximal phalanges on the metacarpals.
- Helps oppose the thumb to the other fingers, and in the various grasping actions of the hand.

Flexor carpi ulnaris:

- Helps flex the wrist on the forearm and incline it on the ulnar side.

Flexor carpi radialis:

- Flexes the wrist and abducts it (inclines it on the radial side).
- Assists pronation of the forearm on the arm.

Pronator teres:

- Pronates and flexes the forearm on the arm. (In normal use, pronation is usually associated with abduction and medial rotation of the shoulder.)

Pronator quadratus:

- Pronates and flexes the forearm on the arm.

Palmaris longus:

- Flexes the wrist on the forearm.

INNERVATIONS

- Pronator teres: median nerve (C6–C7)
- Flexor carpi radialis: median nerve (C6–C7–C8)
- Palmaris longus: median nerve (C6–C7–C8)
- Flexor carpi ulnaris: ulnar nerve (C7–C8–T1)
- Flexor digitorum superficialis: median nerve (C7–C8–T1)
- Flexor digitorum profundus: median nerve and ulnar nerve (C8–T1)
- Flexor pollicis longus: median nerve (C8–T1)
- Pronator quadratus: median nerve (C7–C8–T1)

Fig. 6.49 The medial epicondylar muscles (forearm flexors)

MA: The subject's elbow should be flexed, with his wrist in a neutral position or slightly flexed. His fist should be clenched in a neutral position, neither pronated nor supinated. Place your hand, fingers together, against the medial part of his elbow, with your thenar eminence resting on the medial epicondyle. The position of the practitioner's hand as shown here is as follows.

1. Thumb corresponding to the direction of pronator teres
2. Index finger in line with flexor carpi radialis
3. Middle finger in line with palmaris longus
4. Ring finger in line with flexor digitorum superficialis (tendon going to the fourth finger)
5. Little finger in line with flexor carpi ulnaris

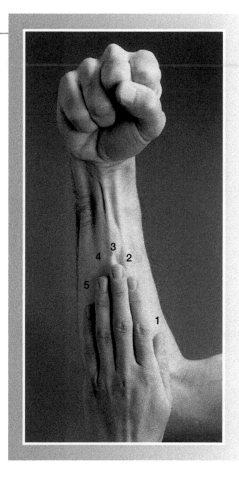

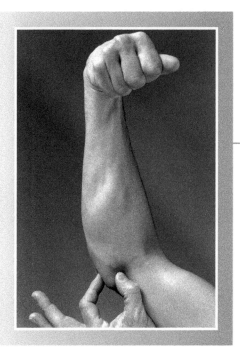

Fig. 6.50 Common tendon of origin of the medial epicondylar muscles (forearm flexors)

MA: Place a thumb-and-finger contact on the subject's medial epicondyle, and ask him to flex his wrist at the same time as inclining it to the ulnar side. You will feel the common tendon contracting beneath your fingers.

CLINICAL NOTE

Medial epicondylitis

This is tendinitis affecting the muscles that attach to the medial epicondyle (pronator teres, flexor carpi radialis, palmaris longus, flexor carpi ulnaris, and flexor digitorum superficialis).

Diagnosis involves isometric testing of each of these muscles, examining stretching of the muscle and using palpation to look for tenderness to pressure. The aim in each of these tests is to find whether it evokes or exacerbates pain.

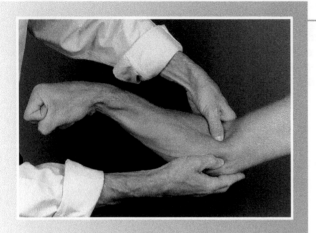

Fig. 6.51 Body of pronator teres

MA: Place your contact just medial to the tendon of biceps brachii. Then ask the subject to pronate his forearm with fist clenched. You will sense the body of this muscle tensing beneath your fingers.

ATTACHMENTS

Pronator teres consists of two heads: the humeral and the ulnar head.

- The humeral head arises from the medial epicondyle of the humerus and the antebrachial fascia.
- The ulnar head arises from the coronoid process of the ulna.
- The two heads join and the muscle is inserted via a short tendon into the middle third of the lateral surface of the radius.

Fig. 6.52 Distal part of pronator teres

MA: Once you have located the body of the muscle, follow it along its oblique course, distally and laterally to its insertion into the middle third of the lateral surface of the radius. Ask the subject to pronate his forearm with fist clenched. This will help you locate the muscle.

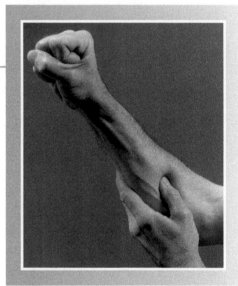

CLINICAL NOTE

Medial epicondylitis

This is the probable diagnosis if pronation against isometric resistance evokes or increases pain at the medial epicondyle. The effect of palpation at this epicondyle is the same, producing tenderness to pressure.

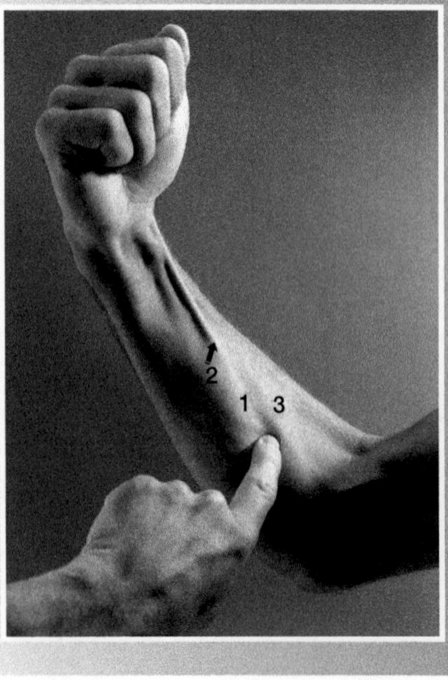

Fig. 6.53 Body of flexor carpi radialis

MA: Ask the subject to flex his wrist, at the same time inclining it radially. You will detect the body of the muscle (1) in continuity with the tendon (2) and medial to pronator teres (3).

ATTACHMENTS

- Flexor carpi radialis arises via a tendon from the anterior surface of the medial epicondyle of the humerus and of the antebrachial fascia.
- It crosses the lateral part of the carpal tunnel and is inserted into the palmar base of the second metacarpal.

CLINICAL NOTE

Pain at the medial epicondyle, evoked or exacerbated by the action of flexing the wrist while inclining it radially, in both cases against isometric resistance, should lead you to suspect **medial epicondylitis.** The effect of palpation at the epicondyle is the same, producing tenderness to pressure.

Fig. 6.54 Tendon of flexor carpi radialis

MA: Ask the subject to perform the same action as that described in Fig. 6.53. The tendon of flexor carpi radialis is the most lateral of the tendons that can be seen in the inferior third of the anterior surface of the forearm.

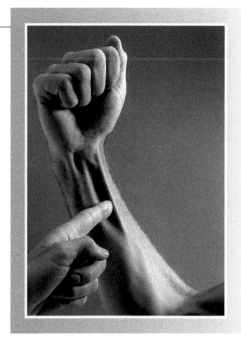

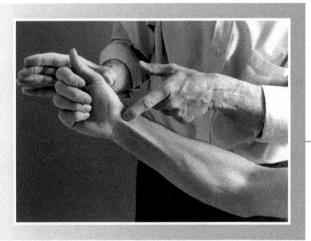

Fig. 6.55 Distal tendon of flexor carpi radialis

MA: Ask the subject to flex his wrist slightly, at the same time inclining it to the radial side. In the adjacent figure the practitioner is resisting the radial inclination.

Note: The tendon is inserted into the anterior surface of the base of the second metacarpal, and sometimes also that of the third metacarpal.

Fig. 6.56 Body of palmaris longus

MA: Ask the subject to flex his wrist. You will detect the body of the muscle (1) in continuity with the tendon (2), shown here by the practitioner's index finger, and medial to flexor carpi radialis (3). This muscle is inconstant.

ATTACHMENTS

- Palmaris longus arises from the anterior surface of the medial epicondyle of the humerus and the antebrachial fascia.
- It is inserted via a tendon at the wrist:
  - median fibers: into the flexor retinaculum and middle palmar aponeurosis;
  - lateral fibers: into the thenar eminence;
  - medial fibers: into the hypothenar eminence.

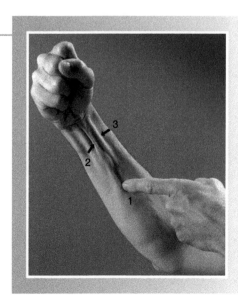

> ### CLINICAL NOTE
>
> Pain at the **medial epicondyle,** evoked or exacerbated by flexion of the wrist against isometric resistance, should lead you to suspect medial epicondylitis. The effect of palpation at the epicondyle is the same, producing tenderness to pressure.

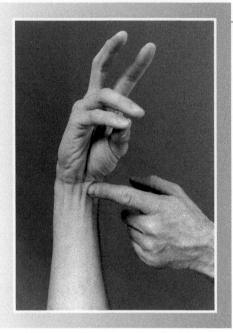

Fig. 6.57 Tendon of palmaris longus

MA: Ask the subject to oppose his thumb to his little finger. This will make the tendon of palmaris longus more prominent. It is a long tendon occupying approximately the inferior two thirds of the anterior surface of the forearm.

Fig. 6.58 Proximal part of flexor carpi ulnaris

MA: Ask the subject to flex his wrist and incline it on the ulnar side. You will detect the body of the muscle (indicated here by the practitioner's index finger) close to the ulna, medial to palmaris longus.

Note: It is very difficult to distinguish the bodies of the medial epicondylar muscles (forearm flexors) on the proximal part of the forearm.

ATTACHMENTS

* Flexor carpi ulnaris arises by two heads:
  - one from the medial epicondyle of the humerus (humeral head);
  - one from the medial border of the olecranon and the superior two thirds of the posterior border of the ulna (ulnar head).
* The tendon is inserted into the anterior surface of the pisiform bone, by means of expansions on the hook of the hamate.

CLINICAL NOTE

Pain at the medial epicondyle, evoked or exacerbated by the action of flexing the wrist while inclining it in the ulnar direction, in both cases against isometric resistance, should lead you to suspect **medial epicondylitis.** The effect of palpation at the epicondyle is the same, producing tenderness to pressure.

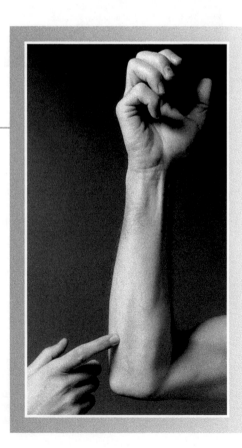

Fig. 6.59 Flexor carpi ulnaris

MA: The two heads of this muscle (described previously, Fig. 6.58) unite into a single muscle body (1) running down the medial surface of the forearm to the distal tendon.

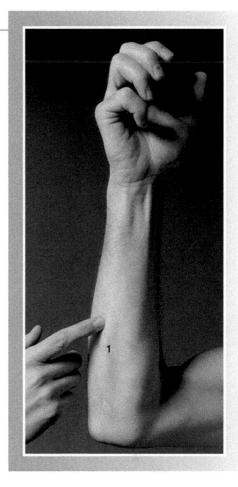

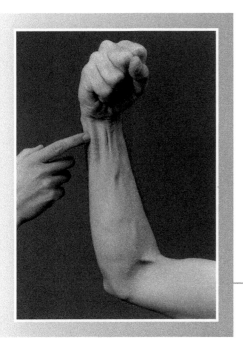

Fig. 6.60 Tendon of flexor carpi ulnaris

MA: This tendon is the most medial of the tendons visible on the anterior surface of the forearm. The action required to make the tendon more prominent is the same as that described for Figure 6.58.

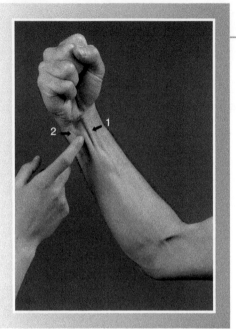

Fig. 6.61 Flexor digitorum superficialis, superficial layer – tendon to the fourth finger

MA: In the adjacent figure, the practitioner's index finger indicates the tendon going to the fourth finger. It lies medial to (on the ulnar side of) the tendon of palmaris longus (1). The practitioner's index finger is against the radial border of the tendon of flexor carpi ulnaris (2). Ask the subject to clench his fist and flex his wrist briefly and repeatedly.

Note: The tendons to the fourth finger and to the third finger belong to the anterior (superficial) layer of flexor digitorum superficialis.

ATTACHMENTS

- Flexor digitorum superficialis consists of two heads: the humero-ulnar and the radial head.
  - The humero-ulnar head arises from the medial epicondyle of the humerus and the coronoid process of the ulna.
  - The radial head arises from the superior half of the anterior border of the radius.
- Muscle fibers arise from a muscular arch between these two heads, and are arranged in two layers:
  - A superficial humero-ulnar layer (or head) runs to the third and fourth fingers.
  - A deep radial layer (or head), which sometimes has two bellies, runs to the second and fifth fingers.
- The four tendons from the body of the muscle pass through the carpal tunnel and are inserted into the palmar surface of the middle phalanx.

> **CLINICAL NOTE**
>
> Pain at the **medial epicondyle,** evoked or exacerbated by the action of flexing the fingers and wrist together, both against isometric resistance, should lead you to suspect medial epicondylitis. The effect of palpation at the epicondyle is the same, producing tenderness to pressure.

Fig. 6.62 Flexor digitorum superficialis, superficial layer – tendon to the third finger

MA: The adjacent figure shows the practitioner's index finger pushing aside the tendon of palmaris longus (1) laterally (to the radial side) to contact the tendon of flexor digitorum to the third finger (2). This lies on the radial border of the tendon of flexor digitorum superficialis going to the fourth finger. Ask the subject to oppose thumb and middle finger (this action is not shown here) and to flex his wrist briefly and repeatedly. This will display the tendon more clearly beneath your fingers. Another method is to ask the subject to clench his fist and flex his wrist briefly and repeatedly, at the same time inclining it slightly to the ulnar side. (See Chapter 7.)

Note: This tendon and the one to the fourth finger belong to the anterior (superficial) layer of the flexor digitorum superficialis.

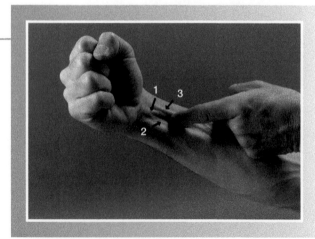

1. Tendon of palmaris longus
2. Tendon of muscle going to the third finger
3. Tendon of flexor carpi radialis

Fig. 6.63 Flexor digitorum superficialis, deep layer – tendons to the fifth finger and index finger

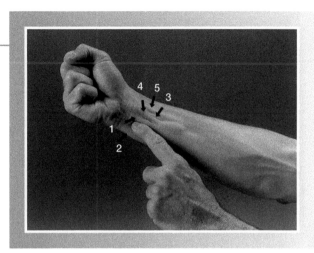

MA: Tendon to the fifth finger: In the adjacent figure, the practitioner's index finger rests on the ulnar border of the tendon going to the fourth finger (1) in order to make contact with the tendon to the fifth finger. This lies between the tendon of flexor carpi ulnaris (2) medially (on the ulnar side) and the tendon to the fourth finger (1) laterally (on the radial side). Ask the subject to oppose thumb and fifth finger while slightly flexing his wrist. This will display the tightening of the tendon more clearly. (See Chapter 7.)

Tendon to the index finger: In the adjacent figure, the tendon to the index finger (3) can also be seen, between the tendon of palmaris longus (4) on the ulnar side and the tendon of flexor carpi radialis (5) on the radial side. Ask the subject to oppose thumb and second finger while slightly flexing his wrist, to display this tendon more clearly. (See Chapter 7.)

Note: The tendons described here belong to the posterior (deep) layer of flexor digitorum superficialis.

Fig. 6.64 Distal body of flexor digitorum superficialis

MA: In the adjacent figure, the practitioner's index finger indicates one belly of the deep (posterior) layer of flexor digitorum superficialis. This layer contains the tendons to the index and little fingers. The superficial (anterior) layer contains the tendons to the ring finger and middle finger. This belly of the muscle can be displayed more clearly if you ask the subject to clench his fist firmly, at the same time flexing his wrist slightly, and to flex his index finger briefly and repeatedly.

Note: This muscle layer cannot be accessed in all subjects.

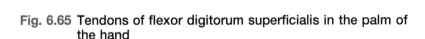

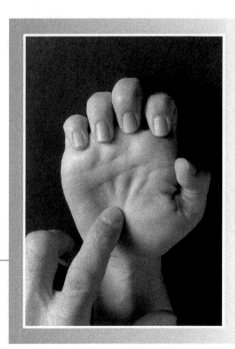

Fig. 6.65 Tendons of flexor digitorum superficialis in the palm of the hand

MA: The tendons are clearly visible on the palm of the subject's hand in the adjacent figure. Ask the subject to hyperextend her metacarpophalangeal joints and at the same time to flex the middle and distal phalanges. Even if the tendons cannot be detected visually as they can here, they are clearly evident to palpation.

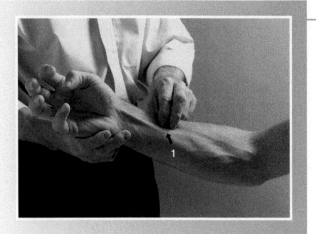

Fig. 6.67 Flexor pollicis longus

MA: Ask the subject to flex the distal phalanx on the first rapidly and repeatedly. You detect the body of the muscle on the distal part of the anterior surface of the radius, laterally to flexor carpi radialis longus.

Fig. 6.66 Body of flexor pollicis longus

MA: Place your contact, using one or two fingers, lateral to flexor carpi radialis (1). Ask the subject for repeated contractions of the distal phalanx of his thumb on the proximal one. You can feel the contraction beneath your fingers.

ATTACHMENTS

- Flexor pollicis longus arises from the superior three quarters of the anterior surface of the radius and from the interosseous membrane of the forearm.
- It is inserted into the palmar surface of the base of the distal phalanx of the thumb.

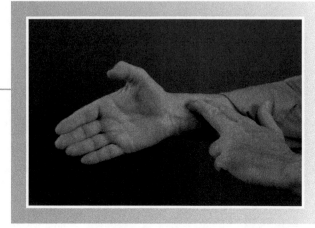

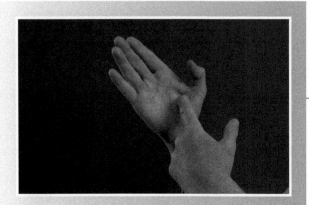

Fig. 6.68 Flexor pollicis longus, tendon at the thenar eminence

MA: This tendon can be detected on the distal part of the thenar eminence if you ask the subject to flex the distal phalanx on the first quickly and repeatedly.

Fig. 6.69 Tendon of flexor pollicis longus at the proximal phalanx

MA: This tendon can be detected in the middle of the palmar surface of the proximal phalanx if you ask the subject to flex the distal phalanx on the first quickly and repeatedly.

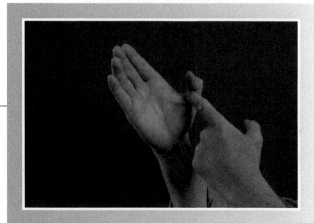

7
The wrist and the hand

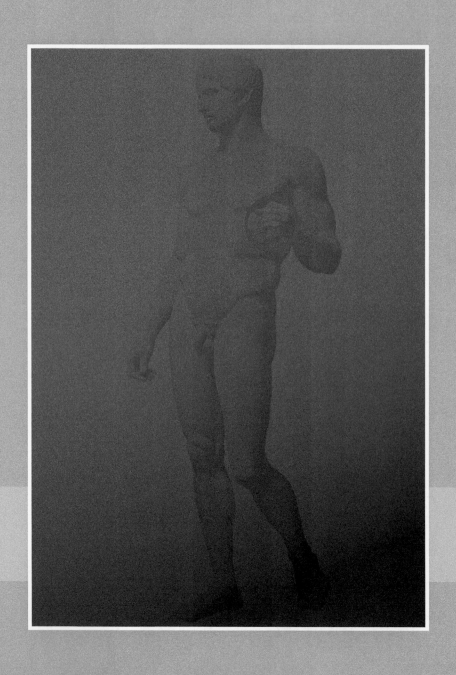

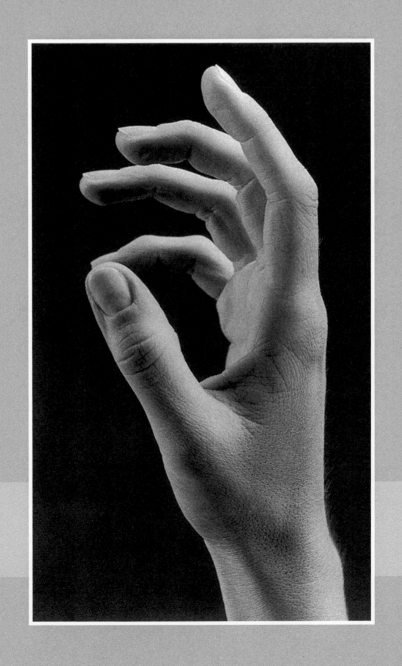

OSTEOLOGY

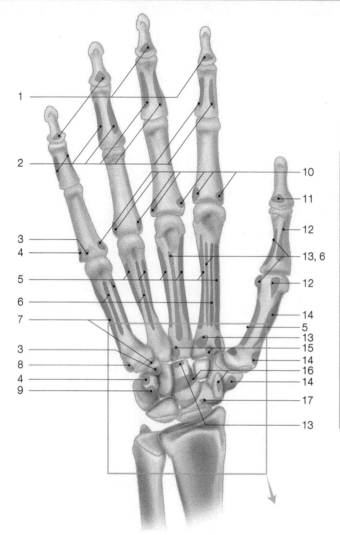

Bones of the hand – anterior (palmar) view

1. Flexor digitorum profundus
2. Flexor digitorum superficialis
3. Flexor digiti minimi brevis
4. Abductor digiti minimi
5. Dorsal interossei
6. Palmar interossei
7. Opponens digiti minimi
8. Extensor carpi ulnaris
9. Flexor carpi ulnaris
10. Interossei
11. Flexor pollicis longus
12. Flexor pollicis brevis and abductor pollicis brevis
13. Adductor pollicis
14. Opponens pollicis
15. Flexor carpi radialis
16. Flexor pollicis brevis
17. Abductor pollicis brevis

Bones of the carpus – anterior view

1. Base of fifth metacarpal	9. Head of ulna
2. Hook of hamate	10. Trapezoid
3. Hamate	11. Trapezium
4. Pisiform	12. Tubercle of trapezium
5. Capitate	13. Scaphoid
6. Triquetrum	14. Tubercle of scaphoid
7. Lunate	15. Radial styloid process
8. Ulnar styloid process	

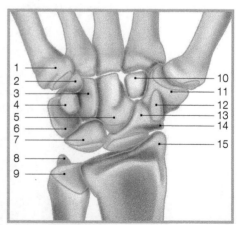

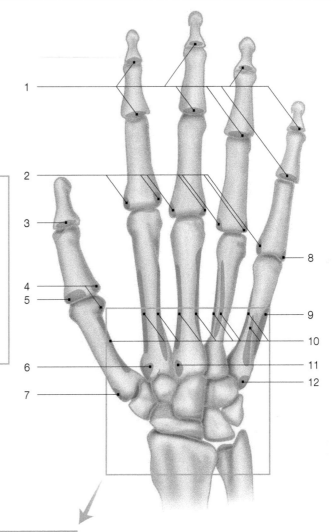

Bones of the hand – posterior view

1. Extensor digitorum muscles
2. Dorsal and palmar interossei
3. Extensor pollicis longus
4. Adductor pollicis
5. Extensor pollicis brevis
6. Extensor carpi radialis longus
7. Abductor pollicis longus
8. Abductor digiti minimi
9. Opponens digiti minimi
10. Dorsal interossei
11. Extensor carpi radialis brevis
12. Extensor carpi ulnaris

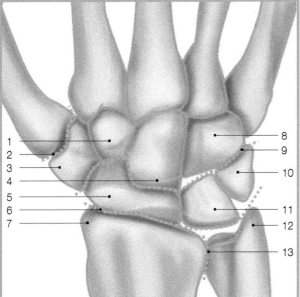

Bones of the carpus – posterior view

1. Trapezoid
2. Carpometacarpal joint of thumb
3. Trapezium
4. Capitate
5. Scaphoid
6. Wrist (radiocarpal) joint
7. Radial styloid process
8. Hamate
9. Midcarpal joint
10. Triquetrum
11. Lunate
12. Ulnar styloid process
13. Distal radioulnar joint

THE INFERIOR EXTREMITY OF THE TWO BONES OF THE FOREARM

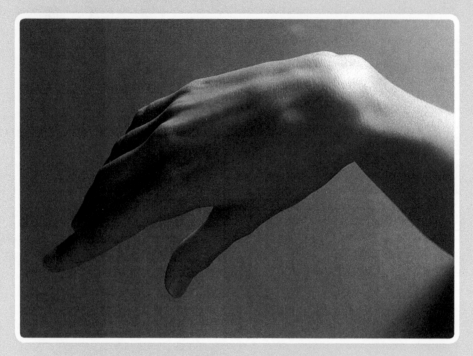

Fig. 7.2 Radial view of the wrist

The notable structures that can be detected by palpation are:

- Head (inferior extremity) of the ulna (Fig. 7.3) and ulnar styloid process (Fig. 7.4)
- Inferior extremity of the radius (Fig. 7.5); medial (ulnar) border (Fig. 7.6); lateral surface and radial styloid process (Fig. 7.7)
- Dorsal tubercle of the radius, posterior view (Fig. 7.8).

Fig. 7.3 Head (inferior extremity) of the ulna

MA: This figure simply shows the position of the head of the ulna (1). It feels like a bulge beneath your fingers, overhanging the medial part of the proximal row of carpal bones. The inferior extremity of the ulna is cylindrical, formed of two raised features separated by a groove. These are the styloid process (Fig. 7.4) and a lateral prominence which articulates with the ulnar notch of the radius.

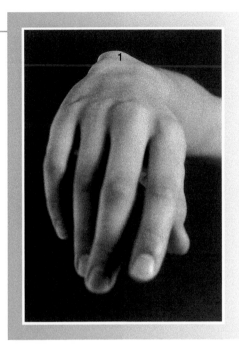

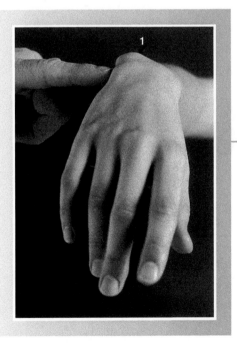

Fig. 7.4 Head (inferior extremity) of the ulna and ulnar styloid process

MA: On the inferior extremity of the ulna (1) is the styloid process, a protuberance that is easy to access using a pincer contact with thumb and index finger. The styloid process is indicated here by the practitioner's index finger. It is separated from the lateral surface, which articulates with the ulnar notch of the radius, by a sagittal groove, through which the tendon of extensor carpi ulnaris passes.

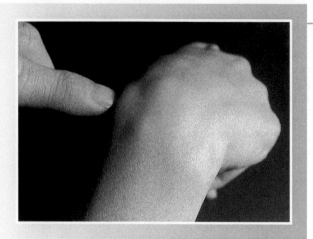

Fig. 7.5 Inferior extremity of the radius

MA: This figure shows the location of the inferior extremity of the radius; it overhangs the lateral part of the proximal row of carpal bones, as well as articulating with them. The inferior surface of the inferior extremity articulates laterally with the scaphoid and medially with the lunate.

> **CLINICAL NOTE**
>
> **The inferior extremity of the radius** can be a site of **fracture.** Examine by palpation, which may detect a point of exquisite pain at various locations on this distal extremity.

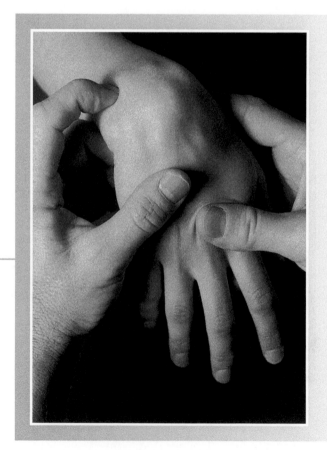

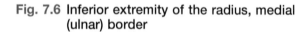

Fig. 7.6 Inferior extremity of the radius, medial (ulnar) border

MA: The ulnar notch is situated at this border. It is a concave surface that articulates with the head of the ulna. The subject's wrist is in a neutral position. Place your index finger on the posterior surface of the head of the ulna, facing the distal end of the radius. Ask the subject to flex her wrist. The medial border will "appear" beneath your finger.

Fig. 7.7 Inferior extremity of the radius, lateral surface, and radial styloid process

MA: The practitioner's index finger indicates the lateral surface; across this run two vertical grooves. The tendons of abductor pollicis longus and extensor pollicis brevis pass through the anterior groove, and the tendons of the extensor carpi radialis longus and brevis through the posterior one. Distally, the lateral surface terminates in the radial styloid process (1).

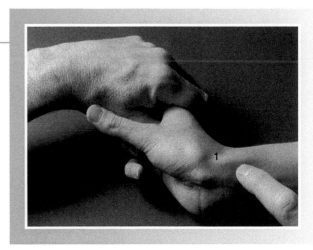

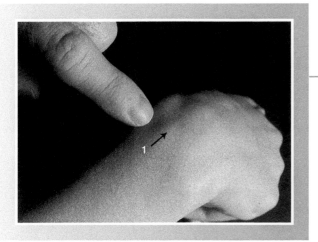

Fig. 7.8 Dorsal tubercle of the radius, posterior view

MA: This tubercle is an important landmark on the posterior part of the wrist. It separates two grooves; the tendon of extensor pollicis longus passes through the lateral groove, and the tendons of the extensor digitorum and extensor indicis through the medial groove. The dorsal tubercle (1) is situated in the middle of the posterior surface of the distal (inferior) extremity of the radius. Its medial limit is marked by the ulnar border of the radius.

THE CARPAL BONES OF THE PROXIMAL ROW

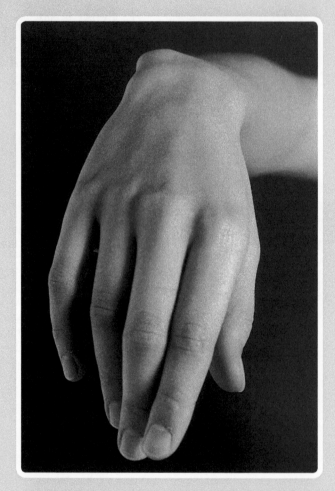

Fig. 7.9 Distal (inferior) view of the proximal row of carpal bones

The notable structures that can be detected by palpation are:

- Anatomic snuffbox (Fig. 7.10)
- Scaphoid (Figs. 7.11–7.19); tubercle of the scaphoid (Fig. 7.16)
- Lunate (Figs. 7.20–7.22)
- Triquetrum (Figs. 7.23–7.25)
- Pisiform (Figs. 7.26 and 7.27).

Fig. 7.10 The anatomic snuffbox

MA: The tendons of extensor pollicis longus (1) and extensor pollicis brevis (2) gradually separate from each other in the region of the wrist, creating a triangular space with its base positioned proximally and its tip distally. This is called the anatomic snuffbox. The scaphoid (proximally) and the trapezium (distally) lie in the floor (3) of the snuffbox. The tendon of abductor pollicis longus, which lies against that of extensor pollicis brevis anteriorly, also forms part of the snuffbox.

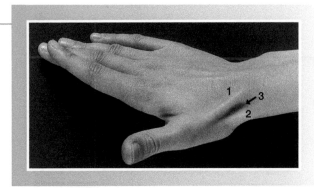

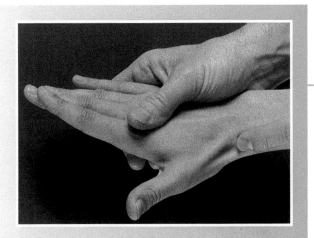

Fig. 7.11 Scaphoid, lateral approach – step 1

MA: The subject's hand is in a neutral position. Once you have located the anatomic snuffbox – the depression between the extensor tendons of the thumb – slide your index finger down into the base of it. The figure alongside shows the practitioner's index finger in a contact that sits between the radial styloid process and the scaphoid.

Fig. 7.12 Scaphoid, lateral approach – step 2

MA: Following the step shown in Figure 7.11, direct your index finger distally farther into the snuffbox. With your other hand, incline the subject's hand in the ulnar direction. The lateral surface of the scaphoid will come into contact with your index finger.

Note: A groove runs across this surface of the scaphoid; the radial artery passes through it.

> **CLINICAL NOTE**
> If palpation here causes exquisite pain in response to pressure, you should suspect **fracture of the scaphoid.**

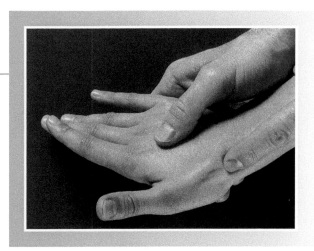

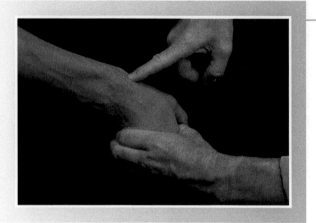

Fig. 7.13 Lateral surface of the scaphoid, another view

MA: Incline the subject's hand in the ulnar direction with one hand. As shown here, the index finger of the practitioner's other hand indicates the lateral surface of the scaphoid in the proximal part of the anatomic snuffbox, close to the radial styloid process.

Fig. 7.14 Scaphoid, anterior approach

MA: Place the subject's wrist in extension, as shown in the adjacent figure. This helps to "disengage" the anterior (palmar) surface of the scaphoid. You should feel a convexity (a bulge) beneath your index finger. This indicates that you have contacted the scaphoid.

> **CLINICAL NOTE**
> Most fractures of the wrist (80% to 90%) involve the scaphoid, and in 75% of such cases the line of fracture runs through the middle part of this bone (the neck of the scaphoid). Fractures of the distal and proximal extremities of the bone are much rarer. The proximal part is less vascularized, and may be the site of complications (such as pseudarthrosis or necrosis). This is more likely if the line of fracture is proximal. Displacement of the two fragments is rare.

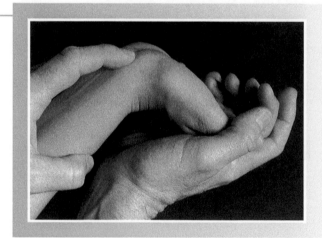

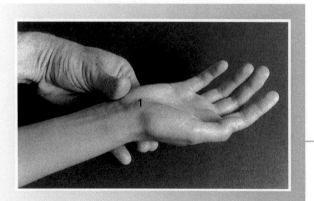

Fig. 7.15 Scaphoid, another anterior approach

MA: Place the interphalangeal joint of your thumb on the radial part of the pisiform, in line with the first cutaneous palmar fold. Flex your interphalangeal joint; the pad of your thumb will come into contact with the palmar surface of the scaphoid (1).

Fig. 7.16 Lateral tubercle of the scaphoid

MA: In the adjacent figure, the practitioner's left thumb is contacting the tubercle of the scaphoid, which is a lateral extension of the anterior (palmar) surface of the scaphoid.

In order to find and palpate this tubercle, position your contact on the anterior part of the tendon of abductor pollicis longus (1). This is made easier if the subject's wrist is repeatedly inclined in the ulnar direction.

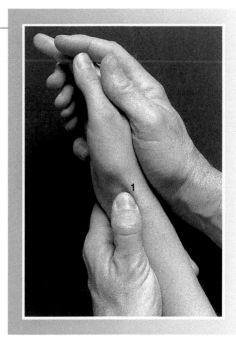

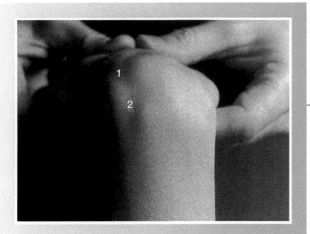

Fig. 7.17 The scaphoid, posterior approach – step 1

MA: Topographical location: To locate the dorsal surface of the scaphoid (1), begin from the lateral side of the inferior extremity of the radius (2) and extend this line distally.

Fig. 7.18 Scaphoid, posterior approach – step 2

MA: Rest your index finger on the joint space of the subject's wrist as shown. With your other hand, draw the subject's hand into palmar flexion. The dorsal surface of the scaphoid can be detected as a convex feature (1) beyond the joint space of the wrist.

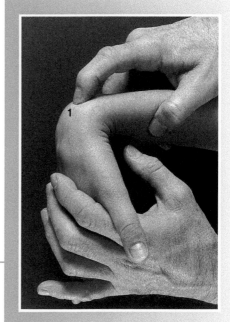

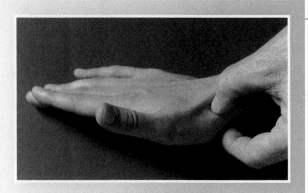

Fig. 7.19 Scaphoid, global approach

MA: The adjacent figure shows an overall approach to the scaphoid. Use a pincer contact with your thumb and index finger to take hold of the palmar and lateral surfaces of the scaphoid. See Figures 7.14 and 7.15 for the location of the palmar surface. The practitioner's thumb is resting on the lateral surface in this photograph. It forms the floor of the anatomic snuffbox.

Note: Another method for the global approach is to take hold of the palmar and dorsal surfaces between thumb and index finger.

Fig. 7.20 Lunate, topographical display

MA: In the adjacent figure, the practitioner's index finger indicates the lunate. It can be made more prominent if you ask the subject to flex her hand. This "disengages" the carpal articular surface at the inferior extremity of the radius.

> **CLINICAL NOTE**
>
> **Necrosis of the lunate** is most commonly post-traumatic, occurring in the absence of fracture or dislocation. The lunate becomes flattened and condenses, and its articular surface becomes irregular. It is extremely rare for this to be primitive necrosis, or for it to occur as a result of deformity such as an ulna that is too short.

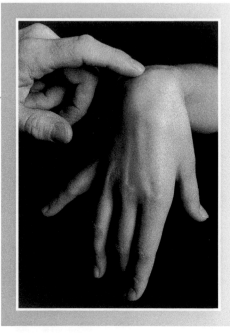

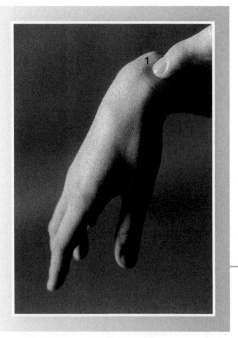

Fig. 7.21 Lunate – proximal approach

MA: The first step is to locate the dorsal tubercle of the radius. Then place your index finger on the medial (ulnar) side of the tubercle, on the wrist joint and pointing toward the fifth metacarpal. Ask the subject to flex her wrist in the palmar direction, and the lunate (1) will present itself to your contact.

Fig. 7.22 Lunate – distal approach

MA: Begin by locating the capitate (Figs. 7.40–7.47). Place your index finger in the depression belonging to the body of the capitate and situated just proximal to the base of the third metacarpal. Then slide your finger over the bulge of the head of the capitate, toward the distal extremity of the radius, between the tendon of extensor digitorum medially (on the ulnar side) and, laterally (on the radial side), a hypothetical line extending distally from the dorsal tubercle of the radius. When the subject's wrist is flexed, the lunate can be detected between the head of the capitate and the posterior border of the radius (toward the ulnar side).

Note:
- If you slide the pad of your finger too far laterally (to the radial side), you will contact the dorsal surface of the scaphoid.
- If you do not slide the pad of your finger far enough toward the radius, you will contact the head of the capitate.

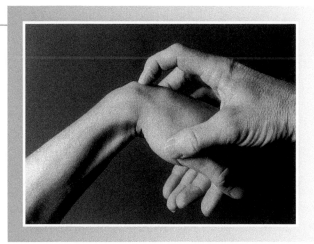

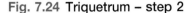

Fig. 7.23 Triquetrum – step 1

MA: The subject's hand needs to be in palmar flexion, with his forearm supinated. Here, the practitioner's index finger indicates the ulnar styloid process, the most distal bony prominence on the medial border of the wrist.

> **CLINICAL NOTE**
>
> You need to be aware of a **supernumerary bone** of the wrist, the triangular bone between the ulnar styloid process and triquetrum. Remember its existence and location when palpating, in order not to mistake it for traumatic detachment of the ulnar styloid process.
>
> **Note:** The shape, size, and location of this sesamoid bone are all variable, and it may be doubled.

Fig. 7.24 Triquetrum – step 2

MA: The position of the subject's forearm and hand is the same as that described for Figure 7.23. Here, the practitioner's index finger indicates the triquetrum, which is the first bony prominence you encounter on the medial border of the wrist, distal to the ulnar styloid process.

> **CLINICAL NOTE**
>
> The **triquetrum** can be a site of fracture if the individual falls onto the dorso-ulnar surface of the wrist. Pain here is cause for suspicion. Palpation of the bone involving pressure produces exquisite pain.

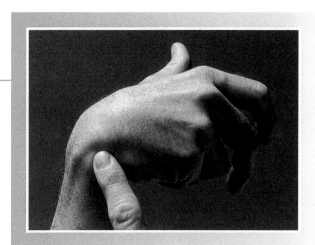

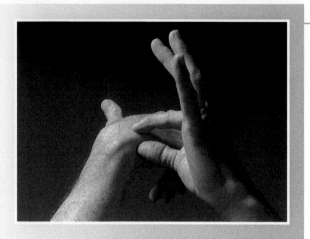

Fig. 7.25 Triquetrum, global approach

MA: Once you have located the bony structures described in Figures 7.23 and 7.24, take an overall hold of the triquetrum. The practitioner's thumb is on the medial (ulnar) surface of the triquetrum and his index finger on the dorsal surface.

> **CLINICAL NOTE**
>
> The triquetrum can also be involved in **transverse synostosis** (fusion of two bones of the same row; in this case the triquetrum and lunate). Palpation to mobilize it will detect if this is the case.

Fig. 7.26 Pisiform

MA: In the adjacent figure, the practitioner's index finger indicates the tendon of flexor carpi ulnaris, which is important for locating the pisiform because the tendon is inserted into the anterior surface of the bone. An additional guide to location is the fact that the pisiform is situated at the base of the hypothenar eminence.

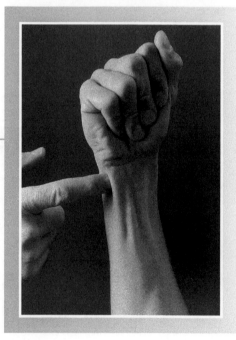

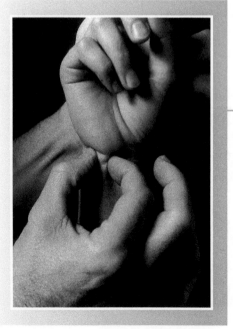

Fig. 7.27 Pisiform

MA: The posterior surface of the pisiform articulates with the triquetrum. Its anterior surface can be felt as a prominence under the skin. In the adjacent figure, the practitioner has taken hold of the pisiform between thumb and index finger.

Note: The subject's wrist should be allowed to fall naturally into a position of palmar flexion. This relaxes the tendon of the flexor carpi ulnaris, and makes the pisiform easier to mobilize and examine.

> **CLINICAL NOTE**
>
> **Fracture of the pisiform** should be considered following a direct fall onto the hypothenar eminence, with wrist extended. (Fracture of the hamate should also be considered.) Palpation causes exquisite pain in response to pressure in that case. Another possibility is dislocation of this bone; this is clearly detected on palpation.

THE CARPAL BONES OF THE DISTAL ROW

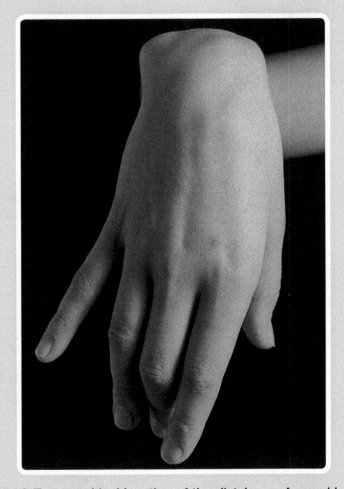

Fig. 7.28 Topographical location of the distal row of carpal bones

The notable structures that can be detected by palpation are:
- Trapezium (Figs. 7.29–7.32)
- Tubercle of the trapezium (Figs. 7.33–7.36)
- Trapezoid (Figs. 7.37–7.39)
- Capitate (Figs. 7.40–7.47)
- Hamate (Figs. 7.48 and 7.49)
- Hook of the hamate (Figs. 7.50–7.52).

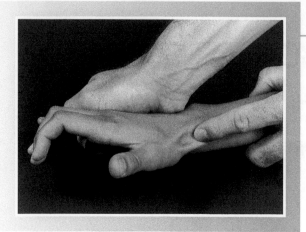

Fig. 7.29 Trapezium – step 1: Locating the anatomic snuffbox

MA: Begin by locating the anatomic snuffbox. Place your thumb into the snuffbox (position indicated here by the practitioner's index finger), the floor of which is formed by the scaphoid.

Fig. 7.30 Trapezium – step 2

MA: Following the step shown in Figure 7.29, shift your thumb distally until you contact the base of the first metacarpal. You will detect the trapezium beneath your thumb.

CLINICAL NOTE

Osteoarthritis between the trapezium and the base of the first metacarpal (osteoarthritis of the base of the thumb, sometimes called trapeziometacarpal or basal thumb arthritis or root arthrosis) is quite common. Palpation finds deformation of the trapezium and radial subluxation of the first metacarpal, and increased distance between the bases of the first and second metacarpals.

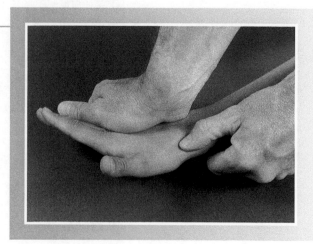

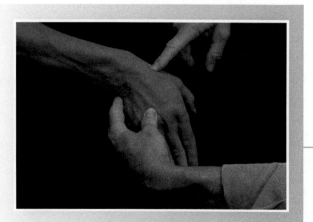

Fig. 7.31 Lateral surface of the trapezium, another view

MA: In this figure, the practitioner has inclined the subject's hand in the ulnar direction with one hand. The index finger of his other hand indicates the lateral surface of the trapezium, at the distal end of the anatomic snuffbox and close to the base of the first metacarpal.

Fig. 7.32 Trapezium, global approach

MA: In the adjacent figure, the practitioner has taken hold of the trapezium as a whole, between his thumb and index finger. Position your contact just proximal to the base of the first metacarpal. Ask the subject to mobilize the first metacarpal; this will help confirm that you have made contact with the trapezium, as it remains immobile when the metacarpal is moved.

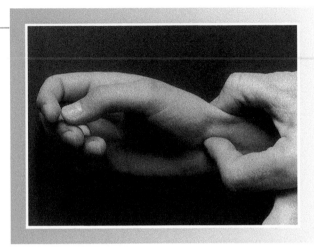

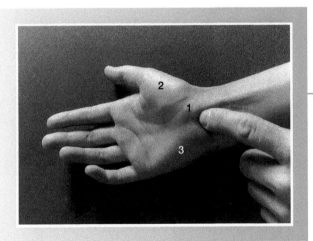

Fig. 7.33 Tubercle of the trapezium, step 1

MA: Begin by locating the scaphoid (1), and the space between the thenar (2) and hypothenar (3) eminences at the fold created by the flexion of the wrist. The practitioner's index finger indicates the convexity on the anterior surface of the wrist created by the scaphoid.

Fig. 7.34 Tubercle of the trapezium, step 2

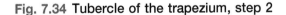

MA: Place the interphalangeal joint of your thumb between the thenar and hypothenar eminences on the anterior part of the subject's wrist, in contact with the scaphoid, and with your thumb in line with the column of the subject's thumb, as shown.

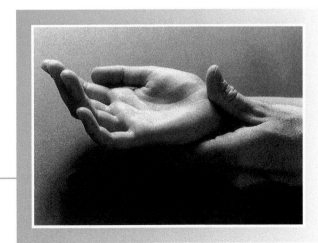

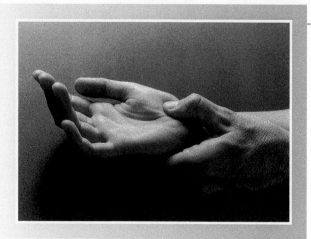

Fig. 7.35 Tubercle of the trapezium, step 3

Once you have completed steps 1 and 2 (Figs. 7.33 and 7.34), set down your thumb in line with the column of the subject's thumb, just proximal to the base of the first metacarpal. The tubercle of the trapezium is directly beneath the pad of your thumb.

Fig. 7.36 Tubercle of the trapezium, distal approach – another view

MA: Palpate this ridge or tubercle directly between the palmar surface of the scaphoid (which is shaped like a rounded tubercle) and the base of the first metacarpal. It feels like a ridge beneath your fingers. Ask the subject to circumduct the first metacarpal; this will help you make sure that you have located the correct structure. (You can either ask the subject to do this, or circumduct it passively, yourself.) Maintain your contact in the same position as you do so.

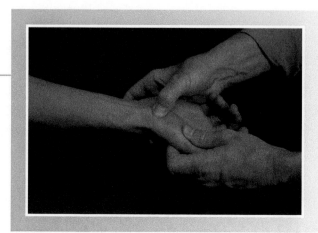

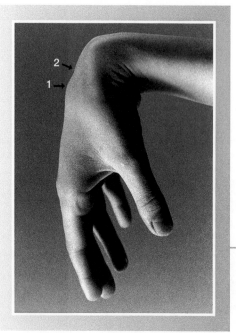

Fig. 7.37 Trapezoid, topographical location

MA: The adjacent figure shows the location of the base of the second metacarpal (1) and of the trapezoid (2) on the back of the hand.

Note: These two structures on the dorsal surface of the hand should not be confused. The bony prominence is the base of the second metacarpal; the dorsal surface of the trapezoid is recessed.

Fig. 7.38 Trapezoid, step 1

MA: Place your index finger as shown in the adjacent figure – flat against the base of the second metacarpal, the bony prominence indicated above (Fig. 7.37).

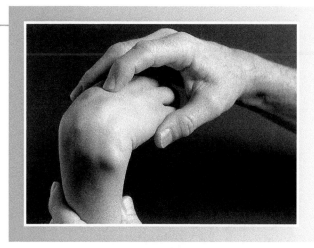

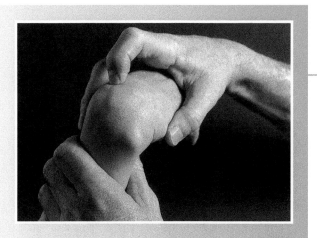

Fig. 7.39 Trapezoid, step 2

MA: From the position shown in Figure 7.38, slide your index finger into the depression that lies proximal to it, slipping your contact in between the tendons of extensor carpi radialis longus and extensor carpi radialis brevis.

Note: Contact with the dorsal surface of the trapezoid is not always easy to achieve, because the bone is set back considerably relative to the base of the second metacarpal.

Fig. 7.40 Capitate, form and location – dorsal view

MA: This is the largest of the bones of the wrist, and its main axis lies in line with that of the hand. It consists of:

- an enlarged, rounded superior part or head (1);
- an inferior part or body (2);
- a transitional region between them, the neck.

Note: Proximally, the capitate articulates with the scaphoid and the lunate, fitting in against these two bones. Distally, it lies opposite the articular surfaces of the second, third, and fourth metacarpals. Its lateral (radial) surface articulates with the scaphoid proximally and with the trapezoid distally. Its medial (ulnar) surface articulates with the hamate.

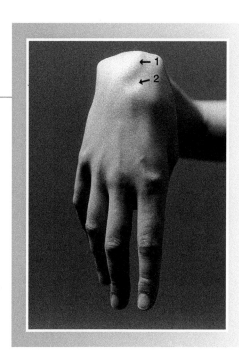

> **CLINICAL NOTE**
>
> The capitate can also be involved in **transverse synostosis** (fusion of two bones of the same row: proximal or distal). In this case, fusion would be between the capitate and the hamate. Palpation to mobilize it will detect if this is so.

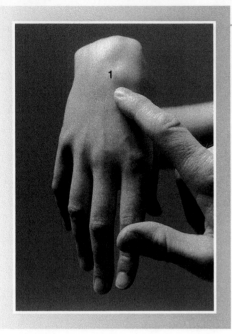

Fig. 7.41 Capitate, dorsal view – step 1

MA: The first step is to place a contact at the base of the third metacarpal (1). The capitate is situated proximally in line with this bone.

Fig. 7.42 Capitate, dorsal view – step 2

MA: Following the step shown in Figure 7.41, slide your index finger along from the base of the third metacarpal in the proximal direction. You will find a depression (1) just beyond it, belonging to the body of the capitate. The rounded feature (2) beyond that, rising above the depression, is the head of the capitate.

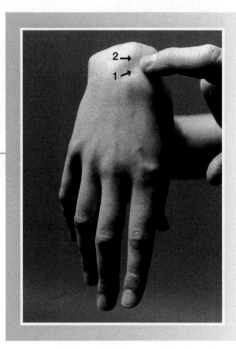

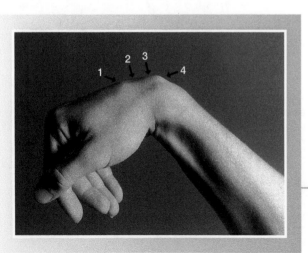

Fig. 7.43 Display of the bony landmarks needed when palpating the capitate, lateral view

MA: In this profile view, the base of the third metacarpal (1), the depression in the capitate (2), the head of the capitate (3), and the lunate (4) can all be clearly distinguished. The lunate becomes accessible if you flex the subject's wrist.

Fig. 7.44 The depression on the dorsal surface of the capitate, lateral view

MA: Place your index finger in the depression that lies in line with the base of the third metacarpal, on the radial side of the tendon of the extensor digitorum.

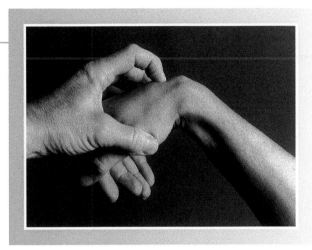

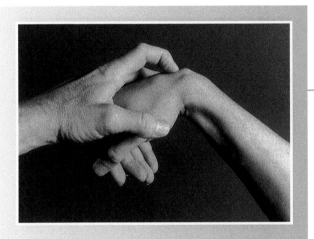

Fig. 7.45 Head of the capitate, lateral aspect

MA: Once you have located the depression as described above (Fig. 7.44), shift your index finger proximally (but without sliding it over the skin) until you contact a convex structure. This is the head of the capitate.

Note: Do not confuse this structure with the lunate.

Fig. 7.46 The capitate and lunate

MA: The adjacent figure shows a global contact, between the practitioner's index fingers. The practitioner's two index fingers are in contact with the head of the capitate and the more proximally situated lunate. Do not confuse the capitate and the lunate.

> **CLINICAL NOTE**
> One of the most commonly found fusions of the carpal bones involves the **triquetrum** and the **lunate.**

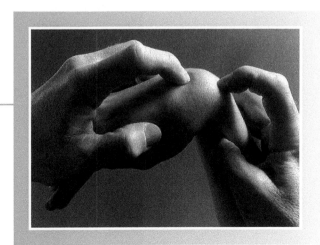

233

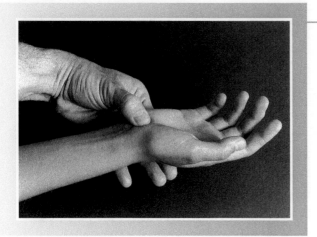

Fig. 7.47 Capitate, global approach

MA: Begin by locating the pisiform. Then place the interphalangeal joint of your thumb on the pisiform, with your thumb pointing transversely, following the direction of the first palmar fold. Your index finger should rest on the back of the subject's hand, in the depression of the capitate, which is in line with the base of the third metacarpal. Now flex the interphalangeal joint of your thumb. This contact provides an overall approach to the capitate.

Fig. 7.48 Hamate, medial approach (i.e., from the ulnar side)

MA: Begin by locating the ulnar styloid process (1) (see also Fig. 7.4) and triquetrum (2). Next, position your index finger on the medial surface of the hamate, between the base of the fifth metacarpal (3) and the triquetrum (2).

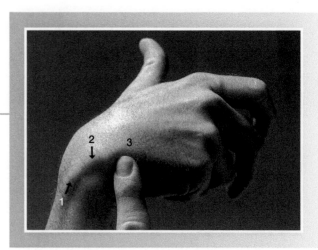

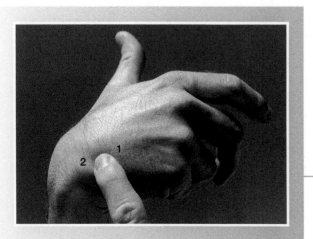

Fig. 7.49 Hamate, dorsal approach

MA: Begin with the contact described in Figure 7.48; then slide your index finger on to the dorsal surface of the hamate, between the bases of the fourth and fifth metacarpals (1) and the dorsal surface of the triquetrum (2).

Fig. 7.50 Hook of the hamate, step 1

MA: Begin by locating the pisiform (indicated here by the practitioner's index finger), which lies at the base of the hypothenar eminence (1), at the ulnar extremity of the first anterior palmar fold (2).

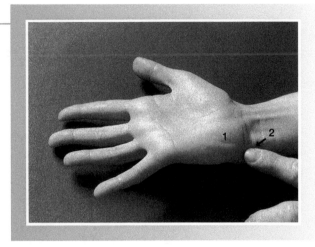

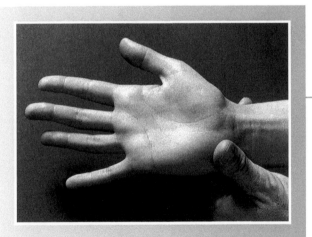

Fig. 7.51 Hook of the hamate, step 2

MA: Once you have located the pisiform, place the interphalangeal joint of your thumb on it.

Note: As shown here, your thumb should point toward the subject's index finger or the first commissure.

Fig. 7.52 The hook of the hamate, step 3

MA: From the thumb position described above (Fig. 7.51), flex the distal phalanx of your thumb on the proximal one, directing the movement toward the subject's index finger or the first commissure. You will make contact with a fullness. This is the hook of the hamate.

> **CLINICAL NOTE**
>
> Fracture affecting this structure can pass unnoticed. It can be diagnosed by palpation: pressure produces exquisite pain, and mobilization, which should be extremely gentle, detects abnormal movement at the **hook of the hamate.** The cause is often sports (e.g., tennis) or a fall onto the hypothenar eminence.
>
> Take care: damage to the ulnar nerve may occur in association with this fracture.

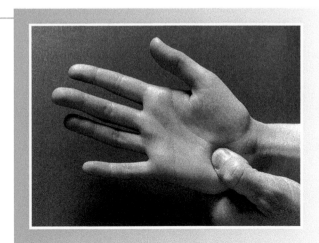

THE METACARPUS AND PHALANGES

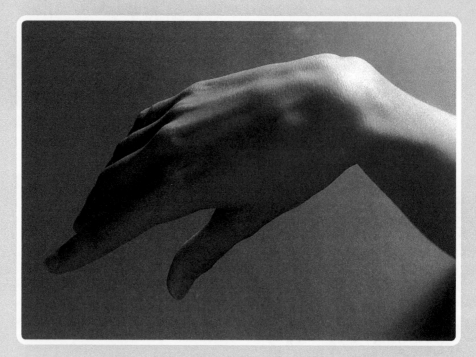

Fig. 7.53 The metacarpals and phalanges: overall radial view

The notable structures that can be detected by palpation are:

- Heads of metacarpals II–V (Figs. 7.54 and 7.55)
- First metacarpal: base (Fig. 7.56), shaft or body (Fig. 7.57), and head (Fig. 7.58)
- Sesamoid bones of the metacarpophalangeal joint (Fig. 7.59)
- Second metacarpal (Fig. 7.60)
- Third metacarpal (Fig. 7.61)
- Fourth metacarpal (Fig. 7.62)
- Fifth metacarpal (Fig. 7.63)
- Proximal phalanx of the thumb (Fig. 7.64)
- Distal phalanx of the thumb (Fig. 7.65).

Fig. 7.54 Heads of metacarpals II–V, dorsal view

MA: The metacarpus is made up of five bones which articulate proximally with the carpal bones and distally with the proximal phalanges of the fingers. The adjacent figure shows how flexing the fingers at the metacarpophalangeal joints causes the heads of the metacarpals (1) to become prominent.

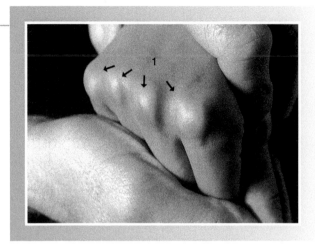

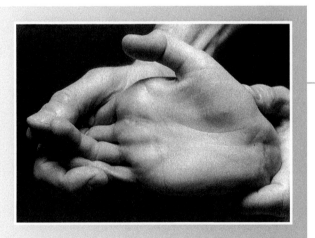

Fig. 7.55 Heads of metacarpals II–V, palmar view

MA: As shown in the adjacent figure, extension of the fingers at the metacarpophalangeal joints causes the palmar part of the heads of the metacarpals to become prominent.

Note: Sesamoid bones can occur here: at the second, third and fourth metacarpophalageal joints, one; at the fifth, one or two. The commonest locations are at the second and fifth.

Fig. 7.56 First metacarpal: the base

MA: The base of the first metacarpal is shaped like a saddle, and articulates only with the trapezium (not with the second metacarpal). Location of the first metacarpal is therefore not only important in its own right, but also when looking for the trapezium.

CLINICAL NOTE

Osteoarthritis of the base of the thumb is the most common type of arthritis affecting the hand. Palpation finds a degree of radial dislocation of the base of the first metacarpal. There is deformation of the trapezium and increased distance between the first and second metacarpals.

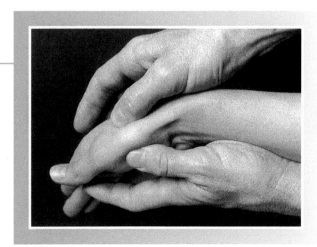

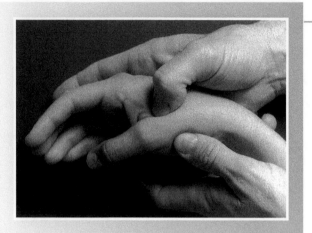

Fig. 7.57 First metacarpal: the shaft

MA: This is the shortest and thickest of the metacarpals. Between the head and base of this bone lies the shaft or body.

Fig. 7.58 First metacarpal: the head (dorsal view) and metacarpophalangeal joint

MA: This articulates with the base of the proximal phalanx. Ask the subject to flex her metacarpophalangeal joint to display the head.

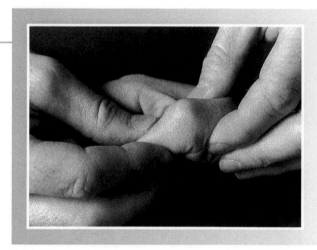

CLINICAL NOTE

Sprain of the metacarpophalangeal joint is fairly frequent. A fall onto the hand that forces the thumb into abduction causes sprain and may rupture the ulnar collateral ligament of the wrist. It is then difficult to maintain stability of the joint or abduct the thumb. Palpation of the ulnar collateral ligament produces a point of extreme pain over a swollen joint.

In addition to sprain, there can be dislocation of the metacarpophalangeal joint, either in the dorsal or the palmar direction.

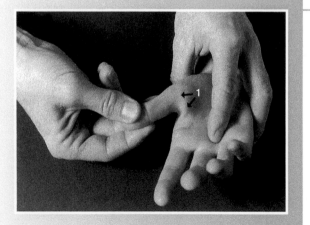

Fig. 7.59 The sesamoid bones of the metacarpophalangeal joint

MA: Anteriorly, the head of the first metacarpal has two horns separated by a groove. The sesamoids are bony nodules that overlie these horns. The sesamoid bones (1) at this joint are always two in number (lateral and medial).

Note: The sesamoid bones may be intratendinous (within the thickness of the tendon) or periarticular (close to the joints, on the palmar side). They appear at the age of 11 years in girls and 13 years in boys. The medial sesamoid appears first, then the lateral one.

CLINICAL NOTE

Increased size of the sesamoids occurs as one of the signs of acromegaly.

Fig. 7.60 Second metacarpal

MA: This is the longest of the metacarpals. Locating the base of this metacarpal is important when palpating the trapezoid. In the adjacent figure, the practitioner's contact spans the second metacarpal; his thumb is at the base and his index finger is at the head of the bone.

Note: The base of this bone articulates with the trapezoid (which is received by the center), with the trapezium on the radial side and with the capitate on the ulnar side.

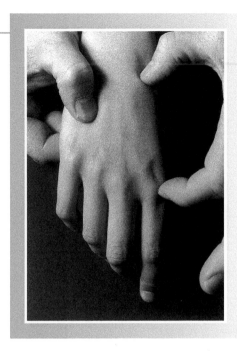

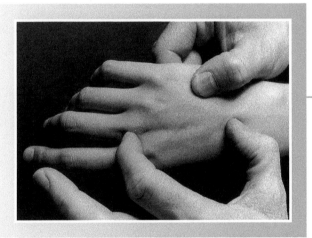

Fig. 7.61 Third metacarpal

MA: The type of contact used for this bone is the same as that described above (Fig. 7.60). The base of this metacarpal, at the position of the practitioner's thumb in the contact shown here, articulates with the capitate.

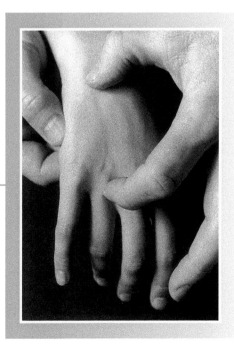

Fig. 7.62 Fourth metacarpal

MA: The type of contact used for this bone is the same as that described for Figure 7.60. The base of this metacarpal articulates with the capitate and with the hamate.

CLINICAL NOTE

Shortness of the metacarpal bone can affect any of the metacarpals, but the fourth metacarpal sign, known as Archibald's sign (**brachymetacarpia of the fourth metacarpal**) is the most frequent. This may be congenital (as in Turner's syndrome) or acquired; the two should be distinguished.

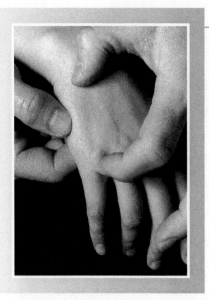

Fig. 7.63 Fifth metacarpal

MA: This is the shortest of the metacarpals. The thumb and index finger contact used for this bone is the same as that described for Figure 7.60. The base of this metacarpal is therefore at the position of the practitioner's thumb in the contact shown here. It articulates with the hamate (see Figs. 7.48–7.52). The practitioner's index finger is at the head of the fifth metacarpal.

Fig. 7.64 The proximal phalanx of the thumb

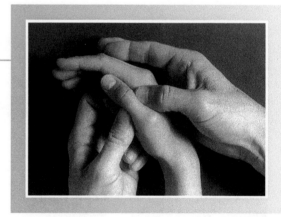

MA: The base of this phalanx has a glenoid cavity articulating with the head of the first metacarpal. The head has a trochlea which occupies the palmar and inferior surfaces and articulates with the base of the distal phalanx.

Note: The head of the proximal phalanx of the other fingers articulates with the base of the middle phalanx.

> **CLINICAL NOTE**
> **Shortness of the proximal phalanx** (brachybasophalangia) is extremely rare, but can affect any finger. The middle phalanges (brachymesophalangia) are more frequently affected.

Fig. 7.65 The distal phalanx of the thumb

The thumb has only two phalanges, while the other fingers have three.

Note: The middle phalanx of the other fingers is shorter and thinner than the proximal one; the shape of each is identical. The distal phalanx is the smallest of the three.

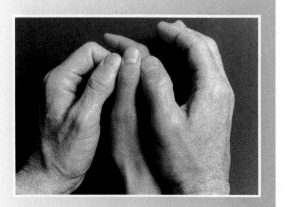

> **CLINICAL NOTE**
> 1. Of the malformations of the distal phalanges (brachytelephalangia), **shortness of the distal phalanx of the thumb** is the most frequently found. This tends to run in families, with females (e.g., mother/daughter) more often affected. Within a family, if only one side is affected, this is always the same side.
> 2. The proximal and distal interphalangeal joints can be affected by **sprains, dislocations** (usually dorsal), and **articular fractures.** (They are more often found at the proximal joint.) Care is needed when palpating, whether looking for tenderness to pressure or mobilizing to look for abnormal frontal or lateral movement. The hand should either be fully extended or slightly flexed when examining these movements in order to test all the ligaments.

MYOLOGY

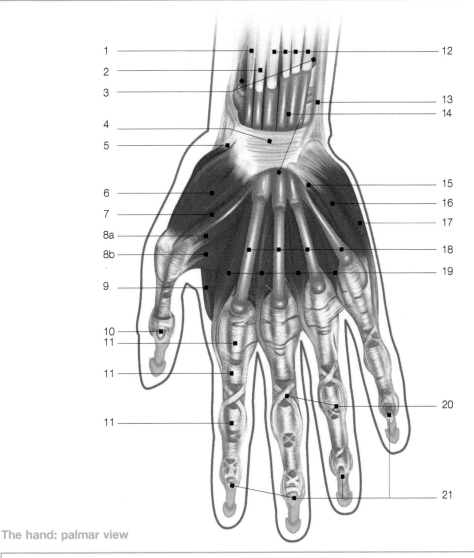

1
2
3
4
5
6
7
8a
8b
9
10
11
11
11
12
13
14
15
16
17
18
19
20
21

The hand: palmar view

1. Flexor carpi radialis
2. Flexor pollicis longus
3. Pronator quadratus
4. Flexor retinaculum (transverse carpal ligament)
5. Opponens pollicis
6. Abductor pollicis brevis
7. Flexor pollicis brevis, superficial head
8a. Adductor pollicis, oblique head
8b. Adductor pollicis, transverse head
9. First dorsal interosseus
10. Flexor pollicis longus

11. Annular ligaments
12. Flexor digitorum superficialis
13. Flexor carpi ulnaris
14. Common flexor sheath
15. Opponens digiti minimi
16. Flexor digiti minimi brevis
17. Abductor digiti minimi
18. Flexor digitorum superficialis
19. Lumbricals
20. Oblique ligaments
21. Flexor digitorum profundus

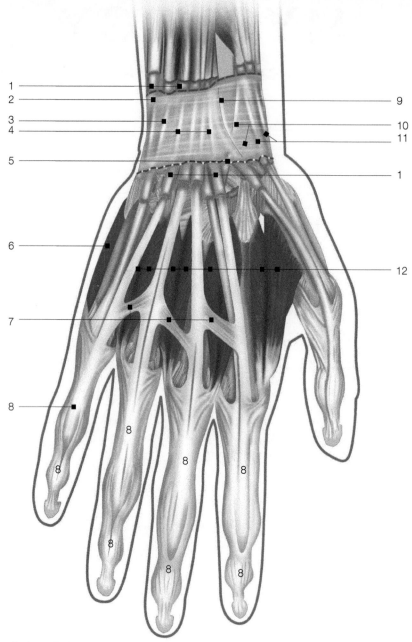

The hand: dorsal view

1. Dorsal carpal tendon sheaths
2. Sixth tendon compartment: extensor carpi ulnaris
3. Fifth tendon compartment: extensor digiti minimi
4. Fourth tendon compartment: extensor digitorum; extensor indicis
5. Extensor retinaculum (*dotted line*)
6. Abductor digiti minimi

7. Intertendinous connections
8. Dorsal aponeurosis
9. Third tendon compartment: extensor pollicis longus
10. Second tendon compartment: extensor carpi radialis longus and brevis
11. First tendon compartment: abductor pollicis longus; extensor pollicis brevis
12. Dorsal interossei

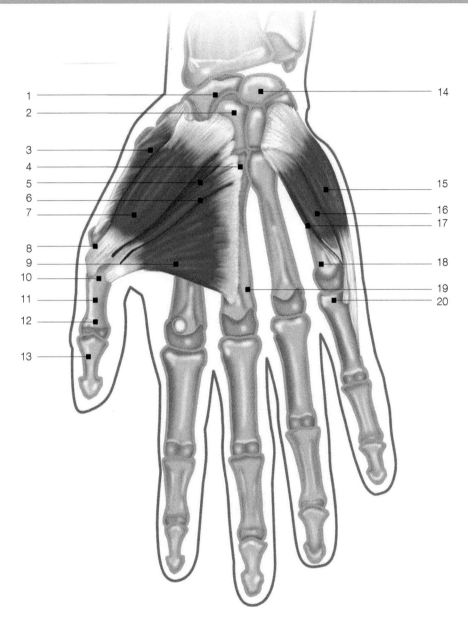

The hand: muscles of the thenar and hypothenar eminences

1. Scaphoid
2. Capitate
3. Opponens pollicis
4. Base of third metacarpal
5. Flexor pollicis brevis, superficial head
6. Adductor pollicis, oblique head
7. Abductor pollicis brevis
8. Head of first metacarpal
9. Adductor pollicis, transverse head
10. Proximal phalanx of thumb, base
11. Proximal phalanx of thumb, shaft
12. Proximal phalanx of thumb, head
13. Distal phalanx of thumb
14. Lunate
15. Abductor digiti minimi
16. Flexor digiti minimi brevis
17. Opponens digiti minimi
18. Fifth metacarpal
19. Third metacarpal
20. Proximal phalanx of little finger, base

THE TENDONS OF THE ANTERIOR PART OF THE WRIST

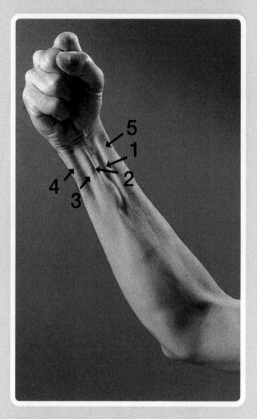

Fig. 7.66 Overall presentation of the tendons on the anterior surface of the wrist

1. Tendon of flexor carpi radialis
2. Tendon of palmaris longus
3. Flexor digitorum superficialis and tendon to the fourth finger
4. Tendon of flexor carpi ulnaris
5. Location of flexor pollicis tendon

The notable structures that can be detected by palpation are:
- Tendon of flexor pollicis longus (Fig. 7.67)
- Tendon of flexor carpi radialis (Fig. 7.68)
- Tendon of palmaris longus (Fig. 7.69)
- Flexor digitorum superficialis:
  - Tendon to the fourth finger (Fig. 7.70)
  - Tendon to the third finger (Fig. 7.71)
  - Tendon to the fifth finger (Fig. 7.72)
  - Tendon to the index finger (Fig. 7.73)
- Tendon of flexor carpi ulnaris (Fig. 7.74).

INNERVATIONS

- Flexor carpi radialis: median nerve (C6–C7–C8)
- Flexor pollicis longus: median nerve (C8–T1)
- Palmaris longus: median nerve (C6–C7–C8)
- Flexor carpi ulnaris: ulnar nerve (C7–C8–T1)
- Flexor digitorum superficialis: median nerve (C7–C8–T1)

Fig. 7.67 Tendon of flexor pollicis longus

MA: Place the pads of one or two fingers just lateral to the tendon of flexor carpi radialis (1). Ask the subject to flex the distal phalanx of her thumb briefly and repeatedly. You will sense the tendon of this muscle beneath your contact.

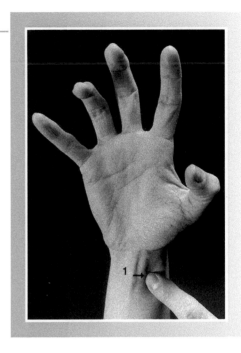

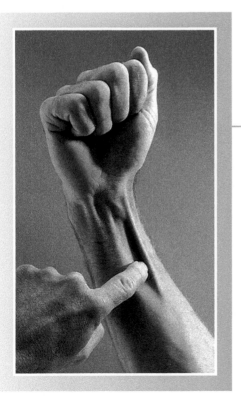

Fig. 7.68 Tendon of flexor carpi radialis

MA: Ask the subject to clench his fist. The tendon will appear on the radial side of the anterior surface of the wrist (indicated here by the practitioner's index finger), just lateral to the tendon of palmaris longus. If it is difficult to display this tendon, ask the subject to flex and abduct his wrist (incline it to the radial side), at the same time slightly pronating his forearm.

CLINICAL NOTE

In patients with **tendinopathy,** palpation of the tendon is painful. Flexion combined with inclination of the wrist to the radial side against resistance is also painful, as is stretching the tendon by extending the wrist and inclining it to the ulnar side.

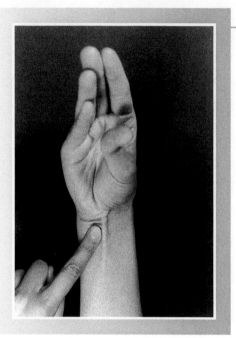

Fig. 7.69 Tendon of palmaris longus

MA: This muscle is inconstant. Ask the subject to oppose her thumb and fifth finger. This will cause the tendon to appear in the middle of the anterior surface of the wrist, between the tendon of flexor carpi radialis, which lies laterally to it, and that of flexor digitorum superficialis medially.

> **CLINICAL NOTE**
>
> In patients with **tendinopathy,** palpation of the tendon is painful. Contraction by flexing the wrist against resistance is also painful, as is stretching the tendon by extending the wrist.

Fig. 7.70 Flexor digitorum superficialis, tendon to the fourth finger

MA: Clenching the fist causes this tendon (1) to become visible, medially to that of palmaris longus (2) (Fig. 7.69). Should this not happen, ask the subject to oppose her thumb and fourth finger, if necessary flexing her wrist at the same time, to enable you to locate the tendon.

Note: In exceptional cases the tendon of flexor digitorum superficialis going to the third finger (3) is also directly visible, as here.

> **CLINICAL NOTE**
>
> **Rupture of the flexor digitorum profundus tendon at its insertion:**
>
> This rupture is seen in sports such as judo. The tendon going to the fourth finger is the one usually affected, although the rupture can occur elsewhere.
>
> - Testing of this muscle at (3) (flexion of the distal phalanx on the middle one) is impossible.
>
> - Testing of flexor digitorum superficialis at (3) (flexion of the middle phalanx on the proximal one) is possible.

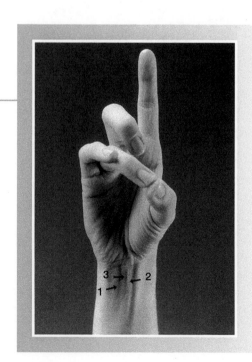

Fig. 7.71 Flexor digitorum superficialis, tendon to the third finger

MA: This tendon (1) can be palpated behind the tendon of palmaris longus (2) and lateral to the tendon of flexor digitorum superficialis going to the fourth finger (3) (Fig. 7.70). This can be done more easily if you ask the subject to oppose her thumb and middle finger, together with slight flexion of the wrist.

Note: Take care not to damage the median nerve, which is very close by.

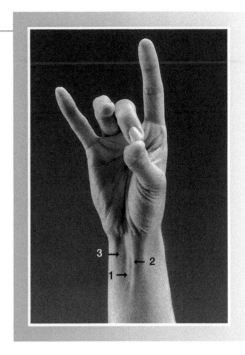

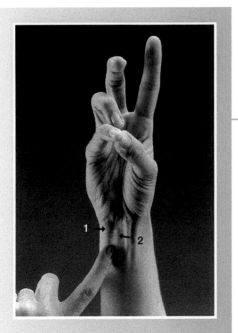

Fig. 7.72 Flexor digitorum superficialis, tendon to the fifth finger

MA: This tendon is situated in the groove indicated here by the practitioner's index finger, between the tendon of flexor carpi ulnaris medially (1) and the tendon of flexor digitorum superficialis going to the fourth finger (2) laterally and anteriorly to it (see also Fig. 7.70). It becomes easier to detect if you ask the subject to oppose her thumb and fifth finger, together with slight flexion of the wrist.

CLINICAL NOTE

Trigger finger

Palpation finds a nodule on the tendon of flexor digitorum superficialis, at the metacarpophalangeal joint. When, from being initially flexed, the finger is extended, the nodule causes it to rebound in a trigger motion. This may cause discomfort or pain. The rebound is caused by the nodule entering the flexor tendon sheath.

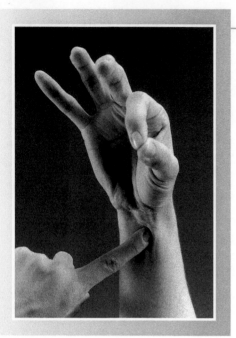

Fig. 7.73 Flexor digitorum superficialis, tendon to the index finger

MA: The tendon going to the index finger is the hardest to detect. It should be apparent if you push aside palmaris longus laterally, as shown here, or if you seek it between palmaris longus and the tendon of flexor carpi radialis. It becomes easier to detect if you ask the subject to oppose her thumb and index finger, together with slight flexion of the wrist.

Note: Take care not to damage the median nerve (see also Fig. 7.94), which is very close by.

> **CLINICAL NOTE**
>
> In patients with **tendinopathy,** palpation of the affected tendon is painful along some part of its route, so you should also palpate the anterior part of the forearm. One or all of the flexor digitorum superficialis tendons may be affected. (There is one tendon going to each of fingers II to V.) Flexing the fingers, combined with flexion of the wrist against resistance, is also painful, as is stretching by extending the wrist and then the fingers.

Fig. 7.74 Tendon of flexor carpi ulnaris

MA: Ask the subject to flex his wrist slightly, inclining it to the ulnar side. The tendon of flexor carpi ulnaris will appear on the part of the anterior surface of the subject's wrist farthest to the medial (ulnar) side.

> **CLINICAL NOTE**
>
> Pain in this tendon, produced by palpation, is the key sign of **tendinopathy** here. Flexing the wrist while inclining it to the ulnar side, against resistance, also produces pain. The diagnosis can be confirmed by stretching the tendon, by extending the wrist and inclining it to the radial side.

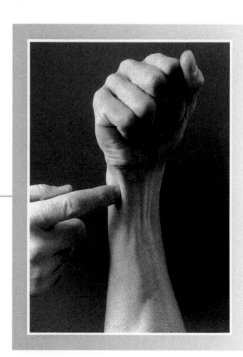

THE TENDONS OF THE LATERAL PART OF THE WRIST

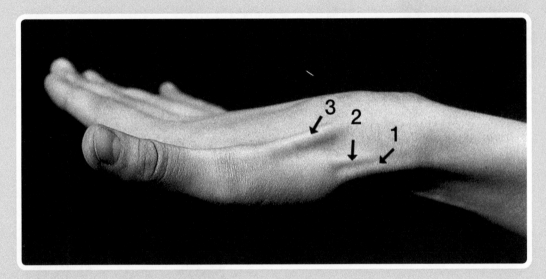

Fig. 7.75 Lateral view of the wrist
1. Tendon of abductor pollicis longus
2. Tendon of extensor pollicis brevis
3. Tendon of extensor pollicis longus

The notable structures that can be detected by palpation are:
- Tendon of abductor pollicis longus (Fig. 7.76)
- Tendon of extensor pollicis brevis (Fig. 7.77)
- Tendon of extensor pollicis longus (Fig. 7.78).

INNERVATIONS

- Abductor pollicis longus: radial nerve (C6–C7–C8)
- Extensor pollicis brevis: radial nerve (C6–C7–C8)
- Extensor pollicis longus: radial nerve (C6–C7–C8)

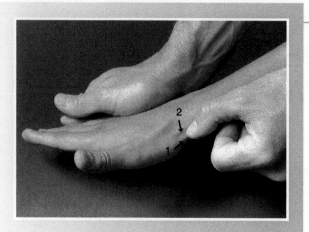

Fig. 7.76 Tendon of abductor pollicis longus

MA: This tendon can be displayed on some subjects as follows. Her wrist should be in a neutral position. As the thumb is drawn away from the plane of the rest of her hand, the tendon of abductor pollicis longus (1) becomes apparent, by the anterior (palmar) part of the tendon of extensor pollicis brevis (2) (Fig. 7.77). Ask the subject to incline her hand to the radial side while you resist this action. This will help you display the tendon.

> **CLINICAL NOTE**
>
> **De Quervain's tenosynovitis**
>
> This is a stenosing type of tenosynovitis, affecting the tendons of abductor pollicis longus and extensor pollicis brevis where they pass through the first osteofibrous tunnel of the wrist, at a point level with the radial styloid process. Palpation evokes exquisite pain on application of pressure at the proximal part of the anatomic snuffbox. Sometimes there is also swelling here.

Fig. 7.77 Tendon of extensor pollicis brevis

MA: The subject's wrist should be in a neutral position. Ask her to draw her thumb away from the plane of the rest of her hand. This usually causes the tendon to appear on the radial part of the wrist, just behind the tendon of abductor pollicis longus.

> **CLINICAL NOTE**
>
> **De Quervain's tenosynovitis** also affects the tendon of this muscle. (See Clinical Note to Fig. 7.76.)

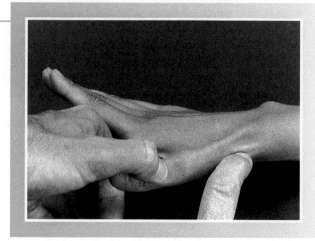

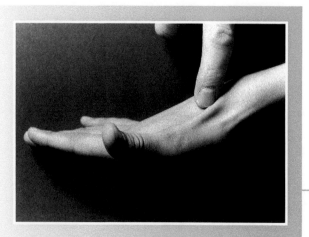

Fig. 7.78 Tendon of extensor pollicis longus

MA: The subject's wrist should be in a neutral position. Ask her to draw her thumb backward from the plane of the rest of her hand. The tendon will appear on the posterolateral part of the wrist.

THE TENDONS OF THE POSTERIOR PART OF THE WRIST

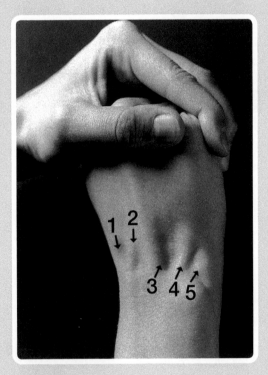

Fig. 7.79 Posterior view of the wrist

1. Tendon of extensor carpi radialis longus
2. Tendon of extensor carpi radialis brevis
3. Tendon of extensor digitorum
4. Tendon of extensor digiti minimi
5. Tendon of extensor carpi ulnaris

The notable structures that can be detected by palpation are:

- Tendon of extensor carpi radialis longus (Fig. 7.80)
- Tendon of extensor carpi radialis brevis (Fig. 7.81)
- Tendon of extensor digitorum (Fig. 7.82)
- Tendon of extensor digiti minimi (Fig. 7.83)
- Tendon of extensor carpi ulnaris (Fig. 7.84).

Note: The tendon of extensor indicis is treated in Chapter 6.

INNERVATIONS

- Extensor carpi radialis longus: radial nerve (C5–C6–C7)
- Extensor carpi radialis brevis: radial nerve (C5–C6–C7)
- Extensor digitorum: radial nerve (C6–C7–C8)
- Extensor digiti minimi: radial nerve (C6–C7–C8)
- Extensor carpi ulnaris: radial nerve (C6–C7–C8)

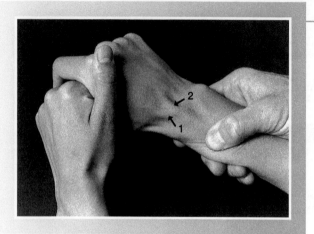

Fig. 7.80 Tendon of extensor carpi radialis longus

MA: This tendon (1) can sometimes be made to appear if the subject simply clenches her wrist tightly. The tendon of extensor pollicis longus (see Fig. 7.78) overlies it. Place the subject's thumb on the palm of her hand; this will separate out the tendon you are looking for. Resist as shown here, as she tries to extend her wrist and incline it to the radial side.

Note: The tendon of extensor carpi radialis brevis (2) lies medially to (on the ulnar side of) this tendon.

CLINICAL NOTE

This tendon can be the site of **tendinopathy** affecting the wrist. Palpation here or at the insertion of the tendon is painful. Pain also results on extension of the wrist, inclining it in the radial direction against resistance, and on stretching the tendon, flexing the wrist and inclining it in the ulnar direction.

Fig. 7.81 Tendon of extensor carpi radialis brevis

MA: This tendon (1) can sometimes be made to appear if the subject simply clenches her wrist tightly. It lies laterally to the tendons of extensor digitorum (2) (Fig. 7.82) and medially to the tendon of extensor carpi radialis longus (Fig. 7.80).

CLINICAL NOTE

This tendon can be the site of **tendinopathy.** Palpation revives the pain. Pain also results on extension of the wrist against resistance, as does stretching the tendon by flexing the wrist.

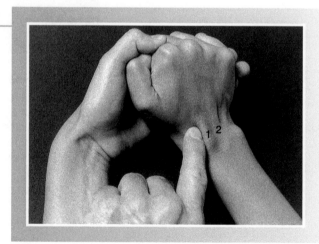

Fig. 7.82 Tendon of extensor digitorum

MA: Ask the subject to extend her wrist and metacarpophalangeal joints against resistance; her proximal and distal interphalangeal joints should remain flexed. This action is usually enough to make the tendon of extensor digitorum prominent on the posterior, middle surface of the wrist.

Note: This tendon groups together the tendons going to the four individual fingers, as well as the tendon of extensor indicis, which lies medially to (on the ulnar side of) the tendon of extensor digitorum going to the index finger.

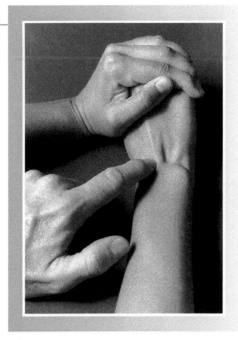

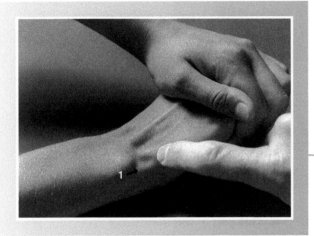

Fig. 7.83 Tendon of extensor digiti minimi

MA: Ask the subject to extend her wrist and little finger while you resist these actions. The practitioner's index finger indicates this tendon, which appears on the posteromedial part of the wrist, laterally to (on the radial side of) the tendon of extensor carpi ulnaris (1) (Fig. 7.84).

Fig. 7.84 Tendon of extensor carpi ulnaris

MA: Ask the subject to incline her wrist to the ulnar side, at the same time extending it. Resist this action. The practitioner's index finger indicates the tendon, which will appear on the posteromedial part of the subject's wrist (on the ulnar side).

> **CLINICAL NOTE**
>
> This tendon can be the site of **tendinopathy:**
>
> - Palpation is painful.
>
> - Extension of the wrist while inclining it to the ulnar side against resistance is also painful.
>
> - Stretching the tendon by flexing the wrist and inclining it to the radial side is similarly painful.

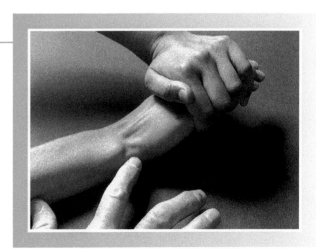

THE INTRINSIC MUSCLES OF THE HAND

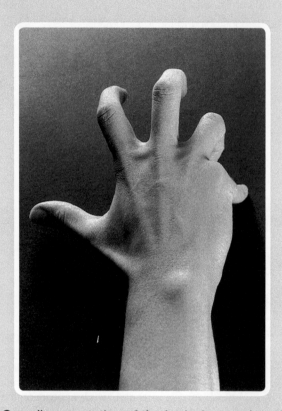

Fig. 7.85 Overall presentation of the intrinsic muscles of the hand

The notable structures that can be detected by palpation are:

- Thenar eminence (Fig. 7.86)
- Hypothenar eminence (Fig. 7.87)
- Flexor tendons of the palm of the hand (Fig. 7.88)
- Lumbricals (Figs. 7.89 and 7.90)
- Lumbricals and dorsal and palmar interossei (Figs. 7.90 and 7.91).

The intrinsic muscles of the hand comprise three groups: the muscles of the thenar eminence, those of the hypothenar eminence, and the muscles of the middle palmar region.

- The muscles of the thenar eminence consist of the following, working from the superficial plane to the deepest:
  - Abductor pollicis brevis
  - Opponens pollicis
  - Flexor pollicis brevis
  - Adductor pollicis.
- The muscles of the hypothenar eminence consist of the following, working from the superficial level to the deepest:
  - Palmaris brevis
  - Abductor digiti minimi

- Flexor digiti minimi brevis
- Opponens digiti minimi.
- The muscles of the middle palmar region belong to three groups arranged one above the other. From palmar to dorsal, these are:
  - Lumbricals
  - Palmar interossei
  - Dorsal interossei.

ACTIONS

The muscles of the thenar eminence:
- Abductor pollicis brevis abducts the thumb.
- Opponens pollicis flexes the thumb and rotates it medially. This action enables the opposition of the thumb to the other fingers.
- Flexor pollicis brevis flexes the proximal phalanx of the thumb and draws it forward and medially, so assisting the opposition of the thumb.
- Adductor pollicis adducts the first metacarpal of the thumb.

The muscles of the hypothenar eminence:
- Palmaris brevis wrinkles the skin on the hypothenar eminence.
- Abductor digiti minimi abducts and flexes the little finger.
- Flexor digiti minimi brevis flexes the proximal phalanx of the little finger on the fifth metacarpal.
- Opponens digiti minimi draws the little finger anteriorly and laterally.

The muscles of the middle palmar region: the actions of the lumbricals and interossei complement each other:
- In the sagittal plane: all flex the proximal phalanx and extend the middle and distal phalanges of the fingers.
- In the frontal plane:
  - The palmar interossei adduct the fingers (draw them together)
  - The dorsal interossei abduct the fingers (draw them apart).

INNERVATIONS

- Abductor pollicis brevis: median nerve (C8–T1)
- Opponens pollicis: median nerve (C8–T1)
- Flexor pollicis brevis: median and ulnar nerves (C8–T1)
- Adductor pollicis: ulnar nerve (C8–T1)
- Palmaris brevis: ulnar nerve (C8–T1)
- Abductor digiti minimi: ulnar nerve (C8–T1)
- Flexor digiti minimi brevis: ulnar nerve (C8–T1)
- Opponens digiti minimi: ulnar nerve (C8–T1)
- Lumbricals: median nerve and ulnar nerve (C8–T1)
- Palmar interossei: ulnar nerve (C8–T1)
- Dorsal interossei: ulnar nerve (C8–T1)

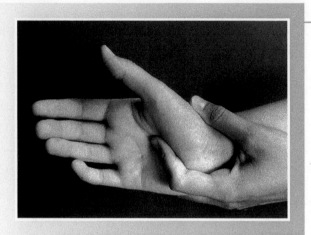

Fig. 7.86 Thenar eminence

MA: This eminence, which the practitioner is shown holding between thumb and index finger, centers on the bony framework provided by the first two metacarpals. It is made up of four muscles, arranged in three layers: the superficial layer, consisting of abductor pollicis brevis; the middle layer, consisting of opponens pollicis and flexor pollicis brevis; and the deep layer, consisting of adductor pollicis.

ATTACHMENTS

Abductor pollicis brevis:

- Origin:
  - Tubercle of the scaphoid
  - The lateral part of flexor retinaculum. (There is sometimes also a fibrous expansion from abductor pollicis longus.)
- Insertion: into the radial border of the base of the proximal phalanx of the thumb and lateral sesamoid.

Opponens pollicis:

- Origin: from the tubercle (ridge) of the trapezium, and from the flexor retinaculum.
- Insertion: into the lateral (radial) border of the first metacarpal.

Flexor pollicis brevis:

- This is composed of two heads: the superficial and deep portions:
  - The superficial portion arises from the tubercle (ridge) of the trapezium and the flexor retinaculum.
  - The deep portion arises from the trapezoid and capitate.
  - The two heads unite, creating a groove that is concave on the medial (ulnar) side and which gives passage to the tendon of flexor pollicis longus. The muscle is inserted on the lateral (radial) part of the base of the proximal phalanx of the thumb and on the lateral sesamoid.

Adductor pollicis:

- This is composed of an oblique head and a transverse head:
  - The oblique head arises from the trapezoid and capitate.
- The transverse head arises from:
  - the third metacarpal; the base of the second metacarpal; the joint capsule of the second, third, and fourth metacarpophalangeal joints.
- The two heads have a common insertion by means of a tendon:
  - into the medial sesamoid;
  - into the medial (ulnar) part of the proximal phalanx of the thumb.

Fig. 7.87 Hypothenar eminence

MA: In this figure, this region is shown held between the practitioner's thumb and index finger. It rests on the skeleton of the fifth metacarpal, and is made up of four muscles. These are arranged as follows, working down from the superficial to the deep layer: palmaris brevis, abductor digiti minimi, flexor digiti minimi brevis, and opponens digiti minimi.

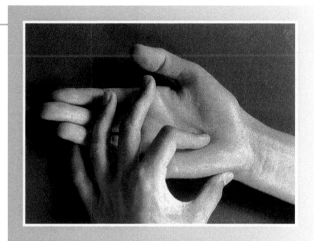

ATTACHMENTS

Palmaris brevis:

- This small cutaneous muscle arises from the ulnar border of the palmar aponeurosis.
- It is inserted into the deep surface of the skin of the hypothenar eminence.

Abductor digiti minimi:

- The abductor muscle of the little finger arises from the inferior side of the pisiform and from the flexor retinaculum.
- It is inserted into the medial aspect of the base of the proximal phalanx of the little finger.

Flexor digiti minimi brevis:

- This arises from the hook of the hamate and the flexor retinaculum.
- It is inserted into the medial aspect of the base of the proximal phalanx of the little finger by a common tendon, together with abductor digiti minimi.

Opponens digiti minimi:

- This arises from the hook of the hamate and the flexor retinaculum.
- It is inserted into the border and ulnar surface of the fifth metacarpal along its entire length.

Note: Abductor digiti minimi can be palpated on the ulnar border of the fifth metacarpal if you ask the subject to abduct her little finger.

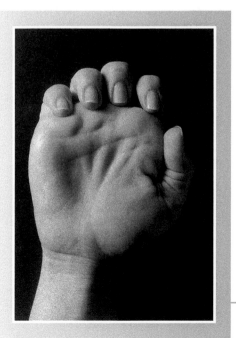

Fig. 7.88 Flexor tendons on the palm of the hand

MA: The tendons of the flexor muscles of the last four fingers are displayed on the palm of the hand as shown.

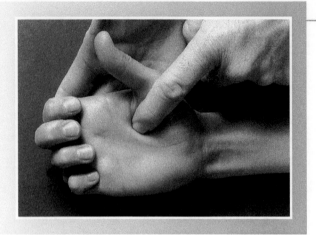

Fig. 7.89 Topographical location of the lumbricals

MA: In the adjacent figure, the practitioner's index finger is seen pushing aside the tendons of flexor digitorum superficialis and profundus going to the index finger. The practitioner's index finger is positioned at the first lumbrical muscle, which arises from the radial side of the tendon of flexor digitorum profundus going to the index finger.

ATTACHMENTS OF THE INTRINSIC MUSCLES OF THE HAND
(MUSCLES OF THE MIDDLE PALMAR REGION)

Lumbricals:

• Origin:
  – The first and second lumbrical muscles arise from the radial border and anterior surface of the tendons of flexor digitorum profundus to the second and third fingers.
  – The third and fourth lumbrical muscles lie between the middle and ring fingers, and the ring and little fingers, respectively. They arise from the radial and ulnar borders and on the anterior surface of the tendons of flexor digitorum profundus going to the adjacent fingers between which that particular lumbrical muscle lies.
• They are inserted into the radial border of the extensor tendon of the corresponding finger, on the proximal, middle, and distal phalanges.

Palmar interossei:

• The palmar interossei arise from the palmar parts of the sides of the metacarpals. At the level of the fingers, these muscles form the so-called dorsal interosseous expansion.
  – The first and second arise from the ulnar (medial) sides of the first and second metacarpals.[1]
  – The third and fourth arise from the radial (lateral) sides of the fourth and fifth metacarpals.
• Each is inserted by means of a deep part and a superficial part (note that there is no palmar interosseous muscle for the middle finger).
  – The deep part is inserted into the ulnar aspect of the base of the proximal phalanx of the first and second finger in the case of the first and second interossei; into the radial aspect of the base of the proximal phalanx of the fourth and fifth finger.
  – The superficial part is inserted into each tendon of extensor digitorum for the corresponding finger at the level of the proximal, middle, and distal phalanges.

Dorsal interossei:

• These arise from the posterior part of the adjacent sides of the metacarpals, and in each of the spaces between those metacarpals. At the level of the fingers, these muscles form the dorsal interosseous expansion.
• Their insertion is by means of a deep part and a superficial part.
  – The deep part is inserted into the radial (lateral) aspect of the base of the phalanges of the index and middle fingers, in the case of the first and second dorsal interossei; into the ulnar (medial) aspect of the base of the phalanges of the middle and ring fingers, in the case of the third and fourth dorsal interossei.
  – The superficial part is inserted into each tendon of extensor digitorum for the corresponding finger, at the level of the proximal, middle, and distal phalanges.

---

[1]Other authors describe three palmar interossei, not four. The first palmar interosseus adducts the thumb, but it is often absent, and tends not to be included in most descriptions of this group of muscles. The muscles are numbered accordingly.

Fig. 7.90 The action of the lumbricals, dorsal interossei, and palmar interossei

MA: In the sagittal plane, this set of muscles (see Note below) is responsible for the flexion of the metacarpophalangeal joints of the last four fingers, and for the extension of the middle and distal phalanges of these fingers (see also Fig. 7.91).

Note: The intrinsic muscles of the hand comprise four lumbricals, four* palmar interossei, and four dorsal interossei.

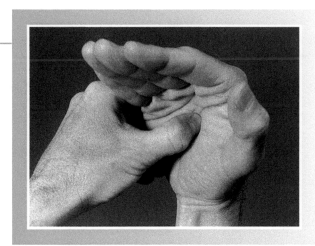

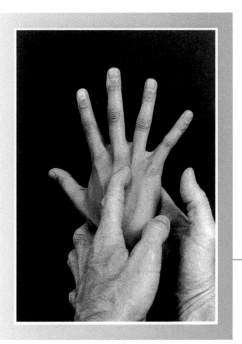

Fig. 7.91 The action of the dorsal and palmar interossei

MA: In addition to the action described above (Fig. 7.90), in the frontal plane, these muscles also abduct (draw apart) the fingers (dorsal interossei) and adduct them (draw them together) (palmar interossei). The contraction of the interossei can be palpated on the back of the hand, in the spaces between the metacarpals.

---

*See footnote to page 258.

NERVES AND BLOOD VESSELS

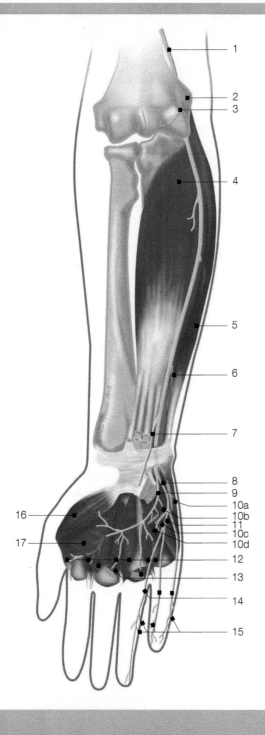

Ulnar nerve

1. Ulnar nerve (C8, T1)
2. Medial epicondyle
3. Articular branch (behind condyle)
4. Flexor digitorum profundus (medial part)
5. Flexor carpi ulnaris
6. Dorsal branch of ulnar nerve
7. Palmar branch
8. Superficial branch
9. Deep branch
10. Hypothenar muscles:
10a. Palmaris brevis
10b. Abductor digiti minimi
10c. Flexor digiti minimi brevis
10d. Opponens digiti minimi
11. Common palmar digital nerve
12. Palmar and dorsal interossei
13. Third and fourth lumbricals
14. Proper palmar digital nerves
15. Dorsal branches
16. Flexor pollicis brevis
17. Adductor pollicis

Cutaneous innervation by the ulnar nerve
Palmar view (A); dorsal view (B)

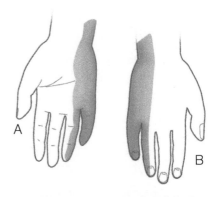

A

B

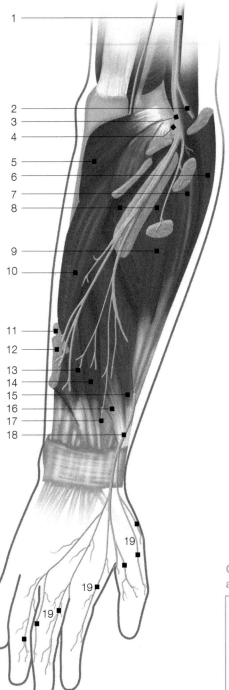

Radial nerve in the forearm (posterior view) and muscles of extensor group and supinator innervated by the radial nerve

1. Radial nerve (C5–C8)
2. Superficial branch
3. Deep branch
4. Lateral epicondyle
5. Anconeus
6. Brachioradialis
7. Extensor carpi radialis longus
8. Supinator
9. Extensor carpi radialis brevis
10. Extensor carpi ulnaris
11. Extensor digiti minimi
12. Extensor digitorum
13. Extensor indicis
14. Extensor pollicis longus
15. Abductor pollicis longus
16. Extensor pollicis brevis
17. Posterior interosseous nerve
18. Superficial branch of radial nerve
19. Dorsal digital nerves

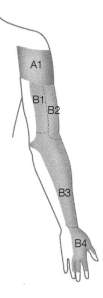

Cutaneous innervation by the axillary and radial nerves

A1. Superior lateral cutaneous nerve of arm (branch of axillary nerve)
 B. Branches of radial nerve:
B1. Posterior cutaneous nerve of arm
B2. Inferior lateral cutaneous nerve of arm
B3. Posterior cutaneous nerve of forearm
B4. Superficial branch of radial nerve and dorsal digital branches

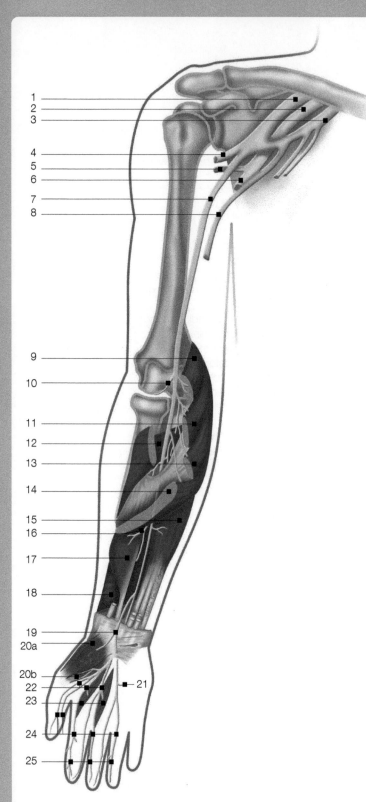

Median nerve (anterior view) and muscles innervated by the median nerve

1. Lateral cord of brachial plexus
2. Posterior cord of brachial plexus
3. Medial cord of brachial plexus
4. Musculocutaneous nerve
5. Axillary nerve
6. Radial nerve
7. Median nerve (C6, C7, C8, T1)
8. Ulnar nerve
9. Pronator teres (humeral head)
10. Articular branch
11. Flexor carpi radialis
12. Pronator teres (ulnar head)
13. Palmaris longus
14. Flexor digitorum superficialis
15. Flexor digitorum profundus
16. Anterior interosseous nerve
17. Flexor pollicis longus
18. Pronator quadratus
19. Palmar branch of median nerve
20. Thenar muscles:
20a. Abductor pollicis brevis
20b. Superficial head of flexor pollicis brevis
21. Anastomosis uniting branch of median nerve and ulnar nerve
22. Common palmar digital nerves
23. First and second lumbricals
24. Proper palmar digital nerves
25. Dorsal branches

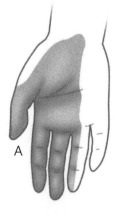
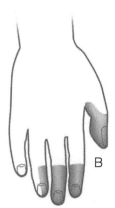

Cutaneous innervation by the median nerve
Palmar view (A); dorsal view (B)

THE PRINCIPAL NERVES AND BLOOD VESSELS

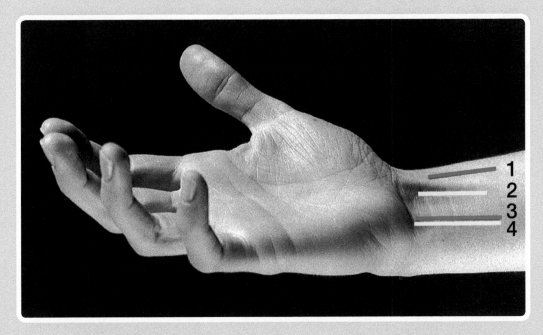

Fig. 7.92 Nerves and blood vessels in the anterior part of the wrist

1. Radial artery
2. Median nerve
3. Ulnar artery
4. Ulnar nerve

The notable structures that can be detected by palpation are:

- The radial pulse: taking the radial pulse at the wrist (Fig. 7.93)
- Median nerve in the anterior part of the wrist (Fig. 7.94)
- The ulnar pulse: taking the ulnar pulse at the wrist (Fig. 7.95)
- Ulnar nerve at the medial extremity of the anterior surface of the wrist (Fig. 7.96).

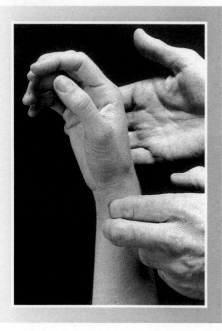

Fig. 7.93 Taking the radial pulse at the wrist

MA: Use a broad two- or three-finger contact on the inferior extremity of the anterior surface of the radius, lateral to (on the radial side of) the tendon of flexor carpi radialis. You will feel the pulse of the radial artery beneath your fingers.

Fig. 7.94 Median nerve in the anterior part of the wrist

MA: From the inferior third of the forearm, this nerve becomes very superficial. It runs behind the antebrachial aponeurosis, between the tendon of flexor carpi radialis laterally, the tendon of flexor digitorum superficialis going to the third finger medially, and the tendon of flexor digitorum superficialis going to the index finger behind. Push aside the tendon of palmaris longus laterally (as shown here) in order to palpate the nerve.

Note: Take extreme care whenever you are palpating a nerve.

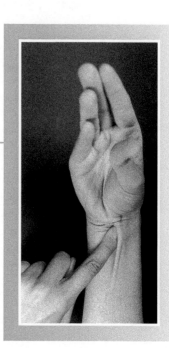

Fig. 7.95 Taking the ulnar pulse at the wrist

MA: Place the pads of two fingers on the medial extremity of the anterior surface of the wrist, at the cutaneous folds. Your fingers should be in contact with the lateral part of the pisiform (i.e., on the radial side of the bone). Slightly extend the subject's wrist in order to detect the pulse of the ulnar artery.

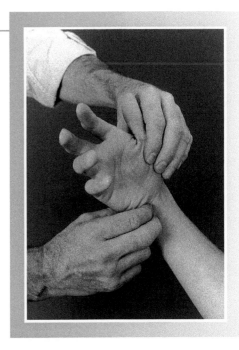

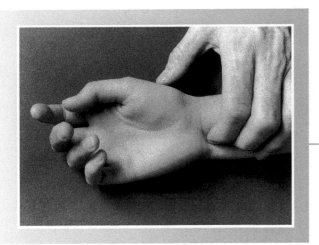

Fig. 7.96 Ulnar nerve at the medial extremity of the anterior surface of the wrist

MA: Access to this nerve can be achieved at the lateral (radial) border of the tendon of flexor carpi ulnaris. It is possible to roll the nerve on top of the tendon of flexor digitorum superficialis going to the fifth finger.

Note: Great care should be taken in this investigation, as at any time when palpating a nerve.

8
The hip

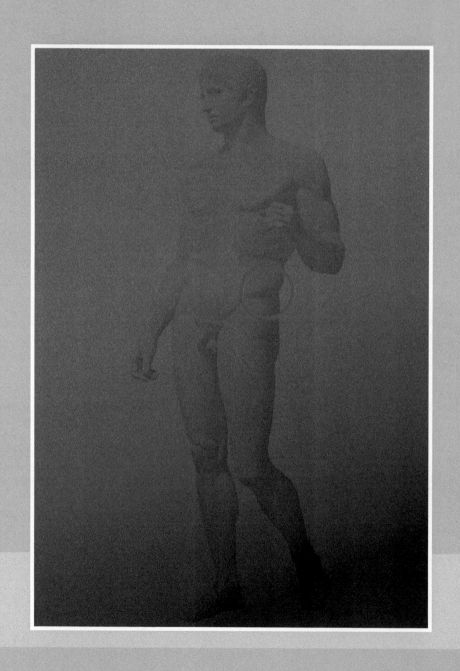

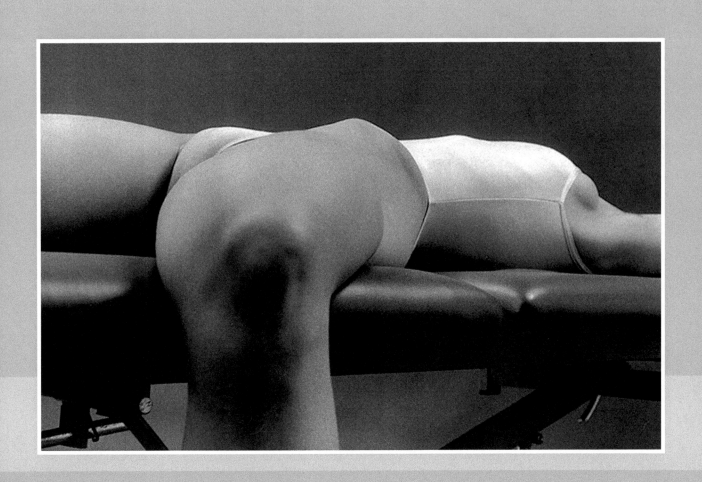

OSTEOLOGY

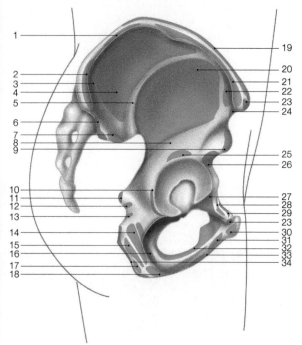

Hip bone (lateral aspect):

1. Latissimus dorsi
2. Gluteus maximus
3. Posterior gluteal line
4. Gluteus medius
5. Anterior gluteal line
6. Sacrotuberous ligament
7. Piriformis
8. Inferior gluteal line
9. Rectus femoris
10. Ischiofemoral ligament
11. Sacrospinous ligament
12. Superior gemellus
13. Inferior gemellus
14. Semimembranosus
15. Biceps femoris
16. Quadratus femoris
17. Semitendinosus
18. Adductor magnus
19. Internal oblique
20. Gluteus minimus
21. External oblique
22. Tensor fasciae latae
23. Inguinal ligament
24. Sartorius
25. Reflected tendon of rectus femoris
26. Iliofemoral ligament
27. Pubofemoral ligament
28. Pectineus
29. Pectinate ligament
30. Adductor longus
31. Adductor brevis
32. Obturator externus
33. Gracilis
34. Sacrotuberous ligament

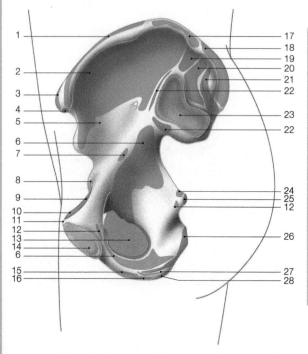

Hip bone (medial aspect):

1. Transversus abdominis
2. Iliacus
3. Internal oblique
4. Inguinal ligament
5. Iliac fossa
6. Obturator internus
7. Psoas minor and the arcuate line
8. Iliopubic eminence
9. Pectinate ligament
10. Lacunar ligament
11. Pubic angle
12. Levator ani
13. Obturator membrane
14. Articular surface of pubic symphysis
15. Corpus cavernosum
16. Ischiocavernous
17. Quadratus lumborum
18. Erector spinae muscles
19. Iliolumbar ligament
20. Interosseous sacroiliac ligament
21. Iliac tuberosity and posterior sacroiliac ligaments
22. Anterior sacroiliac ligaments
23. Auricular surface
24. Coccygeus
25. Sacrospinous ligament
26. Sacrotuberous ligament
27. Transversus abdominis (deep fibers)
28. Transversus abdominis (superficial fibers)

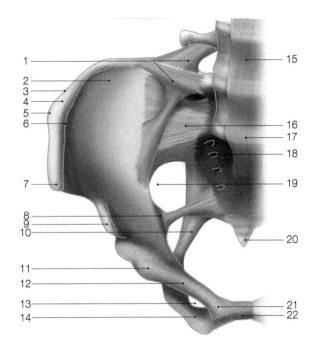

Pelvic bones and ligaments (anterior view)

1. Iliolumbar ligament
2. Iliac fossa
3. External lip of iliac crest
4. Intermediate zone of iliac crest
5. Tubercle of iliac crest
6. Internal lip of iliac crest
7. Anterior superior iliac spine
8. Ischial spine
9. Antero-inferior iliac spine
10. Sacrotuberous ligament
11. Iliopubic eminence
12. Superior pubic ramus
13. Obturator foramen
14. Inferior pubic ramus
15. Anterior longitudinal ligament
16. Anterior sacroiliac ligament
17. Sacral promontory
18. Anterior sacral foramina
19. Greater sciatic notch
20. Coccyx
21. Pubic tubercle
22. Pubic symphysis

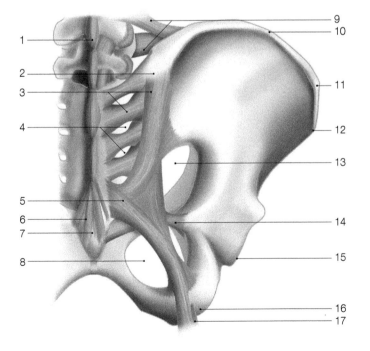

Pelvic bones and ligaments (posterior view)

1. Supraspinous ligament
2. Posterior superior iliac spine
3. Posterior sacroiliac ligaments
4. Posterior sacral foramina
5. Sacrotuberous ligament
6. Sacrococcygeal ligaments, superficial
7. Sacrococcygeal ligaments, deep
8. Lesser sciatic notch
9. Iliolumbar ligament
10. Iliac crest
11. Tubercle of iliac crest
12. Anterior superior iliac spine
13. Greater sciatic notch
14. Sacrospinous ligament
15. Acetabular margin
16. Ischial tuberosity
17. Tendon of long head of biceps femoris

THE COXOFEMORAL REGION

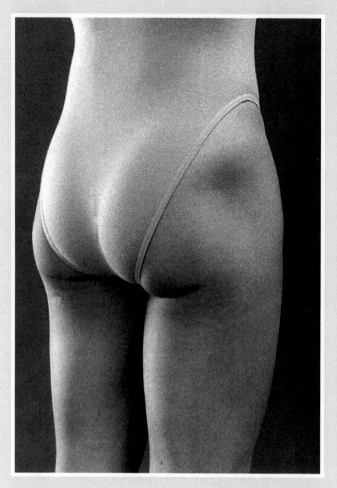 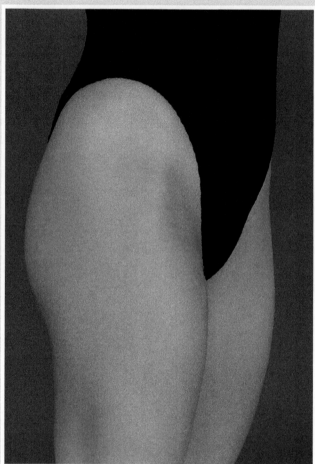

Figs. 8.2 and 8.3 View of the hip region

The palpable bony structures include:

- **The hip bone**
  - The tubercle of the iliac crest (Fig. 8.4)
  - The anterior superior iliac spine (Fig. 8.6)
  - The anterior inferior iliac spine (Fig. 8.8)
  - The iliac tubercle (Fig. 8.5)
  - The greater innominate notch (Fig. 8.7)
  - The pecten pubis (Fig. 8.9)
  - The superior pubic rami (Figs. 8.10 and 8.11)
  - The pubic symphysis (Fig. 8.12)
  - The body of the pubis (Fig. 8.14)
  - The pubic tubercle (Fig. 8.13)

- The posterior superior iliac spine (Fig. 8.15)
- The ischial spine (Figs. 8.18 and 8.19)
- The lesser innominate notch (Fig. 8.16)
- The posterior inferior iliac spine (Fig. 8.17)
- The greater sciatic foramen (Figs. 8.18, 8.20, and 8.21)
- The lesser sciatic foramen (Figs. 8.18 and 8.19)
- The ischial tuberosity (Figs. 8.22 and 8.23)
- The inferior border of the iliac bone (Figs. 8.24 and 8.25)
- **The femur**
  - The femoral head (Figs. 8.26–8.28)
  - The greater trochanter (Figs. 8.29–8.35)
  - The lesser trochanter (Figs. 8.36 and 8.37).

The hip bone

Fig. 8.4 The iliac crest

MA: It is possible to feel the changes in the curvature of this structure:

- a medially concave anterior curve;
- a laterally concave posterior curve;
- a superiorly convex curve, whose apex lies almost midway between its two extremities.

Also visible are its variations in thickness, which are more prominent at both ends, especially at the apex of the anterior curve, i.e., at the level of its tubercle (Fig. 8.5).

To appreciate these two aspects of the iliac crest, just run over it anteroposteriorly, using the pads of two fingers, or grip it between thumb and index finger. You must go over the crest itself as well as its lateral and medial lips.

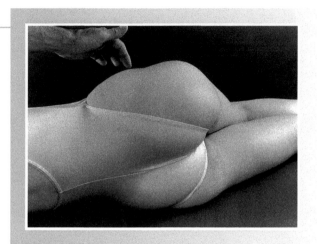

ATTACHMENTS

- The anterior part of the crest receives the insertion of external oblique, internal oblique, and the transverse muscles of the abdomen and gives origin to tensor fasciae latae.
- In its posterior part are inserted latissimus dorsi, quadratus lumborum, and sacrospinalis (or iliocostalis).

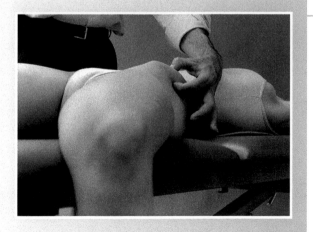

Fig. 8.5 The tubercle of the iliac crest

MA: It lies at the apex of the anterior curve and projects toward the lateral aspect of the iliac fossa. Run over the iliac crest anteroposteriorly between your thumb and index finger to feel the thickening of the superior border of the bone.

Note: In the figure the pad-to-pad grip faces the structure you are looking for, and contact occurs with the index finger.

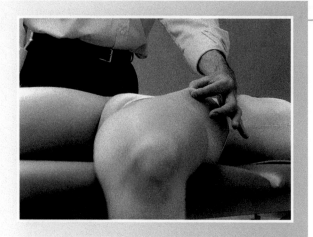

Fig. 8.6 The anterior superior iliac spine

MA: It is easily accessible. You need only localize the most anterior part of the tubercle of the iliac crest, which is precisely where it lies. Then grip it between thumb and index finger to bring it into focus.

ATTACHMENT

Tensor fasciae latae and sartorius arise from the lateral aspect of this structure.

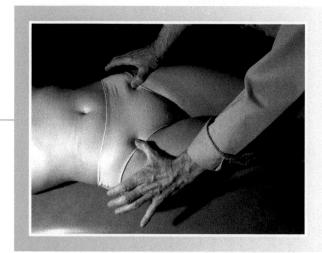

Fig. 8.7 The greater innominate notch

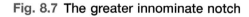

MA: It is partly accessible as it lies below the anterior superior iliac spine.

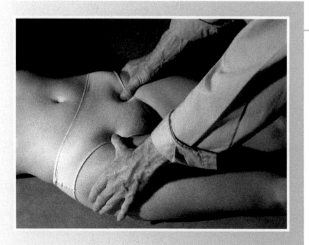

Fig. 8.8 The anterior inferior iliac spine

MA: It is felt by the fingers as a fullness lying about four finger-breadths from the anterior superior iliac spine and at the inferior border of the greater innominate notch. It is fairly accessible depending on the subject's body type. Ask the subject to tilt the pelvis anteriorly to make it easier for you to feel it.

ATTACHMENT

It gives origin to the straight head of rectus femoris.

> **CLINICAL NOTE**
>
> If on palpation you get the impression that this spine is excessively prominent, then consider the possibility of calcification of rectus femoris, which can be confirmed by medical imaging.

Fig. 8.9 The pecten pubis and the pectineal surface

The pecten pubis is the superior boundary of the superior pubic ramus.

MA: The simplest approach is first to localize the pubic tubercle and then to move from it obliquely and laterally toward the anterior superior iliac spine.

Note: During this procedure be careful about the spermatic cord in men and the round ligament in women.

ATTACHMENT

The superficial fibers of the pectineus arise from the pecten, while its deep fibers arise from the pectineal surface along with the pubofemoral ligament.

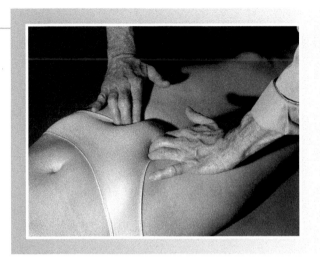

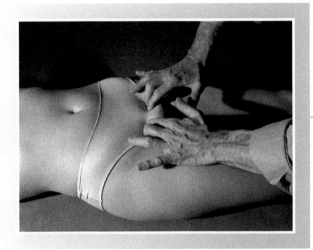

Fig. 8.10 The superior rami of the pubic bones

MA: Place your fingers in hooklike fashion on the superior pubic rami as they lie on either side of the pubic symphysis.

Fig. 8.11 The superior rami of the pubic bones: another approach

MA: Stand at the subject's head and place your thumbs on both superior pubic rami.

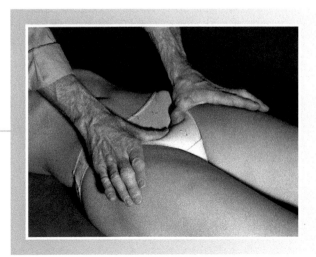

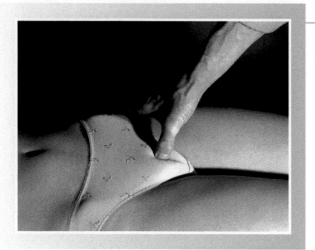

Fig. 8.12 The pubic symphysis

Reminder: It is an amphiarthrosis; the articular surfaces are united by a fibrocartilaginous disc composed of fibers surrounding a gelatinous central core.

MA: The symphysis is felt by the fingers as a depression lying between the two pubic bones and corresponding to the interpubic disc.

ATTACHMENTS

The superior and inferior borders of the symphysis are reinforced by two ligaments (superior and inferior). Anteriorly, the very thick anterior ligament is reinforced by the aponeurotic insertions of latissimus dorsi, of external oblique, and of pyramidalis, and also by the tendons of origin of adductor longus and gracilis. Posteriorly, the symphysis is reinforced by the posterior ligament.

Fig. 8.13 The pubic tubercle

MA: Place your hands on the greater trochanter, and move your thumbs horizontally and medially, looking for a bony spinelike prominence in the pubic region (the mons pubis in women). The tubercle lies at the most medial part of the superior pubic ramus very close to the pubic symphysis or more precisely at the junction of the pecten pubis and the obturator crest.

Note: The pubic tubercle projects anterior to the pubic bone.

ATTACHMENTS

To this tubercle are attached the inguinal ligament and, medial to it, are also attached various fascicles belonging to the abdominal muscles, as well as a portion of adductor longus.

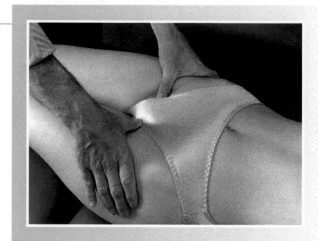

Fig. 8.14 The body of the pubic bone (quadrilateral surface)

MA: The obturator foramen is bounded superiorly by the superior pubic ramus, medially and anteriorly by the quadrilateral surface of the pubic bone, posteriorly by the ischial tuberosity, and inferiorly by the conjoined rami of the ischium and the pubic bone.

The practitioner is holding his thumb on the anterior part of the conjoined rami.

Note: The two pubic bones are united by the pubic symphysis.

ATTACHMENTS

From the most anterior part of the pubic bone arise adductor longus and adductor brevis deep to it; gracilis arises from its inferior border.

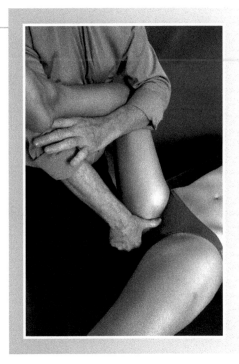

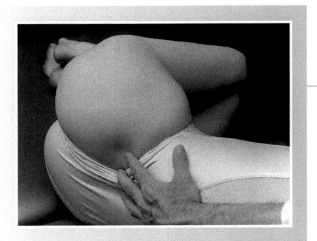

Fig. 8.15 The posterior superior iliac spine

MA: This corresponds on the whole to the skin dimple found more or less in everybody, and it faces the sacroiliac joint. You can also bring it out by finding the most posterior part of the iliac crest and then following it down to its junction with the posterior margin of the hip bone, which forms a shallow depression corresponding to the lesser innominate notch.

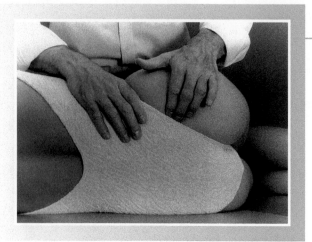

Fig. 8.16 The lesser innominate notch and the posterior inferior iliac spine

The lesser innominate notch

MA: It lies between the posterior superior and the posterior inferior iliac spines, two finger-breadths from the latter, and can be found between these two spines. Alternate forward and backward tilting of the pelvis helps to locate it.

The posterior inferior iliac spine

MA: It lies at the posterior margin of the auricular surface. It can be detected by using the pads of two fingers placed two finger-breadths from the posterior superior iliac spine. You will feel it more easily if you ask the subject to tilt her pelvis forward and backward alternately.

Fig. 8.17 The posterior inferior iliac spine in the prone position: another method of approach

MA: Just follow the lateral border of the sacrum until it joins the iliac bone. At this junction lies the posterior inferior iliac spine.

Note: Just cranial to the spine lies the lesser innominate notch.

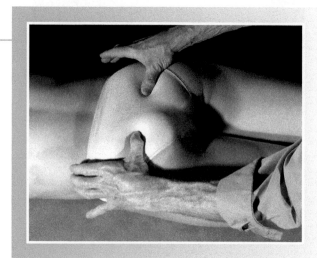

Fig. 8.18 The ischial spine and the lesser sciatic notch

The ischial spine

MA: The subject lies on one side with her hip flexed. First, using the pads of two fingers, locate the ischial tuberosity and keep your fingers fixed on the subject's skin while they slide into the lesser sciatic notch. (This is the same as making the subject's skin slide over the underlying tissues.)

The ischial spine lies at the proximal end of this notch.

Note: Gluteus maximus must be in a relaxed state.

It is at this point that obturator internus is reflected.

ATTACHMENTS

• Its lateral surface gives origin to superior gemellus.
• To its apex is attached the sacrospinous ligament.

The lesser sciatic notch

MA: First locate the ischial tuberosity with the pads of two fingers (see Fig. 8.22). The fossa that lies cranial to it and runs toward the sacrum is the lesser sciatic notch, where obturator internus is reflected.

Gluteus maximus must be in a relaxed state. In some cases it is better to have the subject's hip less flexed than shown in Fig. 8.17, since it lets you palpate the muscle more easily through the body of gluteus maximus, which is now in a more relaxed state.

Note: This notch lies between the ischial spine and the ischial tuberosity.

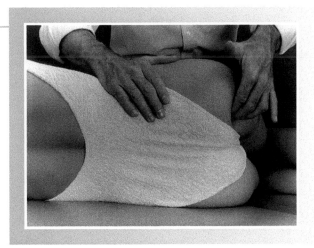

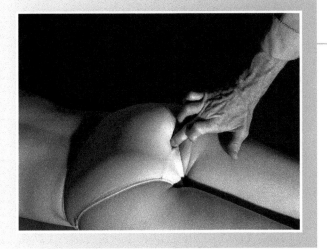

Fig. 8.19 The ischial spine and the lesser sciatic notch in the prone position: another method of approach

MA: First locate the most distal part of the greater sciatic notch (as indicated in Fig. 8.21) and maintain the same contact. Then, without letting your fingers slide on the subject's skin, move them up and down repeatedly and you will feel under your fingers a fullness corresponding to the ischial spine.

The lesser sciatic notch is continuous with the greater sciatic notch and the ischial spine. You can also approach it from the ischial tuberosity by placing your fingers just cranial to the superior margin of the tuberosity.

Note: In the adjacent figure the mode of approach uses only one hand.

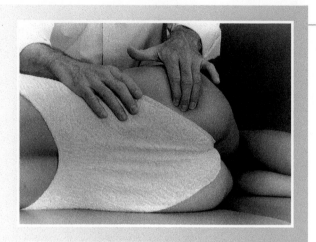

Fig. 8.20 The greater sciatic notch

MA: First use the pads of two fingers to locate the posterior inferior iliac spine. Then press on the gluteal surface of the iliac fossa and "dive" toward the greater sciatic notch and the lateral border of the sacrum.

Note: The wide and deep greater sciatic notch is bounded by the posterior inferior iliac spine and the ischial spine. You can reach it through the body of gluteus maximus.

You must not forget that it is concave posteriorly and that piriformis and the sciatic nerve both exit through it. These observations should influence the way you investigate this notch.

Fig. 8.21 The greater sciatic notch in the prone position: another method of approach

MA: Using the fingers of both your hands placed very flat on the relaxed buttock, try to identify a straight sharp border.

Note: In the adjacent figure the method of approach uses only one hand.

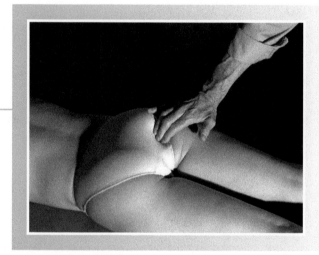

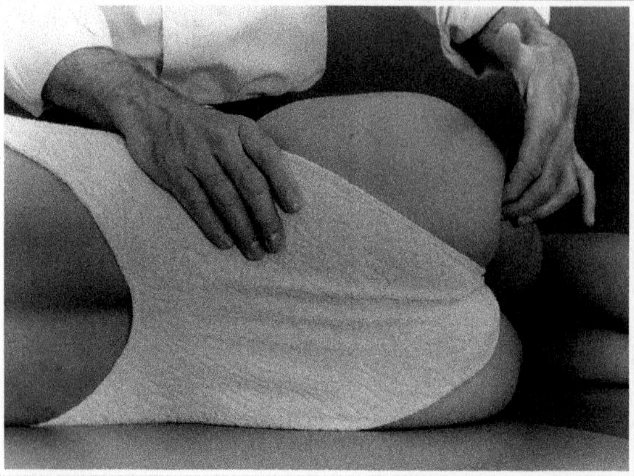

Fig. 8.22 The ischial tuberosity

MA: It is oval in shape with a bulky posterosuperior extremity and a narrow inferior extremity continuous with the inferior border of the hip bone. When the hip is flexed, it is freed from gluteus maximus.

You can also palpate it in the prone subject in the middle of the gluteal fold, which serves as a cutaneous landmark.

Note: It is on the ischial tuberosities that we sit most of the time.

ATTACHMENTS

- Inferior gemellus arises from the superior part of the ischial tuberosity just superior and lateral to the insertion of the sacrotuberous ligament.
- It is the site of origin of the hamstring muscles (semimembranosus, semitendinosus, and biceps femoris).
- Adductor magnus arises from it.
- The sacrotuberous ligament is attached to its medial border.

Fig. 8.23 The ischial tuberosity in the prone position: another method of approach

MA: Place your thumb over the cutaneous landmark provided by the gluteal fold in order to make contact with the ischial tuberosity where the hamstrings take their origin.

> **CLINICAL NOTE**
>
> **Ischial bursitis:** Palpation with pressure applied to the tuberosity will cause an exquisite pain.
>
> **Tendinopathy of the hamstrings:** Palpation with pressure applied to these tendons will be painful, and any investigation of these muscles may cause pain and reveal some degree of weakness. Stretching these muscles will also cause pain.
>
> **Disinsertion of the hamstrings:** It is very rare. On palpation your fingers will feel a notch opposite the disinserted tendons, and knee flexion will be seriously compromised.

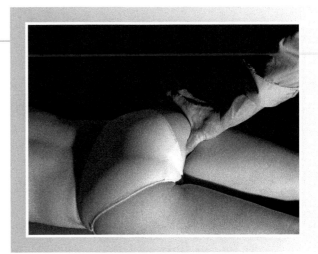

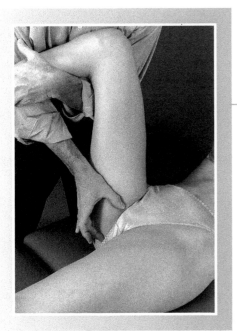

Fig. 8.24 The inferior border of the hip bone

MA: Locate the ischial tuberosity (Fig. 8.22) and the most anterior and medial part of the inferior pubic ramus.

The inferior border of the hip bone has two parts:
- anteriorly, an articular surface in contact with that of the contralateral pubic bone to form the pubic symphysis;
- posteriorly, a rugged surface with two lips (internal and external) and a groove.

ATTACHMENT

Gracilis arises from the external lip.

Fig. 8.25 The inferior border of the hip bone

MA: Place your hand on the body of adductor longus and follow the muscle proximally until it reaches the inferior border of the hip bone. You will make contact using the lateral border of your index finger or with your thumb.

ATTACHMENT

Gracilis arises from the inferior and anterior parts of this border.

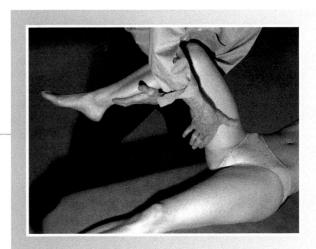

The femur

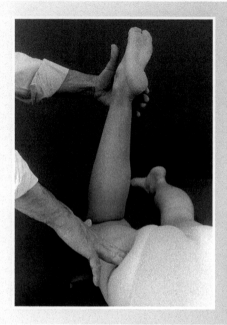 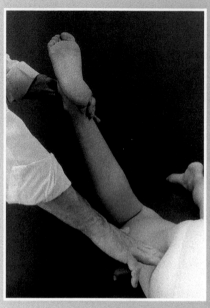

Figs. 8.26 and 8.27 Posterior approach to the femoral head

MA: Rotate the subject's hip medially so as to displace the femoral head posteriorly. It can then be felt through the body of gluteus maximus between the greater trochanter and the lateral aspect of the hip bone.

In order to get a better feel of the femoral head, keep rotating the hip several times. Slightly distal and posterior to its center the femoral head has a dimple – the fovea capitis, which has a rough surface and is pierced by numerous blood vessels.

ATTACHMENT

The ligament of the head of femur is inserted into the fovea.

Fig. 8.28 Anterior approach to the femoral head

MA: With the subject lying on her side, stand behind her and use your hip to stabilize her pelvis in the anteroposterior plane.

Place your proximal hand on the anterolateral part of her hip and use the pads of your fingers to hold the anterior part of her hip.

With your distal hand cradle the anteromedial part of the thigh being examined and gently extend her lower limb while keeping her pelvis steady with your hip. Your proximal hand will gradually feel a fullness, which is the femoral head as it projects anteriorly.

Note: During this procedure you will be able to feel the femoral pulse as it is displaced anteriorly by the protrusion of the femoral head.

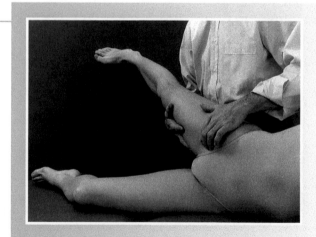

Fig. 8.29 Approach to the greater trochanter with the subject lying on her side

MA: In this position the greater trochanter normally juts out on the lateral surface of the hip.

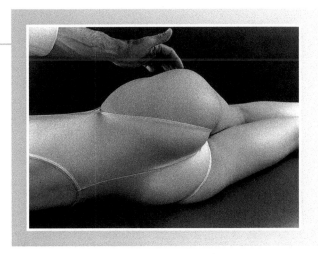

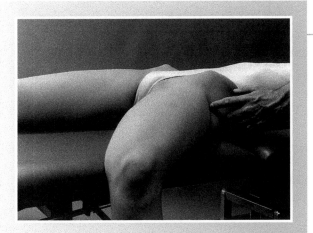

Fig. 8.30 Approach to the greater trochanter with the subject supine

MA: In this position, with the lower limb slightly abducted, the greater trochanter is directly accessible in the skin dimple produced by hip abduction. This position provides optimal relaxation of the surrounding muscles and facilitates access to the different parts of the greater trochanter, i.e., its superior, inferior, anterior, and posterior borders and its lateral and medial aspects.

ATTACHMENTS

- Superior border: piriformis
- Anterior border (or anterior aspect): gluteus minimus
- Posterior border: quadratus femoris
- Lateral aspect: gluteus medius
- Medial aspect:
  - obturator externus inserted into the trochanteric fossa
  - obturator internus and the gemelli inserted superior and anterior to the trochanteric fossa
- Its inferior border limits its lateral aspect inferiorly and is also called the crest of vastus lateralis, which is inserted here.

CLINICAL NOTE

If palpation induces pain in any of its borders (superior, anterior, posterior, lateral, and inferior), consider the possibility of a tendinopathy or of a tenobursitis related to the inserted muscle. Also, investigation of the muscle will cause pain and/or reveal some degree of weakness. Passive movements at the hip joint should not be restricted or painful.

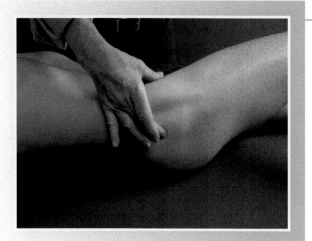

Fig. 8.31 The greater trochanter: superior border

Piriformis is inserted here.

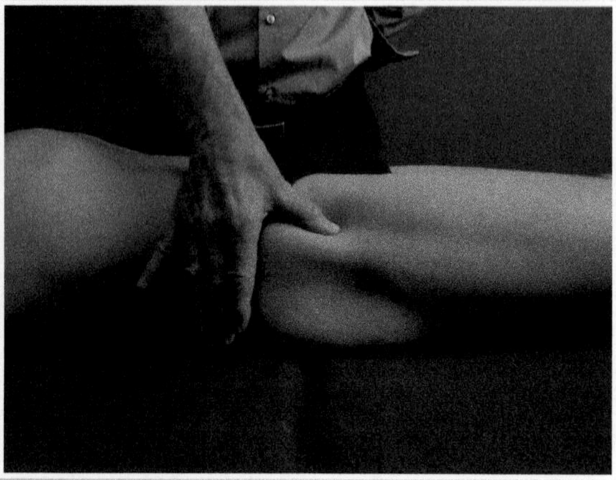

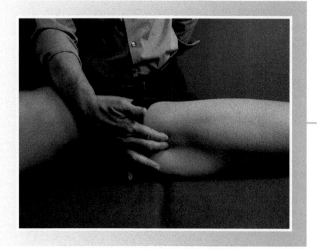

Fig. 8.32 The greater trochanter: anterior border

Gluteus minimus is inserted here.

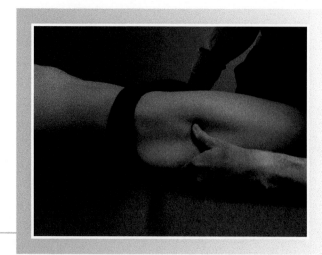

Fig. 8.33 The greater trochanter: lateral aspect

Gluteus medius is inserted here.

Fig. 8.34 The greater trochanter: inferior border

Vastus lateralis is inserted here.

Fig. 8.35 The greater trochanter: posterior border

Quadratus femoris is inserted here.

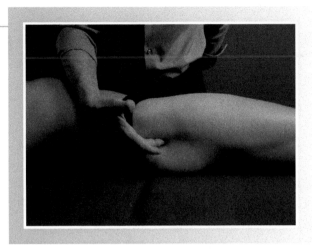

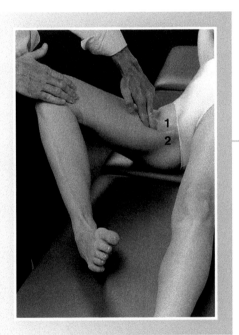

Fig. 8.36 The lesser trochanter – stage 1: demonstration of the "hiatus" between adductor longus (1) and gracilis (2)

MA: The adjacent illustration shows a posteromedial view of gracilis (2) and adductor longus (1). The subject is supine with hip and knee flexed: by preventing the subject from adducting the thigh horizontally, you can bring out the two muscles you are looking for.

You can make contact with the lesser trochanter directly in the gap between these two muscles.

Fig. 8.37 The lesser trochanter – stage 2: direct contact

MA: While the dorsal part of your hand cradles the medial aspect of the subject's leg, you can displace the lesser trochanter anteriorly by laterally rotating her hip. Slide the thumb of your other hand deep into the soft tissues between adductor longus and gracilis and look for a relatively perceptible fullness.

ATTACHMENT

• Insertion of iliopsoas either by a common tendon or by two tendons separated by a synovial bursa.

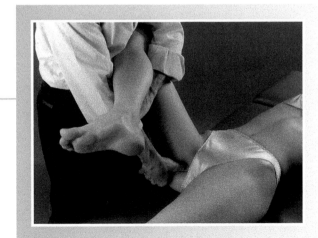

MYOLOGY

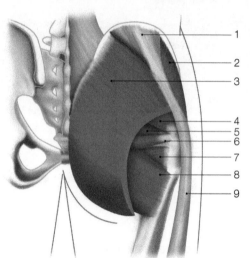

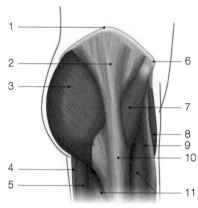

Gluteal region (superficial plane)

1. Iliac crest
2. Gluteal fascia
3. Gluteus maximus
4. Semitendinosus
5. Biceps femoris
6. Anterior superior iliac spine
7. Tensor fasciae latae
8. Sartorius
9. Rectus femoris
10. Iliotibial tract
11. Vastus lateralis

Iliotibial tract (superficial plane)

1. Gluteal fascia
2. Tensor fasciae latae
3. Gluteus maximus
4. Gluteus medius
5. Piriformis
6. Tendons of obturator internus and gemelli
7. Quadratus femoris
8. Gluteus maximus (deep bundle)
9. Gluteus maximus (superficial bundle)

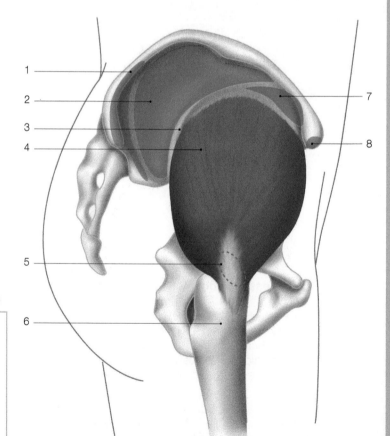

Gluteal region (deep plane)

1. Gluteus maximus
2. Gluteus medius
3. Anterior gluteal line
4. Gluteus minimus
5. Synovial bursa
6. Greater trochanter
7. Tensor fasciae latae
8. Sartorius

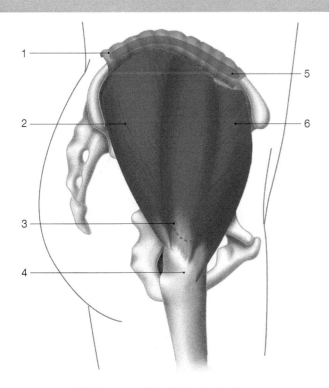

Gluteus medius (lateral view)

1. Gluteal fascia
2. Posterior bundle
3. Synovial bursa
4. Greater trochanter
5. Insertion of gluteus medius
6. Anterior bundle

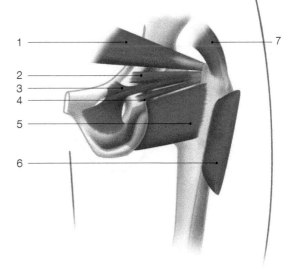

Pelvitrochanteric muscles (posterior view)

1. Piriformis
2. Superior gemellus
3. Obturator internus
4. Inferior gemellus
5. Quadratus femoris
6. Gluteus maximus
7. Gluteus medius

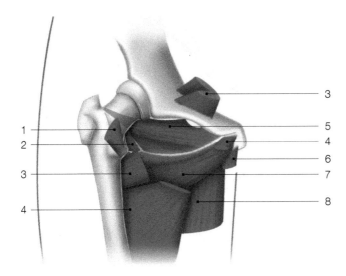

Medial pelvitrochanteric muscles (anterior view)

1. Iliopsoas
2. Quadratus femoris
3. Pectineus
4. Adductor longus
5. Obturator externus
6. Gracilis
7. Adductor minimus
8. Adductor magnus

THE LATERAL INGUINOFEMORAL REGION

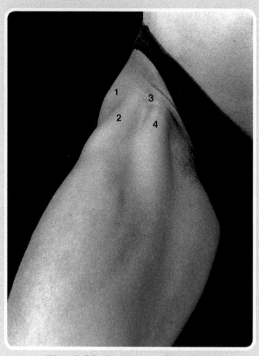

Fig. 8.38 Anteromedial view
1. Gluteus medius
2. Tensor fasciae latae

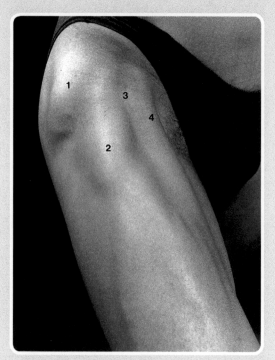

Fig. 8.39 Anterolateral view
3. Rectus femoris
4. Sartorius

With its apex located superiorly this triangular region is bounded:

- proximally by its apex, consisting of the anterior superior iliac spine;
- laterally by tensor fasciae latae;
- medially by sartorius;
- deeply by its "floor," supplied by rectus femoris, whose proximal extremity slips in between the two above-mentioned muscles.

Note: The muscles demarcating this region belong topographically to the femoral region.

ACTIONS OF THE MUSCLES OF THE LATERAL INGUINOFEMORAL REGION

- Tensor fasciae latae (Fig. 8.40):
  - It flexes, abducts, and medially rotates the thigh on the pelvis.
  - It extends the leg on the thigh and laterally rotates the leg on the thigh when the knee is flexed.

  - It stabilizes the knee transversely in equilibrium with the anserine muscles.
- Sartorius (Fig. 8.41):
  - It flexes, abducts, and laterally rotates the thigh on the pelvis.
  - It flexes and medially rotates the leg on the thigh.
  - It stabilizes the pelvis in the sagittal plane.
  - It tilts the pelvis forward.
  - It stabilizes the knee laterally with the help of the other two anserine muscles (semitendinosus and gracilis).
- Rectus femoris (Fig. 8.42):
  - It extends the knee and flexes the hip.

INNERVATIONS

- Sartorius: femoral nerve (L2, L3)
- Quadriceps: femoral nerve (L2–L4)
- Tensor fasciae latae: superior gluteal nerve (L4, L5)

Fig. 8.40 Tensor fasciae latae

MA: Resistance applied on the anteromedial surface of the flexed thigh (not shown in the illustration) prevents further flexion of the thigh and brings out two muscular bodies in the proximal part of the thigh.

The more lateral is that of the tensor fasciae latae, which runs between the anterior superior iliac spine and the greater trochanter.

ATTACHMENTS

The tensor arises from the lateral aspect of the anterior superior iliac spine and from the anterior extremity of the lateral lip of the iliac crest.

1. Tensor fasciae latae
2. Sartorius
3. Rectus femoris

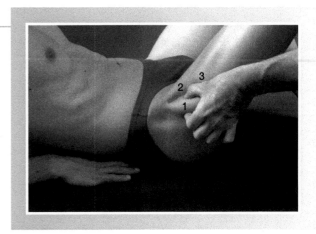

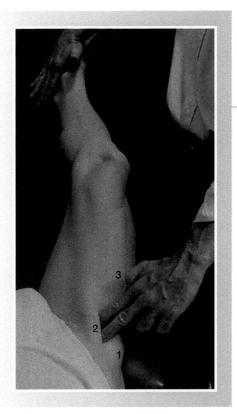

Fig. 8.41 Close-up of sartorius

MA: Use the same procedure as for tensor fasciae latae. Sartorius is the more medial of the two muscular bodies that stand out in the proximal part of the thigh when resistance is applied to the anteromedial aspect of the thigh in order to oppose flexion of the thigh on the pelvis. The anterior superior iliac spine is the bony landmark, since the muscle arises from it.

Note: Sartorius is the medial border of the lateral inguinofemoral region. It is also the lateral border of the medial inguinofemoral region (the femoral triangle).

ATTACHMENTS

These muscles arise from the anterior superior iliac spine:

1. Tensor fasciae latae
2. Sartorius
3. Rectus femoris

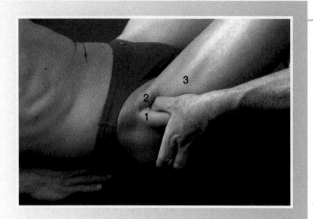

Fig. 8.42 Close-up of rectus femoris

MA: In the fossa between tensor fasciae latae laterally and sartorius medially you will be able to look for the most proximal part of rectus femoris.

Even when it is in a state of relaxation you can easily feel its proximal extremity under your fingers. You can also ask the subject to contract and relax the muscle repeatedly to allow you to get a better feel of its fibers. Apart from the hip flexion already asked for, the only other muscular action required of the subject is knee extension.

The straight head of the muscle arises from the anterior inferior iliac spine and the reflected head from the floor of the supra-acetabular groove.

ATTACHMENTS

It arises from the anterior inferior iliac spine and from the supra-acetabular groove and inserts into the base of the patella and into the tibial tuberosity.

1. Tensor fasciae latae
2. Sartorius
3. Rectus femoris

THE MEDIAL INGUINOFEMORAL REGION OR FEMORAL TRIANGLE

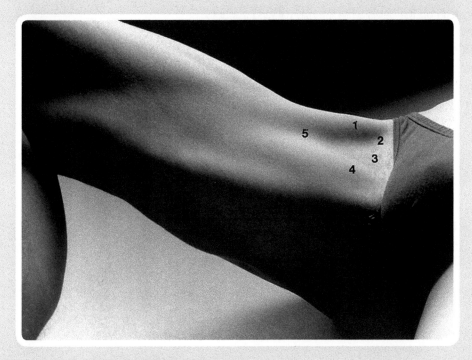

Fig. 8.43 Medial view

1. Sartorius
2. Iliopsoas
3. Pectineus
4. Adductor longus
5. The apex of the femoral triangle (Scarpa's triangle), where sartorius meets adductor longus

Triangular in shape with its apex located inferiorly, this region, known as the femoral triangle is bounded:

- proximally, by its base consisting of the inguinal ligament, which extends from the anterior superior iliac spine to the pubic tubercle;
- laterally by sartorius;
- medially by adductor longus;
- distally at its apex, by the junction of sartorius and adductor longus;
- by its "floor," consisting of the pectineus medially and iliopsoas laterally. This arrangement of muscles forms a distally concave gutter that harbors the blood vessels and nerves for the lower limb.

Note: Sartorius, adductor longus, and pectineus belong to the femoral region.

ACTIONS OF THE MUSCLES OF THE MEDIAL INGUINOFEMORAL REGION

- **Actions of Sartorius (Fig. 8.41):**
  - It flexes, abducts, and laterally rotates the thigh on the pelvis.
  - It flexes and medially rotates the leg on the thigh.
  - It stabilizes the pelvis in the sagittal plane.
  - It tilts the pelvis anteriorly.
  - It laterally stabilizes the knee with the other anserine muscles (semitendinosus and gracilis).
- **Actions of Iliopsoas (Figs. 8.48–8.50):**
  - When its fixed end is at the level of the trunk:
    - It flexes the thigh on the pelvis while laterally rotating it slightly.
    - It has a small component of adduction.
  - When its fixed end is on the femur:
    - Iliacus flexes and tilts the pelvis anteriorly.
    - Psoas produces anterior flexion, ipsilateral flexion, and contralateral rotation of the lumbar spine.
- **Actions of the adductors (pectineus and adductor longus) (Figs. 8.44–8.47):**
  - They adduct the thigh on the pelvis.
  - They laterally rotate the thigh on the pelvis, excepting the medial part (the inferior bundle or the vertical bundle) of adductor magnus, which helps in producing medial rotation.
  - Apart from the vertical bundle, all these muscles contribute to flexion of the thigh on the pelvis, and they can become extensors beyond a certain degree of flexion (45°).
  - They stabilize the pelvis in equilibrium with the abductors.
- **Actions of Gracilis:**
  - It flexes and medially rotates the leg on the thigh.
  - It adducts and medially rotates the thigh on the pelvis.

INNERVATIONS

- Sartorius: femoral nerve (L1–L3)
- Psoas: lumbar flexus (L1–L3)
- Iliacus: femoral nerve (L2–L4)
- Pectineus: femoral nerve and obturator nerve (L2–L4)
- Adductor longus: femoral nerve and obturator nerve (L2–L4)
- Gracilis: obturator nerve (L2–L4)
- Iliacus: femoral nerve (L2–L4)
- Psoas: ventral rami of lumbar nerves (L1–L3)

Fig. 8.44 Adductor longus

MA: With the subject's hip and knee flexed, abduct the lower limb you are investigating, using a cradling hold. Ask her to adduct her thigh and resist her movement in order to make adductor longus stand out in relief in the superomedial corner of the thigh.

ATTACHMENTS

See Figure 8.31.

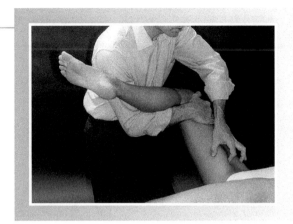

> **CLINICAL NOTE**
>
> If this procedure reveals some weakness and is painful, consider some form of muscular injury. Since evaluation of the adductors is global, only pain elicited on palpation will identify specifically the injured muscle.

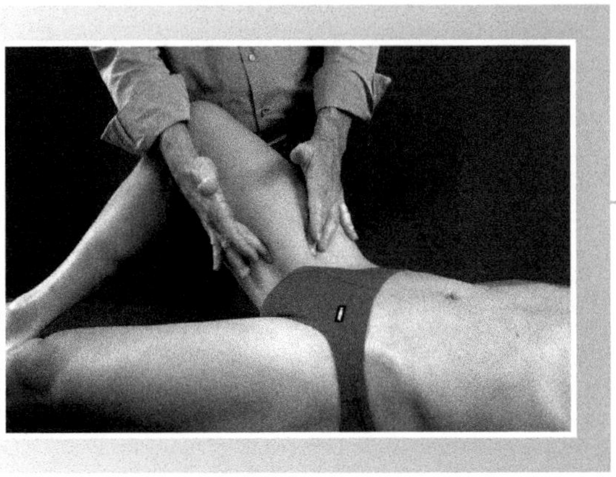

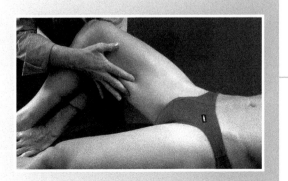

Fig. 8.45 Adductor longus: another method of approach

MA: Ask the subject to adduct his thigh, and resist this movement with your right forearm. You can then grip the body of the muscle between your two hands.

Fig. 8.46 Pectineus

MA: Look for this muscle lateral to adductor longus in the fossa that is continuous with it. It forms the medial portion of the "floor" of the femoral triangle. In the adjacent picture sartorius lies between the index and middle fingers of your left hand, i.e., the hand that is resisting the flexion and adduction of the hip. Your right hand will lie on pectineus.

ATTACHMENTS

See Fig. 8.30 (femoral region).

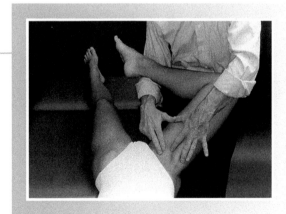

Fig. 8.47 Pectineus: another method of approach

MA: Place your hand in the depression that lies between adductor longus and sartorius; this corresponds to the muscle you are looking for.

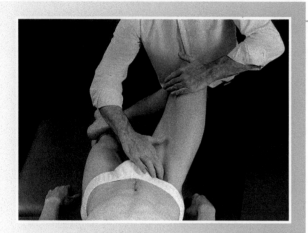

Fig. 8.48 Iliopsoas

MA: Place your contact medial to the proximal portion of sartorius near its origin from the anterior superior iliac spine. Iliopsoas is accessible at this point, since it is reflected over the iliopectineal surface and then courses over the anterior aspect of the hip joint beyond that point of reflection. It is bordered medially by pectineus. Make the muscle contract by opposing the subject's hip flexion with your distal hand, and your fingers can feel the contraction of the muscle fibers as they pass over the iliopubic eminence.

Note: This is a sensitive region and must be approached with caution.

CLINICAL NOTE

Bursitis

You must palpate medial to sartorius. In case of bursitis, palpation will exacerbate the pain, and you will feel a mass under your fingers. During testing hip flexion against resistance will be weaker and elicit pain.

ATTACHMENTS

- Psoas arises from:
  - the intervertebral discs of T12–L5;
  - the lateral and adjacent surfaces of the vertebral bodies T12–L5;
  - the fibrous arches located on the lateral aspects of the vertebral bodies and running from the superior borders of these same vertebrae (each arch and its corresponding vertebra bounds an orifice through which course the lumbar vessels and the rami communicantes of the sympathetic nervous system);
  - the anterior surfaces of the transverse processes of the lumbar vertebrae.
  - It inserts into the apex of the lesser trochanter.
- Iliacus arises from:
  - most of the concavity of the iliac fossa;
  - the medial lip of the iliac crest;
  - the iliolumbar ligament and the base of the sacrum posteriorly.
- The iliac and psoas muscles are inserted into the lesser trochanter by a common tendon or by two tendons separated by a synovial bursa.

Fig. 8.49 Iliopsoas in its proximal part – stage 1: looking for landmarks

MA: When you resist the subject by placing a hand on his forehead, the straplike abdominal muscles stand out along with the lateral border of the rectus abdominis.

Place your thumb on his navel, your middle finger on the anterior superior iliac spine, and your index finger at the midpoint of the line corresponding to the lateral border of rectus abdominis.

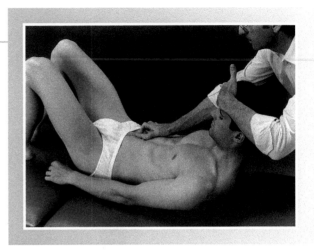

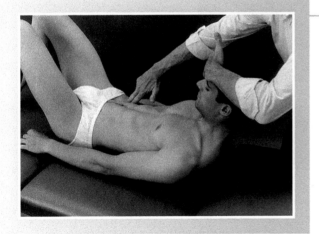

Fig. 8.50 Iliopsoas in its proximal part – stage 2

MA: The point you have specifically identified in the lateral border of rectus abdominis (see Fig. 8.49), is the best point from which to approach iliopsoas.

Once the landmark is identified, the subject should rest his head on a cushion to relax the abdominal muscles. You can change your position and stand at the level of his hip in order to proceed. It is essential for you to "penetrate" the abdominal muscles with care and by stages so as to overcome the defense mechanisms of the abdominal wall, which will certainly come into play. Active flexion of the hips will tighten the iliopsoas muscle, and you will get a better appreciation of the body of the muscle you are looking for.

Note: The contact shown in the adjacent figure illustrates the "point of entry" into the abdominal muscles and not the method of palpation.

THE GLUTEAL REGION

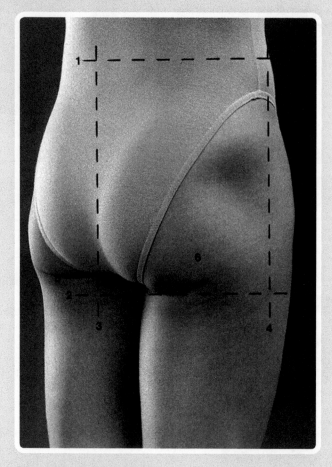

Fig. 8.51 Posterolateral view

1. Superior border: iliac crest
2. Inferior border: gluteal fold
3. Medial border: iliac crest and coccyx in continuity
4. Lateral border: it is an imaginary vertical line running down from the anterior superior iliac spine to the greater trochanter intersecting the most lateral part of the gluteal fold or its extension.

Note: This imaginary line has the remarkable property of corresponding more or less to the posterior border of tensor fasciae latae.

5. Gluteal fold
6. Gluteus maximus

The superficial plane

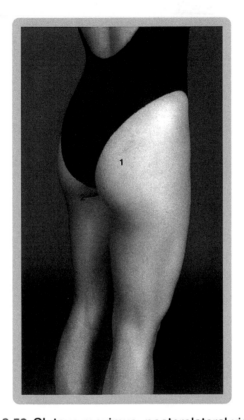

Fig. 8.52 Gluteus maximus, posterolateral view
1. Gluteus maximus
2. Gluteal fold

The superficial plane of the gluteal region is represented by one muscle: gluteus maximus (Fig. 8.53).

ACTIONS

- It extends the thigh over the pelvis.
- It laterally rotates the thigh on the pelvis.
- It stabilizes the pelvis in the sagittal plane.
- It tilts the pelvis posteriorly.

INNERVATION

- Inferior gluteal nerve (L5, S1, S2)

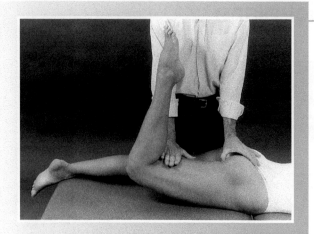

Fig. 8.53 Gluteus maximus

MA: The maneuver illustrated in this figure aims at visualizing gluteus maximus.

The iliac crest, the greater trochanter, and the ischial tuberosity are the essential bony landmarks that demarcate the gluteal region. The gluteal fold is virtually horizontal and corresponds roughly to the inferior border of the muscle as it runs obliquely and inferomedially.

Ask the subject to lift the anterior part of her thigh from the table with her knee flexed without any compensation in the lumbar region.

Putting pressure on the postero-inferior part of the thigh prevents the mobilization of an intermediate joint (in this case, the knee) and allows you to bring out the body of the muscle and to assess the quality of its contraction relative to that of the contralateral muscle.

Note: Knee flexion "shortens" the hamstrings and favors the specific activity of gluteus maximus as extensor of the hip joint.

The middle plane

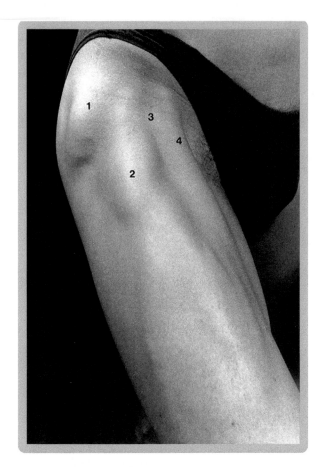

Fig. 8.54 Anterolateral view of the hip
1. Gluteus medius (Figs. 8.55 and 8.56)
2. Tensor fasciae latae (Fig. 8.56)
3. Rectus femoris
4. Sartorius

The middle plane of the gluteal region is represented by one muscle: gluteus medius.

ACTIONS OF GLUTEUS MEDIUS

- When its fixed end is at pelvic level:
  - It abducts the thigh on the pelvis.
  - Its anterior fibers flex and medially rotate the thigh on the pelvis.
  - Its posterior fibers extend and laterally rotate the thigh on the pelvis.
- When its fixed end is at femoral level:
  - It stabilizes the pelvis in the frontal plane.

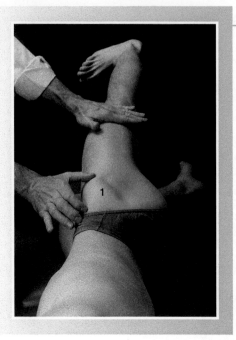

Fig. 8.55 Gluteus medius

MA: The essential bony landmarks are the anterior part of the iliac crest and the superior border of the greater trochanter.

Ask the subject to abduct his slightly extended lower limb against resistance: the body of the muscle will tense up under your fingers.

Ask him to keep his hip abducted and flexed, and then rotate it medially in rapid successive bursts. Do not forget that tensor fasciae latae lies inferior and anterior to gluteus medius.

Note: Your resisting hand is placed on the inferior and lateral part of the thigh above the knee in order to prevent recruitment of the intermediate joint (in this case, the knee). The body of the muscle (1) visible in the adjacent illustration is that of gluteus medius. It lies posterior and superior to tensor fasciae latae.

ATTACHMENTS

- This muscle arises from the gluteal surface of the iliac fossa between the iliac crest and the anterior and posterior gluteal lines and from the lateral lip of the iliac crest.
- It is inserted into the lateral surface of the greater trochanter.

INNERVATION

- Superior gluteal nerve (L5, S1)

Fig. 8.56 Gluteus medius and tensor fasciae latae

MA: Try to distinguish gluteus medius (1) from tensor fasciae latae (2).

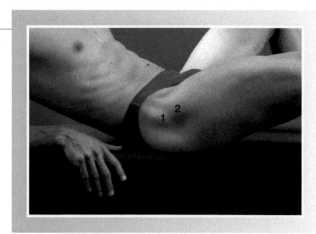

The deep plane

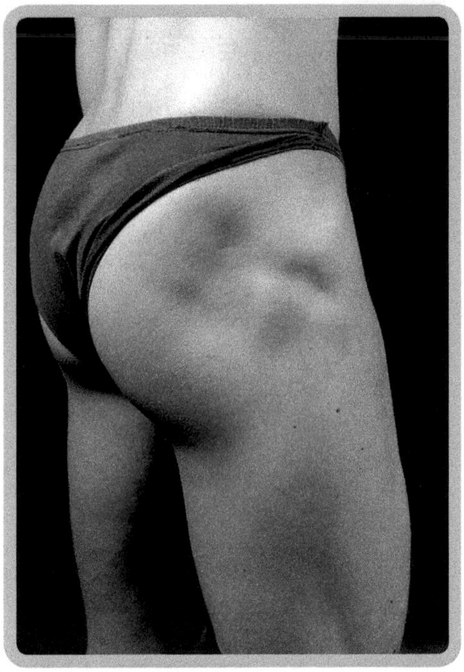

Fig. 8.57 Posterolateral view of the hip

The deep plane of the gluteal region contains the following:

- Gluteus minimus (Figs. 8.58 and 8.59)
- The pelvitrochanteric muscles:
  - Piriformis (Figs. 8.60–8.62)
  - Inferior and superior gemelli (Figs. 8.64 and 8.65)
  - Obturator internus (Figs. 8.63–8.65)
  - Quadratus femoris (Fig. 8.66)
  - Obturator externus (Fig. 8.67)

Note: Gluteus minimus is covered by the body of gluteus medius.
To approach the other muscles of the deep plane you must go through gluteus maximus.

ACTIONS

- **Actions of gluteus minimus:**
  - It medially rotates the thigh on the pelvis.
  - It abducts the thigh on the pelvis.
  - It stabilizes the pelvis in the coronal plane.
  - It takes part in flexion of the thigh on the pelvis.
- **Actions of the pelvitrochanteric muscles:**
  - They all laterally rotate the hip.
  - Piriformis abducts and stabilizes the hip when its fixed end is on the femur.
  - Quadratus femoris is an adductor.

Note: The pelvitrochanteric muscles are lateral rotators when the hip is extended. They are horizontal abductors when the hip is flexed.

INNERVATIONS

- Gluteus minimus: superior gluteal nerve (L4, L5, S1)
- Inferior gemellus and quadratus femoris: nerve to inferior gemellus and nerve to quadratus femoris (L4, L5, S1)
- Obturator externus: obturator nerve (L3–L5)
- Piriformis: nerve to piriformis (L5, S1, S2)
- Obturator internus and superior gemellus: nerve to obturator externus and nerve to superior gemellus (L5, S1, S2)

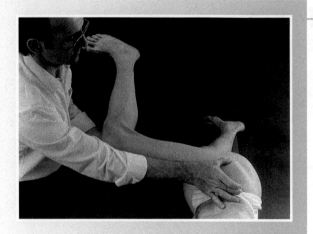

Fig. 8.58 Gluteus minimus

MA: Place your proximal hand (your palpating hand) between the superior border of the greater trochanter and the most anterior part of the iliac crest.

In this position your grip will straddle tensor fasciae latae between your thumb and your other fingers. In the palm of your distal hand, cradle the medial part of the subject's knee and support her entire leg.

From this starting position (hip and knee flexed at 90°) ask the subject to rotate her hip medially. In effect this movement results in the "elevation" of her leg. Under your fingers you will feel an undifferentiated muscle mass corresponding to tensor fasciae latae. Gluteus minimus and gluteus medius lie posterior and superior to this muscle mass.

Note: You cannot gain direct access to this muscle because it is overlain by the anterior fibers of gluteus medius, whose action is similar to that of gluteus minimus.

ATTACHMENTS

- Gluteus minimus arises from the gluteal surface of the iliac fossa anterior and distal to the curved semicircular anterior gluteal line.
- It is inserted into the anterior border of the greater trochanter.

Fig. 8.59 Another mode of approach

MA: The subject lies on her side with her contralateral hip and knee in the flexed position. Place one of your hands on the distal part of the lateral aspect of the leg (in order to resist any medial rotation of her hip). Your other hand will pick up the contraction of gluteus minimus through the body of gluteus medius.

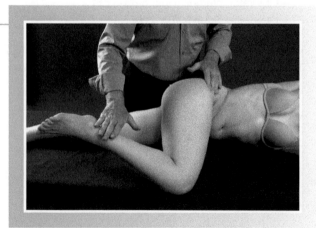

Fig. 8.60 Piriformis

ATTACHMENTS

- It arises from the anterior aspect of the second and third sacral vertebrae.
- It adheres to superior gemellus and is inserted into the superior border of the greater trochanter.

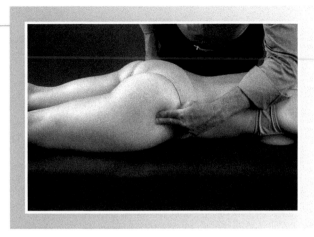

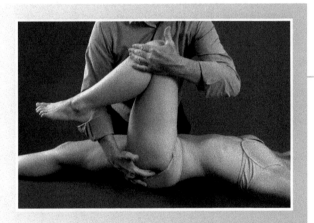

Fig. 8.61 Piriformis

MA: You can palpate piriformis in the gluteal region. To locate precisely the direction of this muscle, which lies deep to the gluteal muscles, you must keep in mind the following two bony landmarks: the superior border of the greater trochanter and the lateral border of the sacrum. Piriformis connects these two landmarks.

Fig. 8.62 Piriformis in a relaxed state

MA: With the subject lying prone and your hand placed facing the superior border of the greater trochanter, you can palpate piriformis transversely, just lateral to the lateral border of the sacrum.

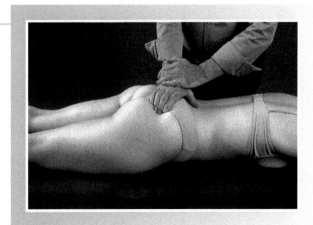

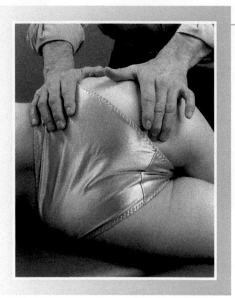

Fig. 8.63 Obturator internus

MA: When you palpate the lesser sciatic notch with the pads of two fingers, you will make contact with obturator internus, since it is at the level of the notch that the muscle is reflected.

ATTACHMENTS

The muscle arises from the medial surface of the obturator membrane, from the medial surface of the ischiopubic ramus, posterior to the insertion of the obturator membrane, and from the internal surface of the ilium between the obturator foramen and the arcuate line. It is inserted with the two gemelli anterior and superior to the trochanteric fossa, where obturator externus is also inserted.

Fig. 8.64 Inferior and superior gemelli and obturator internus

MA: Use both hands and a powerful grip at the level of the lesser sciatic notch. From this reference point you can move your grip toward the greater trochanter in order to contact the muscles you are looking for, i.e., the gemelli, which accompany the obturator internus right down to its femoral insertion.

ATTACHMENTS

- Superior gemellus arises from the lateral surface of the iliac spine.
- Inferior gemellus arises from the superior pole of the ischial tuberosity.
- These two muscles join the tendon of obturator internus before inserting together into the medial aspect of the greater trochanter.

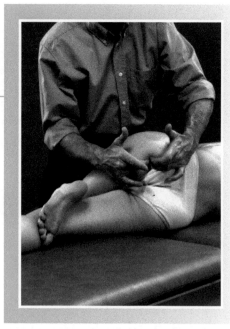

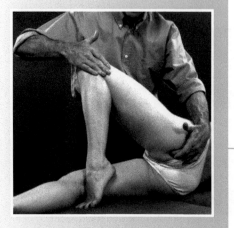

Fig. 8.65 Inferior and superior gemelli and obturator internus

MA: In the adjacent figure the practitioner's grip has moved into the gluteal region looking for the contraction of the muscles under investigation. These muscles are made to contract by applying resistance on the lateral surface of the subject's knee while she abducts her flexed hip horizontally.

Note: These three muscles lie caudal (distal) to piriformis.

Fig. 8.66 Quadratus femoris

MA: This muscle cannot be studied directly, for it lies deep to gluteus maximus. The essential bony landmarks are the ischial tuberosity medially and the greater trochanter laterally. The essential muscular landmark is the inferior border of gluteus maximus.

Place the subject on her side with her hip slightly flexed and prevent her from laterally rotating and abducting her hip by applying resistance on the lateral aspect of her knee. The body of the muscle you are looking for tightens under your fingers and is felt through the body of gluteus maximus, which must be perfectly relaxed, near its inferior border and between the two notable bony landmarks mentioned above.

Palpation is difficult in normal subjects.

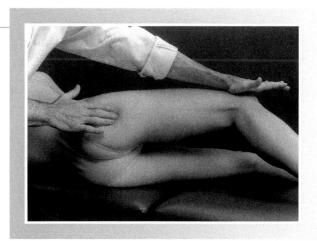

ATTACHMENTS

This muscle arises from the lateral aspect of the ischial tuberosity and is inserted into the posterior aspect of the greater trochanter lateral to the intertrochanteric line.

INNERVATION

• Nerve to quadratus femoris (L5, S1)

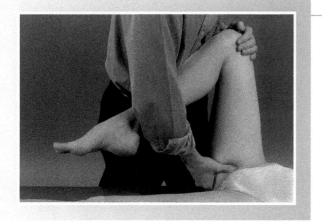

Fig. 8.67 Obturator externus

MA: With the subject's hip and knee flexed at 90°, place the thumb of your palpating hand between adductor longus and gracilis. With your right forearm, resist her lateral hip rotation, which you have asked her to perform as successive waves of contraction and relaxation. This muscular activity tightens the muscle in question, and you can feel it under your thumb. Your other hand helps maintain her lower limb in position.

ATTACHMENTS

• Obturator externus arises from the hip bone on the lateral surfaces of the bony rim of the obturator fossa and of the obturator membrane and also on the superior border of the ischiopubic ramus.
• It is inserted by a tendon into the trochanteric fossa on the medial aspect of the greater trochanter.

NERVES AND BLOOD VESSELS

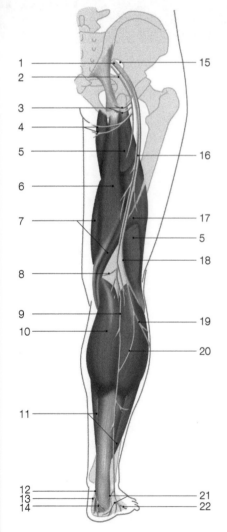

Sciatic and posterior femoral cutaneous nerves

1. Sciatic nerve
2. Posterior femoral cutaneous nerve
3. Inferior clunial nerves
4. Perineal branches
5. Long head of biceps femoris
6. Semitendinosus
7. Semimembranosus
8. Articular branch
9. Sural nerve
10. Medial head of gastrocnemius
11. Soleus
12. Tibial nerve
13. Medial and lateral plantar nerves
14. Medial calcaneal branches
15. Greater sciatic notch
16. Common fibular nerve splitting from sciatic nerve
17. Short head of biceps femoris
18. Common fibular nerve
19. Lateral sural cutaneous nerve
20. Sural communicating branch
21. Lateral calcaneal branches
22. Lateral dorsal cutaneous nerve

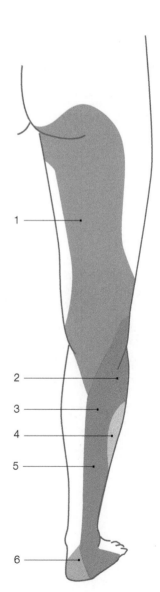

Sciatic and posterior femoral cutaneous nerves

1. Posterior femoral cutaneous nerve

Sciatic nerve:
2. Common fibular nerve via lateral sural cutaneous nerve
3. Medial sural cutaneous nerve
4. Superficial fibular nerve
5. Sural nerve
6. Tibial nerve via medial calcaneal branches

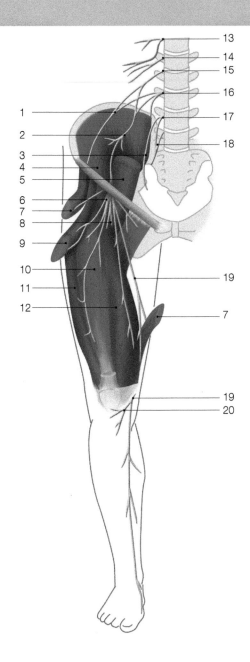

Femoral and lateral femoral cutaneous nerves

1. Lateral femoral cutaneous nerve
2. Femoral nerve
3. Obturator nerve
4. Iliacus
5. Psoas major
6. Articular branch
7. Sartorius
8. Anterior cutaneous branches of femoral nerve
9. Rectus femoris
10. Vastus intermedius
11. Vastus lateralis
12. Vastus medialis
13. T12
14. L1
15. L2
16. L3
17. L4
18. Lumbosacral trunk
19. Saphenous nerve
20. Infrapatellar branch of saphenous nerve

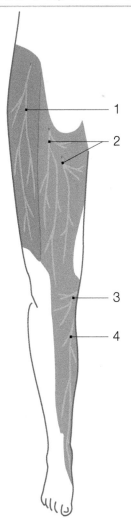

Cutaneous nerves of the thigh

1. Lateral femoral cutaneous nerve
2. Anterior cutaneous branches of femoral nerve
3. Infrapatellar branch of saphenous nerve
4. Medial crural cutaneous nerves (branches of saphenous nerve)

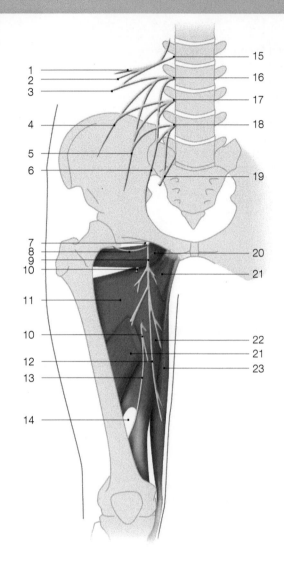

Obturator nerve

1. Iliohypogastric nerve
2. Ilio-inguinal nerve
3. Genitofemoral nerve
4. Lateral femoral cutaneous nerve
5. Femoral nerve
6. Obturator nerve
7. Posterior branch
8. Articular branch
9. Anterior branch
10. Posterior branch
11. Adductor brevis
12. Cutaneous branch
13. Articular branch of the knee
14. Opening in adductor magnus
15. L1
16. L2
17. L3
18. L4
19. Lumbosacral trunk
20. Obturator externus
21. Adductor longus
22. Adductor magnus
23. Gracilis

- The posterior part of adductor magnus is supplied by the sciatic nerve.
- Pectineus (an adductor) is supplied by the femoral nerve.

Obturator nerve
Cutaneous innervation

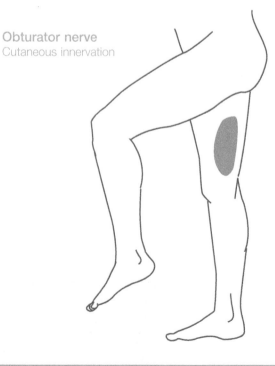

Dermatomes of the lower limb

Anterior view

Posterior view

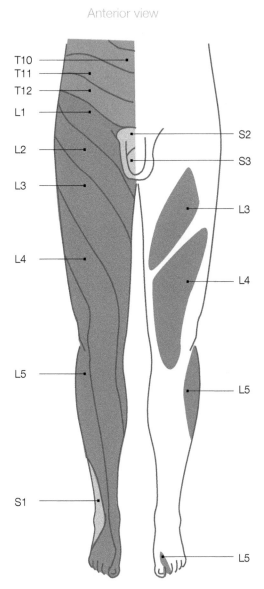

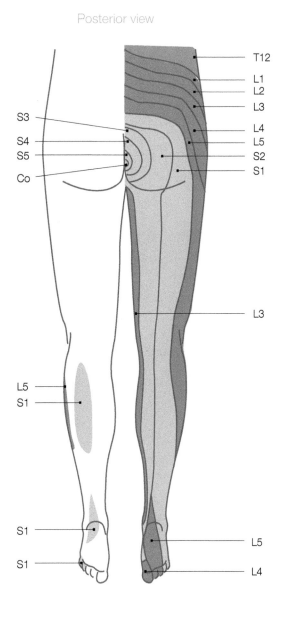

Co – Coccygeal

THE MEDIAL INGUINAL REGION

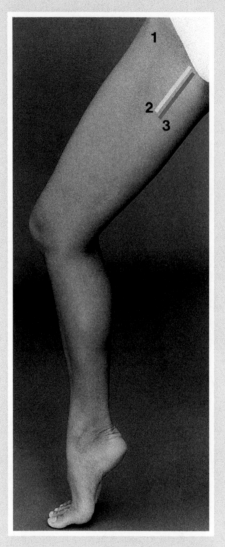

Fig. 8.68 Medial view of the thigh

1. Sartorius
2. Femoral nerve (Figs. 8.70–8.72)
3. Femoral artery (Fig. 8.69)

Fig. 8.69 The femoral artery

MA: Place two fingers along the artery and lightly compress it at the midpoint of an imaginary line running from the anterior superior iliac spine to the pubic tubercle. You can feel the arterial pulse better when the subject's hip is in the neutral position or is slightly extended.

Note: Adjacent to the artery and medial to it your finger can also feel under the skin two small and more or less round structures: they are the superficial inguinal lymph nodes.

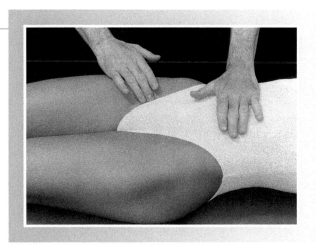

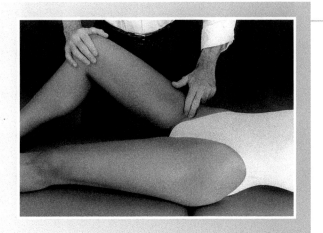

Fig. 8.70 The femoral nerve: stage 1

MA: This nerve is of mixed origin consisting of the roots of L2–L4. Just as you did for the femoral pulse (see Fig. 8.69), place the pads of two fingers at the midpoint of an imaginary line running from the anterior superior iliac spine to the pubic tubercle.

To stretch the nerve: as the subject lies supine, gradually and passively extend her hip on her pelvis while keeping her knee flexed, and place your other hand on the sacrum to stabilize her pelvis.

Note: The subject can keep her lower limb in the neutral position for hip flexion-extension, i.e., lying flat on the table and not with hip and knee flexed, as shown in the adjacent figure.

CLINICAL NOTE

Femoral nerve lesions

Its dermatome includes the anteromedial aspect of the thigh and of the knee as well as the medial part of the leg and the medial border of the foot (with the exception of the big toe).

Its myotome includes iliopsoas, sartorius, pectineus, and quadriceps.

Any abnormal sensitivity in its dermatome and/or any detection of weakness in one or more of the muscles in its myotome will indicate a lesion in the nerve. A weaker knee-jerk reflex will confirm the presence of a lesion.

Causation: Two examples include cycling (prolonged sitting with the trunk flexed) and a hip prosthesis.

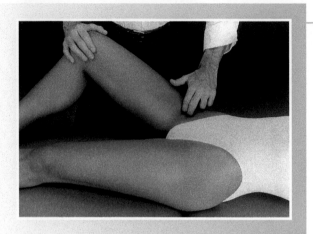

Fig. 8.71 The femoral nerve: stage 2

MA: Next you need only move your grip laterally by one finger-breadth toward sartorius to reach the structure you are after. You must approach it cautiously with the pads of your fingers, using a hooklike grip as shown in the figure, with all the care needed for such a structure. Your fingers will feel the nerve as a full cylindrical cord.

Fig. 8.72 The lateral femoral cutaneous nerve

MA: This is a sensory nerve that arises from the roots of L2 and L3 and then exits the abdominal cavity by passing under the inguinal ligament medial to sartorius, which it then crosses mediolaterally at the level of the greater innominate notch (the space between the two anterior iliac spines). In order to palpate the nerve, tighten sartorius (1) by resisting the subject as she flexes her hip, and roll the nerve (2) under your fingers as it crosses the anterior surface of that muscle before supplying the gluteal region on the posterior aspect of the thigh and the anterolateral aspect of the thigh down to the knee.

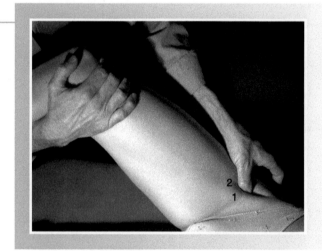

CLINICAL NOTE

Lesions of the femoral cutaneous nerve

Its dermatome includes the anterolateral aspect of the thigh from the anterior superior iliac spine down to the superolateral portion of the patella.

In taking a clinical history, look for sensory disturbances (hypo-/hyper sensitivity, sensation of pins and needles) and discomfort in wearing clothes radiating atypically to the thigh, the buttocks, the scrotum, or the labium maius.

To stretch the nerve: with the subject lying on her side, extend and posteriorly adduct her lower limb while you stand behind her.

Palpation with pressure applied inferior and medial to the anterior superior iliac spine will elicit sensory disturbances.

Causation:

- direct blows to the anterior superior iliac spine (soccer and rugby);

- compression of the nerve by a belt;

- hypertonicity of the abdominal muscles;

- gynoid type of obesity: excessive amounts of fat compressing the nerve.

THE GLUTEAL REGION

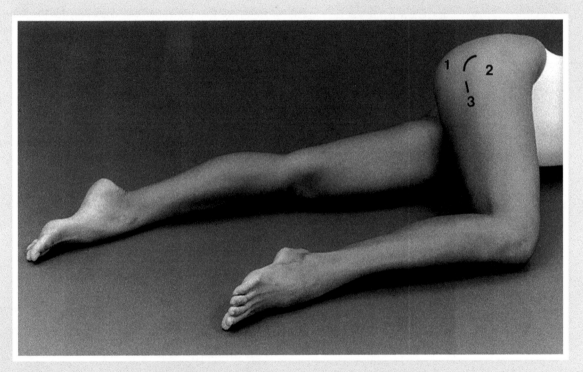

Fig. 8.73 The sciatic nerve in the gluteal region

1. Ischial tuberosity (Fig. 8.74)
2. Greater trochanter (Fig. 8.75)
3. Sciatic nerve (Figs. 8.74–8.77)

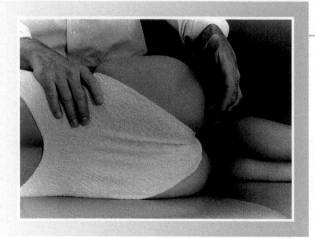

Fig. 8.74 Locating the sciatic nerve – stage 1: looking for the ischial tuberosity

MA: The sciatic nerve is a composite nerve originating from the roots of L4, L5, S1, and S2. It exits the pelvis via the greater sciatic notch and passes between the inferior border of piriformis and the superior border of the sacrospinous ligament. Stuck as it is to the ischial spine, it lies anterior to the inferior gluteal nerve.

The following are the four zones of vulnerability for the nerve (where you will need to look for pain elicited by palpation with pressure):

• its passage through the sciatic notch;
• when it runs deep to piriformis;
• when it runs close to the ischial tuberosity;
• at the bottom of the buttock between gluteus maximus and the long head of biceps femoris.

MA: In the position shown, the subject's hip is flexed and the ischial tuberosity is normally free of gluteus maximus. Place the pads of your middle and ring fingers as indicated in the adjacent figure.

Fig. 8.75 Locating the sciatic nerve – stage 2: looking for the greater trochanter

MA: While still keeping your fingers in the same position, place your thumb on the greater trochanter.

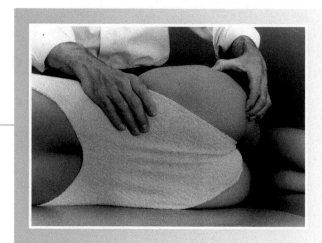

Fig. 8.76 Locating the sciatic nerve – stage 3

MA: Imagine a line running from the two bony structures you have located and position your index finger roughly at the midpoint. This is the location of the sciatic nerve.

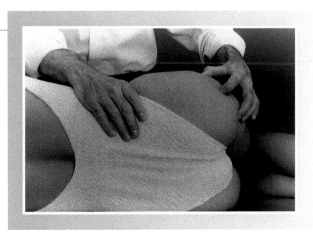

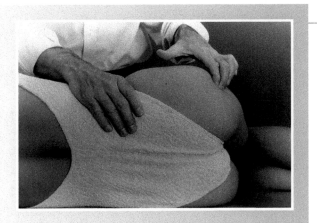

Fig. 8.77 The sciatic nerve: stage 4

MA: At this level the nerve has a diameter of about one finger-breadth. You must approach it cautiously crosswise using the pads of two fingers.

Note: You can gain access to the nerve only if the body shape of the subject is favorable and through a perfectly relaxed gluteus maximus. Then your fingers will be able to feel the nerve as a full cylindrical cord.

CLINICAL NOTE

Lesions of the sciatic nerve

Its dermatome is the posterior part of the thigh. Investigate this region using palpation with pressure so as to elicit possible sensory disturbances.

Its myotome includes semitendinosus, semimembranosus, the vertical or posterior bundle of adductor magnus, and biceps femoris.

Any testing revealing weakness in one or all of these muscles is significant. Do not forget to stretch the nerve by passively flexing the subject's hip. Knee extension (with the patient lying prone) will cause a sharp pain in the posterior aspect of the thigh.

9

The thigh

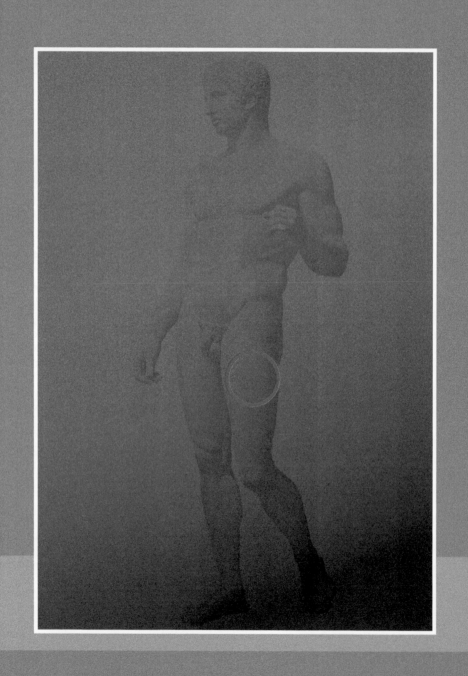

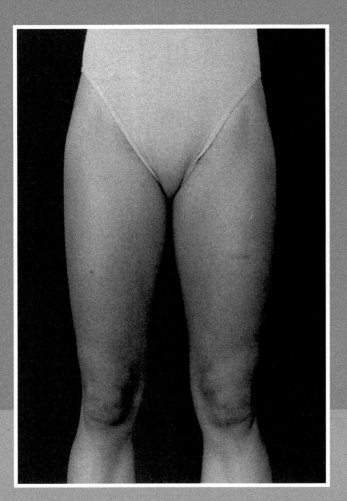 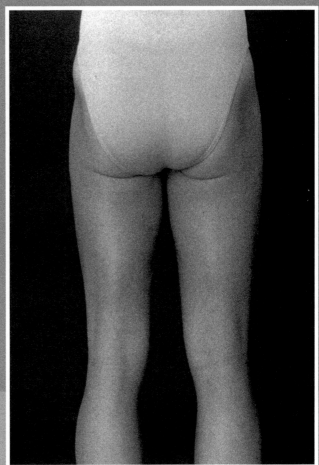

MYOLOGY

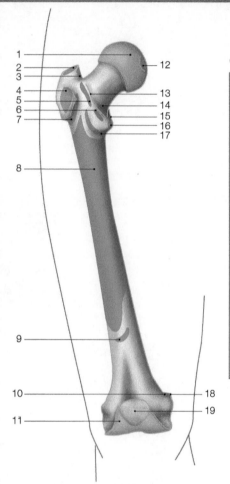

Osteology of the femur (anterior view)

1. Femoral head
2. Piriformis
3. Obturator internus and superior and inferior gemelli
4. Gluteus minimus
5. Iliofemoral ligament
6. Pubofemoral ligament
7. Vastus lateralis
8. Vastus intermedius
9. Articularis genus
10. Adductor magnus
11. Patellar surface
12. Fovea capitis
13. Intertrochanteric line
14. Femoral neck
15. Lesser trochanter
16. Psoas major
17. Vastus medialis
18. Tubercle of adductor magnus
19. Patella

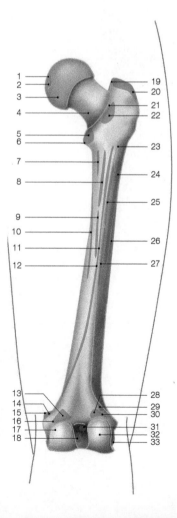

Osteology of the femur (posterior view)

1. Fovea capitis
2. Ligament of head of femur
3. Femoral head
4. Femoral neck
5. Iliopsoas
6. Lesser trochanter
7. Pectineus
8. Adductor brevis
9. Adductor longus
10. Vastus medialis
11. Adductor magnus
12. Medial supracondylar line

13. Medial head of gastrocnemius
14. Adductor magnus
15. Adductor tubercle
16. Supracondylar tubercle
17. Medial condyle
18. Posterior cruciate ligament
19. Obturator externus
20. Gluteus medius
21. Intertrochanteric crest
22. Quadratus femoris
23. Gluteal tuberosity

24. Vastus lateralis
25. Gluteus maximus
26. Vastus intermedius
27. Short head of biceps femoris
28. Lateral head of gastrocnemius
29. Plantaris
30. Lateral supracondylar tubercle
31. Anterior cruciate ligament
32. Lateral condyle
33. Popliteus

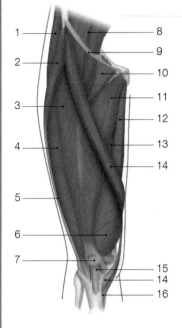

Anterior muscles of thigh

1. Gluteus medius
2. Tensor fasciae latae
3. Rectus femoris
4. Vastus lateralis
5. Iliotibial tract
6. Vastus medialis
7. Patella
8. Iliopsoas
9. Inguinal ligament
10. Pectineus
11. Adductor longus
12. Gracilis
13. Adductor magnus
14. Sartorius
15. Patellar ligament
16. Semimembranosus

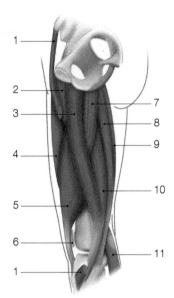

Medial muscles of thigh

1. Sartorius
2. Adductor longus
3. Gracilis
4. Rectus femoris
5. Vastus medialis
6. Patella
7. Adductor magnus
8. Semitendinosus
9. Biceps femoris
10. Semimembranosus
11. Gastrocnemius

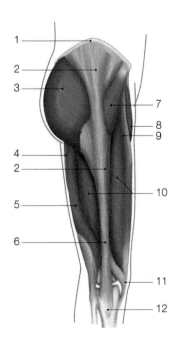

Iliotibial tract (lateral view)

1. Iliac crest
2. Gluteal aponeurosis
3. Gluteus maximus
4. Semitendinosus
5. Biceps femoris
6. Iliotibial tract
7. Tensor fasciae latae
8. Sartorius
9. Rectus femoris
10. Vastus lateralis
11. Patella
12. Lateral tibial condyle

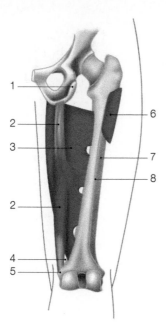

Adductor magnus (posterior view)

1. Ischial tuberosity
2. Posterior bundle
3. Anterior bundle
4. Adductor hiatus
5. Adductor tubercle
6. Gluteus maximus
7. Femur
8. Linea aspera

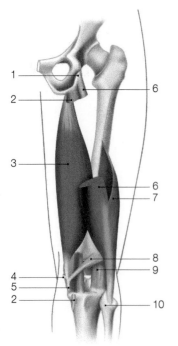

Hamstring muscles (semitendinosus and rectus femoris partially resected)

1. Ischial tuberosity
2. Semitendinosus
3. Semimembranosus
4. Medial expansion
5. Main tendon of insertion
6. Long head of biceps femoris
7. Short head of biceps femoris
8. Lateral expansion
9. Articular capsule
10. Fibular head

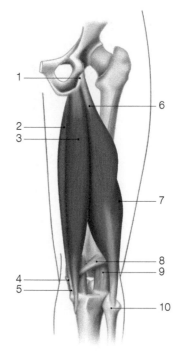

Hamstring muscles

1. Ischial tuberosity
2. Semimembranosus
3. Semitendinosus
4. Medial expansion
5. Main tendon of insertion
6. Long head of biceps femoris
7. Short head of biceps femoris
8. Lateral expansion
9. Articular capsule
10. Fibular head

THE ANTERIOR FEMORAL REGION: THE MUSCLES OF THE ANTERIOR COMPARTMENT

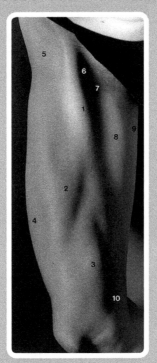

Fig. 9.3 Anteromedial view of the thigh

1. Sartorius (Figs. 9.4–9.8)
2. Rectus femoris (Figs. 9.18–9.20)
3. Vastus medialis (Figs. 9.13 and 9.14)
4. Vastus lateralis (Figs. 9.15–9.17)
5. Tensor fasciae latae (Figs. 9.21 and 9.26)
6. Iliopsoas
7. Pectineus
8. Adductor longus
9. Gracilis
10. The distal tendon of adductor magnus inserting into the adductor tubercle on the medial condyle and running between vastus intermedius and sartorius when the knee is flexed.

This region comprises the following muscles of the anterior compartment:

- Sartorius
- Quadriceps femoris, consisting of:
  - vastus medialis
  - vastus lateralis
  - rectus femoris
  - vastus intermedius and the articularis genus (neither mentioned further in this book)
- Tensor fasciae latae and iliotibial tract

Note: This last muscle can be classified equally as belonging to the superficial plane of the muscles of the gluteal region with gluteus maximus.

319

Sartorius

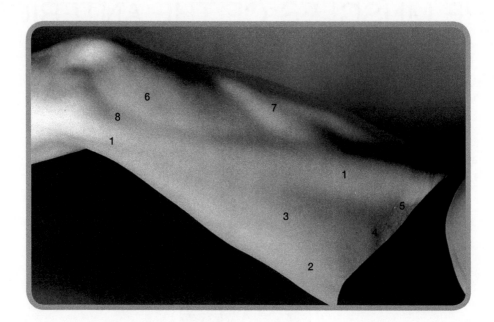

Fig. 9.4 Sartorius: medial view of sartorius and visualization of its relations with other thigh muscles

1. Sartorius (Figs. 9.5–9.8)
2. Gracilis
3. Adductor longus
4. Pectineus
5. Iliopsoas
6. Vastus medialis
7. Rectus femoris
8. Distal tendon of adductor magnus inserted into the medial condyle on the adductor tubercle

ACTIONS OF SARTORIUS

- It flexes, abducts, and laterally rotates the hip.
- It flexes and medially rotates the knee.
- It stabilizes the pelvis in the sagittal plane.
- It tilts the pelvis anteriorly.
- It stabilizes the knee laterally with the other anserine muscles (semitendinosus and gracilis).

INNERVATION

- Femoral nerve (L1–L3)

Fig. 9.5 Sartorius in its distal part

MA: Ask the subject to maintain an almost complete isometric extension of his knee associated with a slight flexion of the hip.

Then proceed with laterally rotating his hip slightly and applying resistance on the inferomedial extremity of his leg so as to counter hip adduction isometrically.

Note: Your proximal hand is shown "detaching" sartorius from vastus medialis (3). In this particular position of the lower limb, resistance applied to the distal part of the leg makes sartorius stand out at the level of the knee.

ATTACHMENTS

This muscle is inserted into the anteromedial aspect of the tibia along the tibial crest distal to the insertion of the patellar ligament. Its tendon of insertion lies anterior to the tendons of insertion of gracilis and semitendinosus, and together these tendons give rise to what are called the muscles of the pes anserinus.

> **CLINICAL NOTE**
>
> At the insertion of the muscle at the level of the pes anserinus the tendon and the underlying bursa may become inflamed.

1. Rectus femoris
2. Vastus lateralis
3. Vastus medialis
4. Pectineus
5. Tensor fasciae latae
6. Adductor longus
7. Gracilis
8. Sartorius

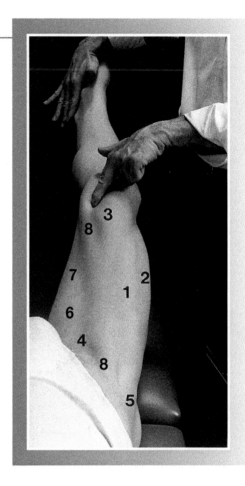

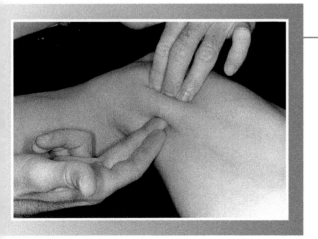

Fig. 9.6 Distal part of sartorius: medial view (knee half-flexed)

MA: By simply keeping the subject's knee in subtotal extension and his hip in slight lateral rotation you can bring out the body of the muscle in order to get hold of it on the medial aspect of the knee using a bimanual grip.

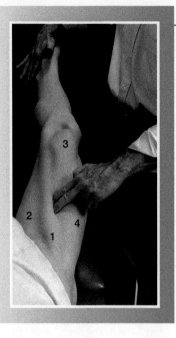

Fig. 9.7 Sartorius (1) in the thigh

MA: Use the method described in the preceding figure to tighten sartorius. When the muscle is not made to stand out, it appears as a flat muscle forming a sort of "depression" at the junction of the anterior and medial compartments of the thigh. It is bordered by the adductor muscles (2) medially, by vastus medialis (3) distally, and by rectus femoris (4) proximally and laterally.

Fig. 9.8 Sartorius (1) in its proximal part

MA: Use the same method as in Figure 9.6 to tighten the muscle. Its proximal part stands out near the anterior superior iliac spine (see Figs. 8.38-8.41).

In order to displace sartorius medially, place your contact in the depression between it and tensor fasciae latae (2). It is bounded medially by iliopsoas (3, not shown in the figure) and by pectineus (4).

ATTACHMENTS

This muscle arises from the lateral aspect of the anterior superior iliac spine anterior to the origin of tensor fasciae latae.

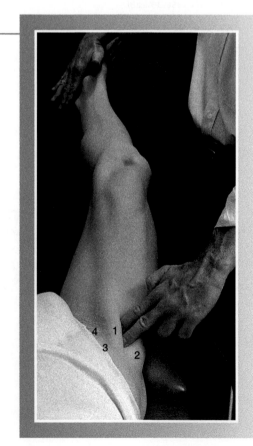

Quadriceps femoris

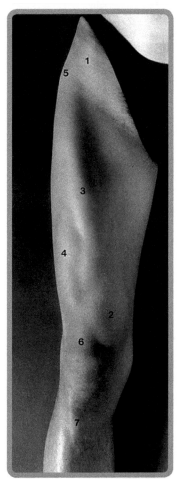

Fig. 9.9 Quadriceps femoris: anterior view of thigh

1. Sartorius
2. Vastus medialis (Figs. 9.10, 9.11, 9.13, and 9.14)
3. Rectus femoris
4. Vastus lateralis (Figs. 9.10, 9.11, 9.13, and 9.15–9.17)
5. Tensor fasciae latae
6. Quadriceps tendon (Figs. 9.10 and 9.11)
7. Patellar ligament (Figs. 9.11 and 9.12)

Note: Vastus intermedius, the deep muscle of the quadriceps, is not visible here.

ACTIONS OF QUADRICEPS FEMORIS

- It extends the knee on the thigh.
- The direct and crossed fibers of the vastus muscles contribute to knee stability in the coronal plane.
- Rectus femoris extends the leg on the thigh and flexes the thigh on the pelvis.

INNERVATION

- Femoral nerve (L2–L4)

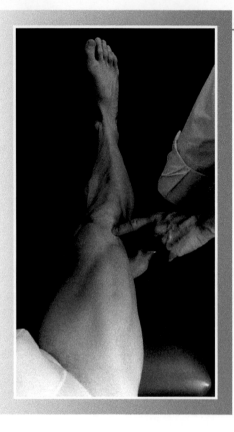

Fig. 9.10 Quadriceps tendon

MA: Place your hand under the subject's knee to make sure that the muscle contracts properly.

Ask him to contract and relax the quadriceps repeatedly, and ensure that he flattens your hand against the table. Then proceed with your investigation of the muscle proximal to the patella and between the vastus muscles.

ATTACHMENTS

This tendon is formed by the meeting of the four heads of the quadriceps: vasti lateralis, medialis, and intermedius, and rectus femoris. It is inserted as a common tendon into the patella. Rectus femoris, forming the superficial plane of this common tendon, and the vasti lateralis and medialis, forming its intermediate plane, contribute to the formation of the patellar ligament, which is inserted into the tibial tuberosity. The tendon of vastus intermedius forms the deep plane of this common tendon and is inserted into the posterior part of the base of the patella.

Fig. 9.11 Quadriceps tendon: close-up

1. Quadriceps tendon
2. Vastus medialis
3. Vastus lateralis
4. Patella
5. Patellar ligament
6. Tibial tuberosity

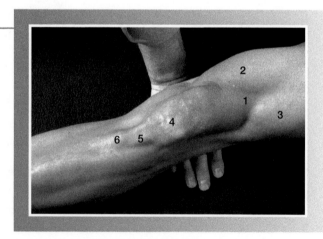

CLINICAL NOTE

Lesions of the quadriceps tendon

The tendon can be ruptured (in exceptional circumstances) above the base of the patella. On palpation you can clearly feel a transverse depression at this level. Clinical examination is more difficult the later it is performed.

On the other hand, overstretching of the quadriceps or microtears at the base of the patella or on its borders are much more frequent. Palpation of these structures will be painful.

Beware: Do not forget that an acutely painful patella may be the seat of a fracture.

Fig. 9.12 The patellar ligament

MA: You can approach it with the subject's knee flexed or extended. Grip its lateral borders between your thumb and index finger. Thus you will be better able to appreciate its slightly oblique course as it runs superoinferiorly and posteroanteriorly.

Note: The patellar ligament is a composite structure made up of both active superficial fibers from the quadriceps and deep passive fibers coming from the patellar apex.

> **CLINICAL NOTE**
> Palpation of this ligament can be painful as a result of a quadriceps tendinitis following an episode of intense biking or running.

1. Patellar apex
2. Patellar ligament
3. Patellar base

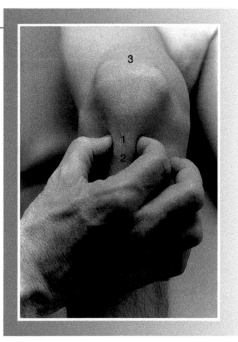

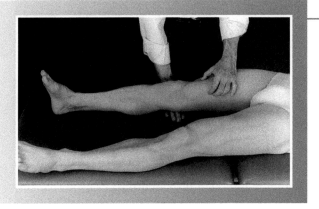

Fig. 9.13 Vastus medialis

MA: To bring out this muscle, ask the subject to extend his knee.

Now place one hand under his knee, with the back of your hand touching his popliteal fossa, and then ask him to flatten your hand against the table.

Use your other hand to investigate vastus medialis, which now stands out in the inferomedial part of the thigh.

Note: The main feature of vastus medialis is that it extends farther distally than vastus lateralis. There is a gap of about four fingerbreadths between their distal ends.

ATTACHMENTS

The site of origin of this muscle is the entire medial lip of the linea aspera and its proximal medial trifurcation, and it extends proximally up to the inferior limit of the intertrochanteric line.

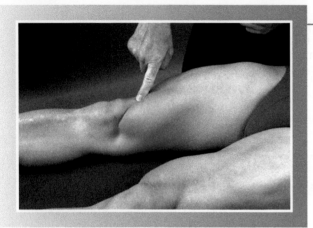

Fig. 9.14 Vastus medialis: close-up

MA: The practitioner's finger indicates vastus medialis, whose tendon takes part in the formation of the quadriceps tendon and has the unique feature of extending farther distally than the vastus lateralis.

Fig. 9.15 Vastus lateralis

MA: It lies on the lateral aspect of the thigh lateral to vastus intermedius, and its lateral aspect is overlain by the iliotibial tract.

To tighten it, use the method described for vastus medialis.

Note: Remember that this muscle extends beyond the posterior border of the iliotibial tract. In this figure the practitioner's hand indicates only the part of the muscle anterior to the iliotibial tract.

ATTACHMENTS

This muscle arises from a crest that bounds the anterior surface of the greater trochanter medially and inferiorly and from the entire lateral lip and the lateral border of the linea aspera.

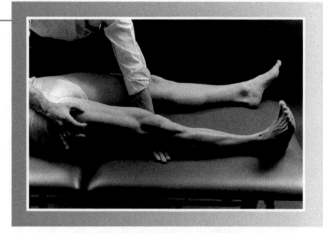

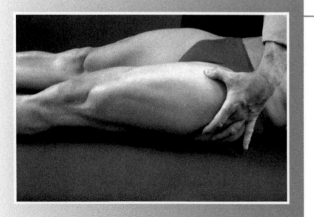

Fig. 9.16 Vastus lateralis: proximal part

MA: Do not forget that the proximal part of vastus lateralis, as indicated by the practitioner's thumb and index finger, extends beyond the margins of the iliotibial tract anteriorly and posteriorly.

Fig. 9.17 Vastus lateralis: distal part

MA: The distal part of vastus lateralis lies anterior to the tendon of the iliotibial tract and joins the common quadriceps tendon.

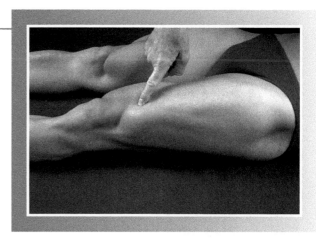

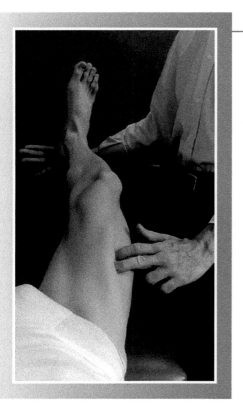

Fig. 9.18 Rectus femoris in the thigh

MA: Ask the subject to flex his hip slightly and to extend his knee partially.

Place your hand under his heel in order to modulate these two movements. Ask the subject to contract his quadriceps isometrically and to maintain this contraction.

In most subjects the muscle stands out in the middle of the thigh between vastus medialis medially and vastus lateralis laterally. In others you must look for the contracted muscle through a rather thick layer of adipose tissue.

CLINICAL NOTE

Of all the quadriceps muscles the rectus is the most often afflicted by injuries: muscle pull, microtears, and especially muscle rupture with hemorrhage.

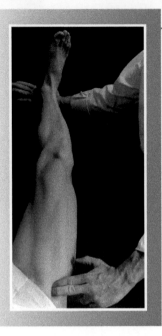

Fig. 9.19 Rectus femoris in its proximal part

MA: Ask the subject to flex his hip and partially extend his knee in order to make the muscle stand out better. Place your distal hand under his heel to control the movements required. Have him raise his heel a little from your supporting hand, and the body of the muscle will contract between sartorius medially and tensor fasciae latae laterally (see Figs. 8.38-8.42).

Note: At this level the body of the muscle slides in between the two above-mentioned muscles to form the floor of the lateral inguinofemoral region.

ATTACHMENT

• It arises from the anterior inferior iliac spine and from the floor of the supra-acetabular groove.
• It is inserted into the base of the patella and the tibial tuberosity.

Fig. 9.20 Rectus femoris, another view

MA: In this figure the muscle is being palpated in the proximal third of the thigh.

1. Rectus femoris
2. Tensor fasciae latae
3. Sartorius

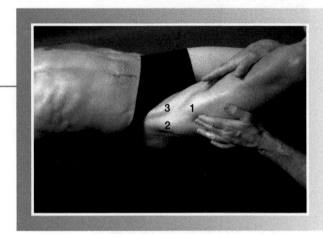

Tensor fasciae latae

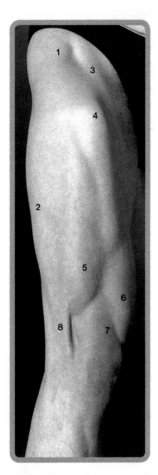

Fig. 9.21 Anterolateral view of the thigh

1. Tensor fasciae latae (Fig. 9.26)
2. Iliotibial tract (Figs. 9.22–9.25)
3. Sartorius
4. Rectus femoris
5. Vastus lateralis
6. Vastus medialis
7. Quadriceps tendon
8. Tendon of iliotibial tract (Figs. 9.24 and 9.27)
9. Gluteus maximus
10. Biceps femoris

ACTIONS OF TENSOR FASCIAE LATAE

- It flexes, abducts, and medially rotates the thigh on the pelvis.
- It extends the leg on the thigh and laterally rotates the leg on the thigh when the knee is flexed.
- It stabilizes the knee in the transverse plane in equilibrium with the anserine muscles.

INNERVATION

- Gluteal nerve (L4, L5, S1)

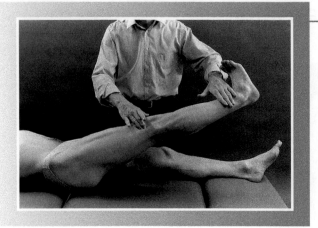

Fig. 9.22 The iliotibial tract in its distal part

MA: With the subject's hip extended and knee slightly flexed, you must resist his hip abduction by placing your hand at the distal end of the lower limb you are investigating proximal to the lateral malleolus. This maneuver will make the space of the lateral femorotibial joint "gap." As a result, the tract is stretched, since it is inserted distal to the joint space mentioned. As it nears the knee, the tract forms a veritable tendon, which stands out prominently, especially in male subjects.

Note: You can also ask the subject to rotate his hip medially as he abducts it, with the effect of making the tract even more visible.

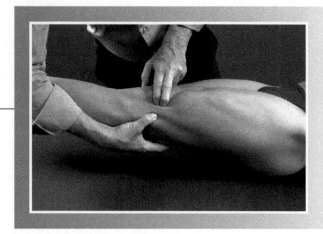

Fig. 9.23 The iliotibial tract: another view

MA: This is a close-up of the distal tendon of the iliotibial tract on its way to its insertion into Gerdy's tubercle.

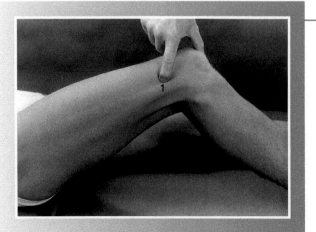

Fig. 9.24 The tendon of the iliotibial tract

MA: With the subject's knee flexed and his foot resting on the table, just ask him to initiate knee extension, and the iliotibial tract (1) will either stand out or become palpable on the lateral part of the knee. Active medial rotation of the leg will bring the tract into further prominence, because it is stretched by this movement. You can likewise ask him to extend his knee fully so as to make the tract stand out even more.

Fig. 9.25 The iliotibial tract in the thigh

MA: Use the same technique as in Figure 9.22.

It is important to remember that the tract lies in the lateral part of the thigh and that vastus lateralis extends beyond its anterior and posterior margins.

Note: Resistance applied by your distal hand on the leg allows the tract to stand out more prominently.

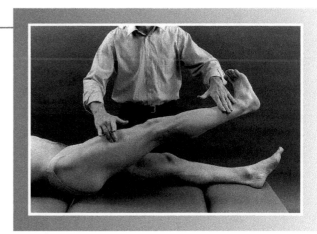

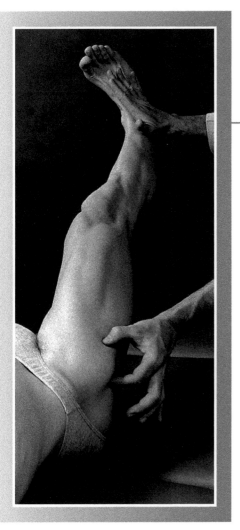

Fig. 9.26 Tensor fasciae latae

MA: With the subject's hip slightly flexed and medially rotated, you need only resist isometrically his hip abduction by applying resistance to the distal extremity of his lower limb proximal to the lateral malleolus. In this position the muscle is preferentially recruited as an abductor and flexor of the hip. As you recruit its third action (as a medial rotator) by asking the subject to alternate his hip rotations repeatedly, the body of the muscle becomes easier to locate. It is felt between the anterior superior iliac spine and the anterior border of the greater trochanter anterior to gluteus medius.

Note: Take care not to mistake tensor fasciae latae for gluteus medius. In the figure the practitioner's grip demarcates the most distal part of the muscle, as it lies deep to gluteus medius.

ATTACHMENTS

- Proximally, it arises from the external surface of the anterior superior iliac spine and from the anterior extremity of the lateral lip of the iliac crest.
- Distally, its body adheres to the proximal quarter of the anterior border of the iliotibial tract, which then becomes its tendon of insertion into Gerdy's tubercle on the lateral tibial condyle.

Note: Do not forget that vastus lateralis arises posterior to the tensor from the lateral border of the linea aspera and can be palpated at this level.

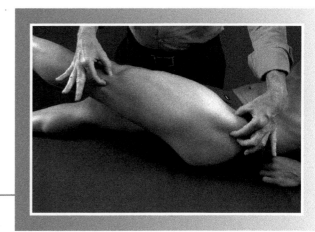

Fig. 9.27 The tendon of the iliotibial tract, global view

MA: The practitioner is seen palpating both tensor fasciae latae (left hand) and the tendon of the iliotibial tract (right hand).

THE POSTERIOR FEMORAL REGION

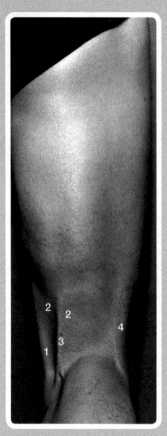

Fig. 9.28 Posterior view of the thigh

1. Gracilis
2. Semimembranosus
3. Tendon of semitendinosus
4. Tendon of biceps femoris

This region comprises the medial and posterior muscle groups.

The medial group includes:

- the five adductor muscles:
  - pectineus (Fig. 9.30)
  - adductor longus (Fig. 9.31)
  - adductor brevis (Fig. 9.32)
  - adductor magnus (Figs. 9.33–9.36)
  - gracilis (Figs. 9.37–9.43)

The posterior group includes:

- the two medial hamstring (ischiocrural) muscles:
  - semitendinosus (Figs. 9.43–9.48, and 9.53–9.55)
  - semimembranosus (Figs. 9.43, 9.44, and 9.46–9.52)
- the lateral hamstring muscle:
  - biceps femoris – long and short heads (Figs. 9.56–9.62)

Note: Only the long head of biceps femoris is a true ischiocrural muscle.

The medial muscle group

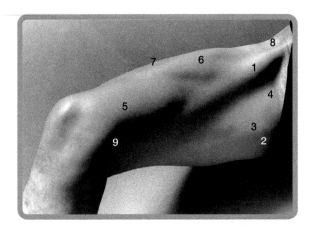

Fig. 9.29 **Medial view of the hip**

1. Sartorius
2. Gracilis (Figs. 9.37–9.43)
3. Adductor longus (Fig. 9.31)
4. Pectineus (Fig. 9.30)
5. Vastus medialis
6. Rectus femoris
7. Vastus lateralis
8. Tensor fasciae latae
9. Distal tendon of insertion of adductor magnus: insertion into the adductor tubercle on the medial tibial condyle (Figs. 9.33–9.36)

This muscle group, located in the posterior femoral region, comprises:

- The four adductors, arranged in three planes:
  - the superficial plane, made up of pectineus and adductor longus
  - the middle plane, containing adductor brevis (Fig. 9.32)
  - the deep plane, containing adductor magnus
- Gracilis.

ACTIONS OF THE ADDUCTOR MUSCLES

- They adduct the thigh on the pelvis.
- They laterally rotate the thigh on the pelvis – except for the medial bundle (also known as the inferior or vertical bundle of adductor magnus), which takes part in medial rotation.
- Apart from the vertical bundle, all these muscles contribute to flexion of the thigh on the pelvis and can become extensors beyond a certain degree of flexion (45°).
- They stabilize the pelvis by balancing out the abductors.

INNERVATIONS

- Pectineus: femoral nerve and obturator nerve (L2–L4)
- Adductor longus: obturator nerve and femoral nerve (L2–L4)
- Adductor brevis: obturator nerve (L2–L4)
- Adductor magnus (Figs. 9.33–9.36):
  - adductor bundles: obturator nerve (L2–L4)
  - vertical bundle: sciatic nerve (L4, L5, S1)

The adductor muscles

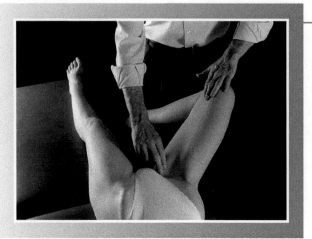

Fig. 9.30 Pectineus

MA: This muscle lies anterior to adductor brevis between iliopsoas laterally and adductor longus medially.

With the subject's knee and thigh flexed, slightly resist her hip adduction isometrically.

A triangular depression with its base lying superiorly will appear in the proximal part of the thigh: it corresponds as a whole to the muscle you are after.

ATTACHMENTS

- The pectineus arises in two planes, superficial and deep:
  - Its superficial fibers arise from the iliopectineal line between the iliopubic eminence and the pubic tubercle.
  - Its deep fibers arise from the anterior lip of the obturator groove.
- It is inserted into the superior part of the intermediate lip of the trifurcated linea aspera.

Fig. 9.31 Adductor longus

MA: First, the subject flexes her knee and hip and abducts her hip horizontally. The practitioner then places his right hand on the medial aspect of her thigh and uses his forearm to resist the subject as she tries to adduct her hip horizontally at his request.

This double maneuver helps to bring out, on the medial aspect of the thigh, a sizable muscular mass, which is none other than the muscle you are looking for.

ATTACHMENTS

- Adductor longus arises from the pubic angle and from the inferior aspect of the pubic tubercle by a narrow, thick, and flattened tendon (medial and inferior to pectineus and superior to adductor brevis).
- It is inserted distal to the middle section of the linea aspera.

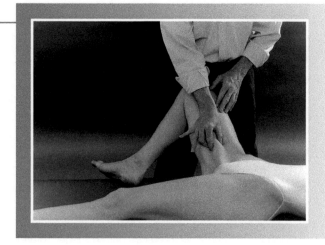

Fig. 9.32 Adductor brevis

MA: Using a cradling hold, progressively abduct the subject's lower limb at the thigh against a slight resistance on her part. Gracilis (1) shows up like a rope along the medial border of the thigh. You must then slide your fingers between this muscle and adductor longus (2) as far proximally as possible in order to come into contact with adductor brevis, particularly its inferior bundle.

Note: In female subjects adipose tissue generally masks the muscular landmark offered by gracilis, but your approach remains the same. First you need only abduct maximally the lower limb you are working on, and after this extreme position is reached, you must then resist her active hip adduction. This modification allows you to locate gracilis better and to slide your fingers between gracilis and adductor longus.

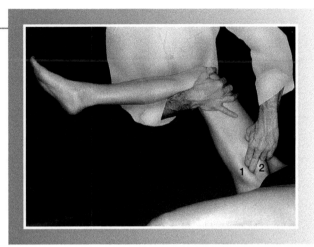

ATTACHMENTS

- Adductor brevis arises anterior and cranial to adductor magnus on the quadrilateral surface of the pubis and the adjoining part of the ischiopubic ramus between the origins of obturator externus and of gracilis.
- It is inserted via two bundles:
  - a superior bundle inserted lateral to the superior intermediate ridge of the linea aspera;
  - an inferior bundle inserted into the superior part of the groove of the linea aspera.

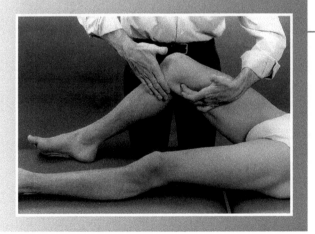

Fig. 9.33 The distal tendon of the posterior or vertical bundle of adductor magnus

MA: The essential bony landmark is the adductor tubercle. The essential muscular landmark is vastus medialis. The tendon you are after lies posterior to that muscle and feels on palpation like a relatively thick, solid, cylindrical cord.

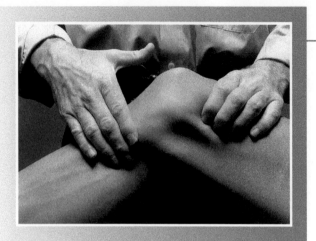

Fig. 9.35 Adductor magnus: external part of its superior bundle

MA: The method of tightening the "landmark" muscles is the same as that described above. You need only slide your proximal hand between adductor longus and gracilis (2) and proceed posteriorly beyond the medial part of the thigh in order to encounter the muscle you are after.

Note: Remember that the superior bundle of adductor magnus arises from the ischial tuberosity, which is a very posterior structure.

ATTACHMENTS

The lateral portion of the muscle splits into two bundles, superior and intermediate. The superior bundle arises from the middle third of the ischiopubic ramus and is inserted into the medial lip of the lateral trifurcation of the linea aspera.

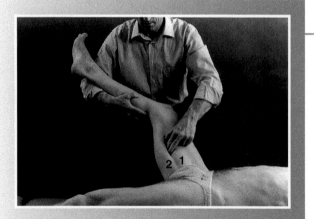

Fig. 9.34 Adductor magnus: posterior or vertical bundle (in its distal part)

MA: The bony landmark is the adductor tubercle (see Fig. 10.21) and the muscular structure of note is vastus medialis.

After locating the posterior part of vastus medialis, look for the tendon of adductor magnus, which your fingers will feel as a full cylindrical cord.

ATTACHMENTS

• It arises from the posterior inferior part of the ischial tuberosity.
• It is inserted into the adductor tubercle.

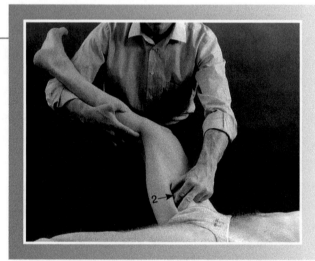

Fig. 9.36 Adductor magnus: the external part of its intermediate bundle

MA: Using a cradling hold, abduct the subject's hip so far as to stretch the adductors you are interested in, in particular adductor longus (1) and gracilis (2).

Slide your palpating hand between these two muscles and, as shown in the adjacent figure, it will encounter the external aspect of the intermediate bundle of adductor magnus, that portion of the muscle that distally overshoots adductor longus and is contiguous with the middle part of the medial portion (the vertical bundle) of adductor magnus.

ATTACHMENTS

The external part of the intermediate bundle (see preceding figure) arises proximally from the ischiopubic ramus and from the external surface of the ischium and is inserted distally into the full length of the groove of the linea aspera.

1. Adductor longus
2. Gracilis

Gracilis

Fig. 9.37 Posteromedial view of the thigh

1. Gracilis
2. Vastus medialis
3. Distal tendon of insertion of adductor magnus into the medial tibial condyle on the adductor tubercle
4. Semitendinosus
5. Semimembranosus
6. Biceps femoris
7. Gluteus maximus

ACTIONS OF GRACILIS

- It flexes and medially rotates the knee.
- It adducts and medially rotates the hip.

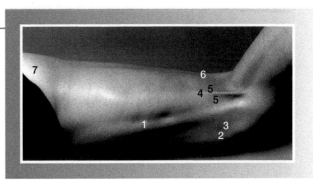

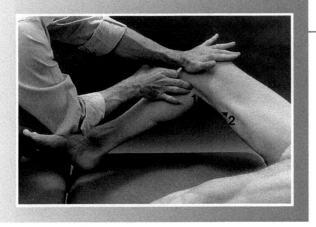

Fig. 9.38 Gracilis: its distal part on the medial tibial border

MA: The subject lies on his back with hip and knees flexed. Ask him to actively rotate his knee medially while isometrically flexing the same joint (by dragging his heel on the table toward his buttocks). Make contact with the posteromedial border of the medial tibial condyle, and your middle finger will lie opposite the tendon you are looking for. Your ring finger now faces semitendinosus (1). Semimembranosus (2) extends on both sides of the semitendinosus tendon and anterior to it.

ATTACHMENTS

Gracilis is inserted into the superior part of the medial aspect of the tibia posterior to sartorius, which lies on top of it, and proximal to semitendinosus.

INNERVATION

- Obturator nerve (L2, L3)

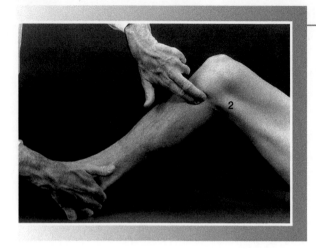

Fig. 9.39 The distal tendon of gracilis

MA: The bony landmark is the same, i.e., the medial border of the tibia, where you have placed your fingers. With your other hand, resist the subject as she flexes and medially rotates his knee by cradling his heel in your palm and pressing your forearm against the medial border of his foot.

You can now feel the tendon you wish to investigate (2) lying proximal to the semitendinosus tendon and posterior to sartorius, which may partially overlap it. The approach may be difficult. Looking for this tendon is relatively easy in a man but much more difficult in a woman because of the amount of adipose tissue present. In this case look for it using a more posterior approach.

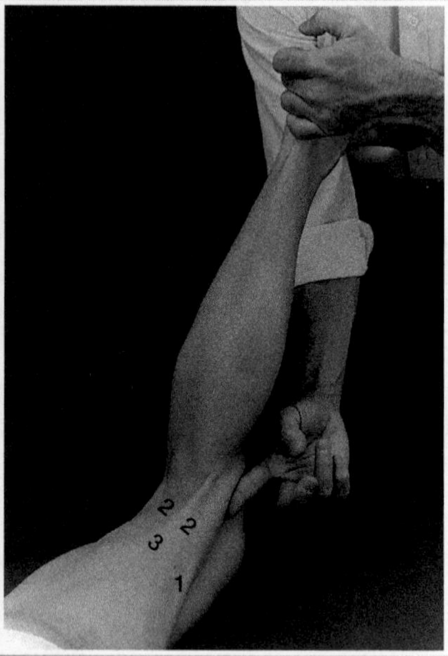

Fig. 9.40 The gracilis tendon

MA: The gracilis tendon stands out anterior and medial to the semitendinosus tendon.

1. Gracilis tendon
2. Semimembranosus tendon
3. Semitendinosus tendon

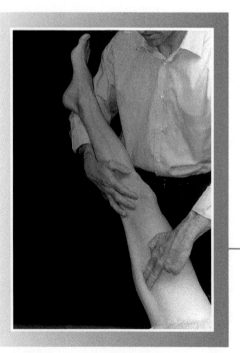

Fig. 9.41 Gracilis in the thigh

MA: Using a cradling hold for your distal hand, grasp the subject's lower limb and passively abduct her hip.

Ask her to adduct her hip against resistance in order to bring out the body of the muscle, which can also be more or less visible depending on the subject. You can then simply "detach" the muscle from the underlying muscle planes by using the pads of two fingers.

Fig. 9.42 Gracilis in its proximal part

MA: The subject's knee is flexed, and her hip is flexed and laterally rotated. Place your distal hand flat on the medial aspect of her knee to resist her horizontal hip adduction. With your proximal hand you can take hold of gracilis on the medial aspect of the thigh.

Note: Adipose tissue, quite abundant in women, can somewhat hamper this approach.

ATTACHMENT

Gracilis arises by a large flat tendon from the body of the pubic bone along the margin of the pubic symphysis.

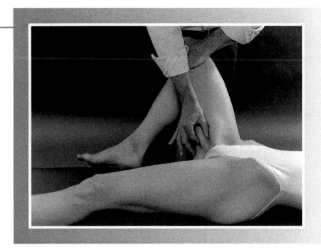

The posterior muscle group

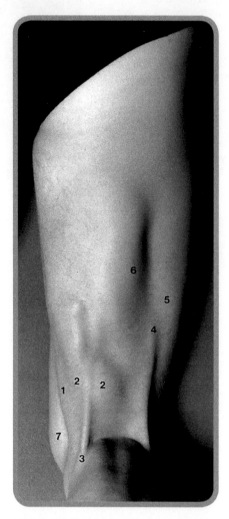

Fig. 9.43 Posterior view of the hip

1. Gracilis
2. Semimembranosus
3. Semitendinosus
4. Tendon of biceps femoris
5. Short head of biceps femoris
6. Long head of biceps femoris
7. Vastus medialis

This group, located in the posterior femoral region, consists of:

- The two medial hamstring muscles:
  - semitendinosus (Figs. 9.44–9.48)
  - semimembranosus (Figs. 9.44, and 9.49–9.52)
- The lateral hamstring muscle – biceps femoris:
  - the long head
  - the short head.

The medial hamstring muscles (semitendinosus and semimembranosus)

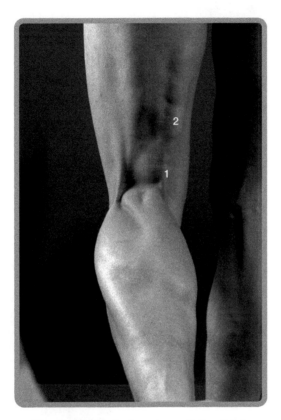

Fig. 9.44 Posterior view of the thigh with the knee half-flexed

1. Semitendinosus
2. Semimembranosus

ACTIONS OF SEMITENDINOSUS AND SEMIMEMBRANOSUS

- On the knee:
    - They flex the leg on the hip.
    - Semitendinosus medially rotates the knee along with the slightly weaker semimembranosus.
    - The hamstring muscles as a group stabilize the knee during rotational movements.
- On the hip:
    - They extend the hip on the pelvis, especially when the knee is extended.
- On the pelvis:
    - They stabilize the pelvis in the sagittal plane.
    - They tilt the pelvis posteriorly.

INNERVATIONS

- Semitendinosus: sciatic nerve (L5, S1, S2)
- Semimembranosus: sciatic nerve (L5, S1, S2)

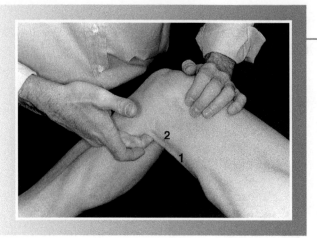

Fig. 9.45 The tendon of semitendinosus on the medial tibial border

MA: As shown in the adjacent figure, apply your finger pads along the medial tibial border, and with your middle finger hook the semitendinosus tendon (1). In this position, with the knee flexed, the tendon of gracilis (2) lies anterior to the semitendinosus tendon.

ATTACHMENTS

- This muscle arises from the posterior aspect of the ischial tuberosity by a common tendon shared with the long head of biceps femoris medial to the origin of semimembranosus.
- It is inserted into the superior part of the medial tibial surface posterior to sartorius and distal to gracilis.

Fig. 9.46 The distal tendon of semitendinosus

MA: The essential bony landmark is the proximal extremity of the medial tibial border. With the subject's knee flexed at about 90°, place one hand flat on the posterior aspect of her calcaneus and on the medial border of her foot, and resist her attempt to flex and medially rotate her knee, while moving your other hand proximally along the medial tibial border until it reaches the tendon you are after. You can also ask the subject to rest her heel firmly against the surface of the table, thereby flexing her knee isometrically and then to perform in rapid succession a series of medial rotations of the leg. Your two hands are now free to investigate.

Technical problem: It is relatively easy to look for this tendon in men but much more difficult in women because of the presence of adipose tissue, in which case you must adopt a more posterior approach.

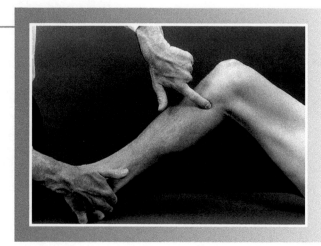

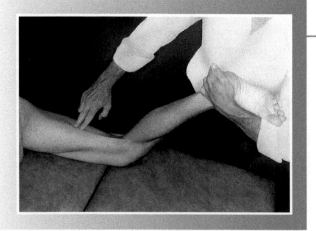

Fig. 9.47 Semitendinosus on the posterior aspect of the thigh

MA: Your distal hand cups the subject's heel and lies flat on the medial border of her foot so as to resist simultaneously her knee flexion and medial rotation. You will find the body of the muscle as the extension of the tendon you have already located in Fig. 9.46.

The muscle lies in the posterior part of the thigh medial to biceps femoris and superficial to semimembranosus.

Note: The peculiar feature of this muscle is the fact that its tendon starts very high proximally on the posterior aspect of the thigh. This is clearly shown in the adjacent figure. Another peculiar feature is the fact that it is fleshy proximally and tendinous distally, the opposite of semimembranosus.

It arises from the ischial tuberosity.

Fig. 9.48 The tendon of semitendinosus

MA: With the subject lying flat on his belly, use your distal hand to cup his heel and resist his attempt to flex his knee. You can also resist his attempt to rotate his knee medially by placing your hand this time flat on the medial border of his foot.

The semitendinosus tendon is the most posterior and the most lateral of the musculotendinous structures observed on the posteromedial aspect of the thigh.

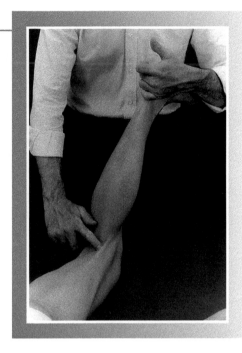

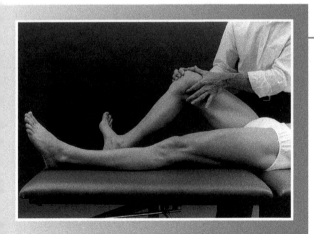

Fig. 9.49 Semimembranosus in its distal part: medial view

MA: With your distal hand, passively rotate the leg laterally so as to free the distal end of the tendon adequately. You will feel the tendon under your fingers as a large cylindrical cord near its insertion into the posteromedial part of the proximal extremity of the medial tibial condyle.

ATTACHMENT

- It is inserted via three tendons:
  - a straight tendon inserted into the posterior part of the medial tibial condyle;
  - a reflected tendon, which under cover of the collateral ligament slides into the horizontal groove on the medial tibial condyle before inserting into the anterior extremity of this groove;
  - a recurrent tendon (also known as the oblique popliteal ligament), which is inserted into the lateral condylar plate, i.e., the thickened portion of the knee capsule.

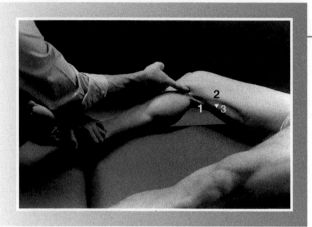

Fig. 9.50 Semimembranosus in its distal part: posteromedial view

MA: In addition to the approach described previously, you may find it useful to ask the subject to flex and medially rotate his knee while you resist these movements, the better for you to feel the tendon under your fingers.

If you place your index finger flat on the semimembranosus at its tibial insertion you will notice, as shown in the adjacent figure, that gracilis (2) crosses it posteriorly in order to come to lie anterior to semitendinosus (1) on the medial tibial border. The body of semimembranosus is labeled as (3).

ATTACHMENTS

Proximally, the muscle arises from the lateral part of the ischial tuberosity medial to quadratus femoris and lateral to the common tendon of the long head of biceps femoris and of semimembranosus.

Fig. 9.51 The tendon of semimembranosus

MA: The essential bony landmark is the angle uniting the medial and posterior aspects of the medial tibial condyle. The subject's knee is kept laterally rotated to bring out fully this bony structure. Use one of your hands to oppose his attempt to flex and medially rotate his knee, while your other hand looks for a tendon that feels like a fairly thick, solid, cylindrical cord under your fingers.

More anteriorly, the reflected tendon of this muscle slides under the collateral tibial ligament to enter the horizontal groove for the insertion of semimembranosus. The approach to this muscle is quite easy if you remember to position the leg properly in lateral rotation, which allows the tendon to stand out adequately.

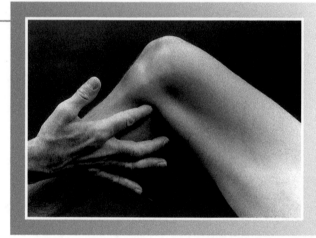

Fig. 9.52 Semimembranosus

MA: Your fingers will feel semimembranosus (3) as a fleshy muscle lying between the tendons of semitendinosus (1) and gracilis (2). You can also observe it lateral to the semitendinosus tendon.

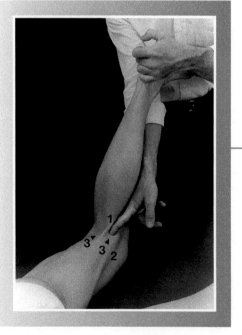

Fig. 9.53 Overall location of the anserine muscles on the medial tibial border

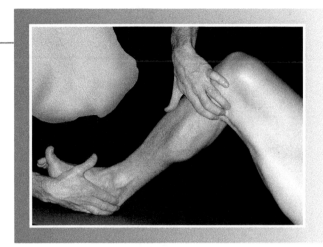

MA: First locate the superior extremity of the medial tibial border and place your fingers as indicated in the adjacent figure. With your other hand resist the subject's attempt to flex and medially rotate the knee isometrically. Ask him to perform a series of movements alternating contraction and relaxation to allow you to better observe the tendons and their topographic locations:

- The semitendinosus tendon is the most distal and is felt under the index finger.
- The gracilis tendon lies just proximal to the previous one and is felt under the middle finger.
- The distal part of sartorius overhangs that of gracilis. As the muscle tightens it is felt under the ring finger, and it is felt even better if the subject is asked to extend his knee slightly.

Note: If you have difficulty identifying the tendons on the medial tibial border, you should palpate them more proximally by slightly moving your fingers posteriorly. This problem can arise in women, where the adipose tissue almost always interferes with palpation of these structures in this location.

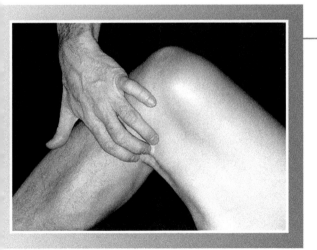

Fig. 9.54 Close-up of the above-mentioned overall location maneuver

MA: This figure is of interest in showing well the respective locations of the various tendons and muscular bodies. The practitioner places his index finger opposite the semitendinosus tendon, his middle finger opposite the gracilis tendon, and his ring finger opposite sartorius, which is not seen in the picture but becomes more obvious if the subject is asked to flex his knee slightly.

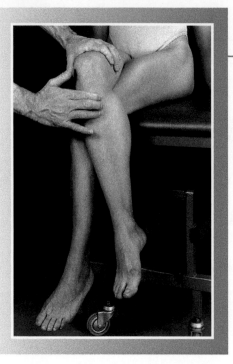

Fig. 9.55 Overall location of the tightened anserine muscles on the anterior and medial parts of the tibia, medial to the tibial tuberosity

MA: Using a wide contact, place your fingers together distal to the medial tibial condyle, and then cup in your palm the tibial tuberosity, along the course of the tendons you have already studied.

Ask the subject to flex her knee isometrically against her contralateral lower limb, and then medially rotate her leg by inverting her foot medially, since the anserine muscles are also rotators of the leg. You can then observe under the skin, directly under your fingers, the tightening of these anserine muscles.

The tendons of the pes anserinus are arranged in two planes:

• a superficial plane consisting of the sartorius tendon, which blends with the superficial fascia of the leg;
• a deep plane lying posteriorly and made up of the gracilis tendon anteriorly and of the semitendinosus tendon posteriorly.

CLINICAL NOTE

When palpation of the anterior aspect of the medial tibial condyle medial to the tibial tuberosity causes pain, and this pain is reproduced when the subject climbs stairs or walks, you must think of an anserine tenobursitis.

The lateral hamstring muscle or biceps femoris (long head)

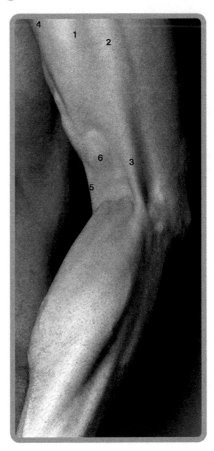

Fig. 9.56 Posterolateral view of the thigh

1. Biceps femoris – long head (Figs. 9.57, 9.59, and 9.62)
2. Biceps femoris – short head (Figs. 9.57, and 9.60–9.62)
3. Biceps femoris tendon (Fig. 9.58)
4. Semitendinosus
5. Semitendinosus tendon
6. Semimembranosus

ACTIONS OF THE BICEPS FEMORIS

- At the knee:
  - It flexes and laterally rotates the knee when flexed.
  - It stabilizes the knee during rotational movements.
- At the hip:
  - It extends the hip, especially when the knee is extended.
- At the pelvis:
  - It takes part in stabilizing the pelvis in the sagittal plane.
  - It tilts the pelvis posteriorly.

INNERVATION

- Sciatic nerve (L5, S1, S2)

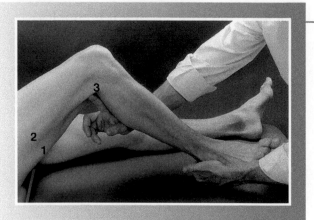

1. Biceps femoris: long head
2. Biceps femoris: short head
3. Tendon of insertion of biceps femoris

Fig. 9.57 Biceps femoris in its distal part

MA: With your hand cupping the subject's heel, resist his knee flexion, and with the anterior surface of your forearm resting on the lateral surface of his foot, resist his lateral knee rotation.

The tendon, shown by the practitioner's index finger, stands out on the lateral part of the subject's knee just before its insertion into the fibular head.

ATTACHMENTS

The muscle is inserted into the fibular head lateral to the insertion of the fibular collateral ligament, from which it is separated by a synovial bursa. It is also inserted into the lateral tibial condyle close to the fibular head and distal to the tibial oblique line.

Fig. 9.58 Location of the biceps femoris tendon in the popliteal fossa – another mode of approach

MA: With the subject in the prone position, cup his heel in your palm and place your forearm on the lateral border of his foot so as to be able to resist his knee flexion and medial rotation simultaneously. The tendon (1) will stand out in the posterolateral part of the popliteal fossa. The body (2) of biceps femoris is also visible.

1. Biceps femoris tendon inserting into the fibular head
2. Body of long head of biceps femoris

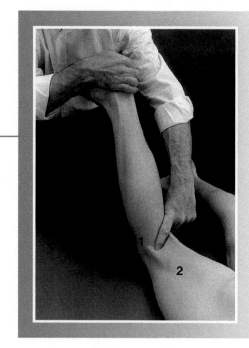

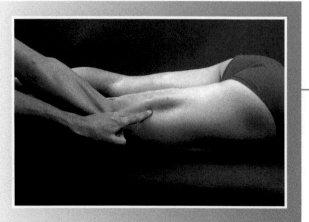

Fig. 9.59 Biceps femoris: long head

MA: From its insertion into the fibular head, the body of the long head of biceps femoris runs an oblique course superiorly and medially to join the medial hamstring muscles (semitendinosus and semimembranosus).

Fig. 9.60 Biceps femoris: short head

MA: From its distal insertion shared with the long head, the body of the short head runs vertically lateral to the long head, since it takes origin from the linea aspera.

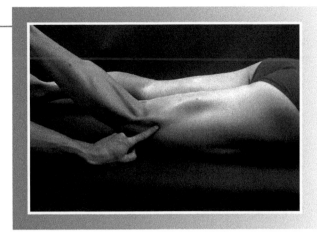

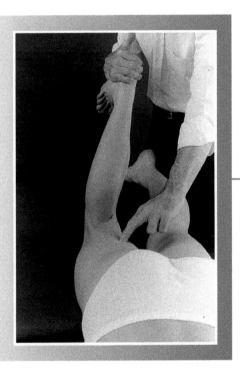

Fig. 9.61 Biceps femoris: short head

MA: The practitioner's index finger points to the junction of the long head of biceps femoris with semimembranosus.

Fig. 9.62 The tendon of origin of the hamstring muscles from the tibial tuberosity

MA: With the subject lying on her belly, the essential cutaneous landmark is the gluteal fold (1). Through it you can palpate the origins of these muscles from the ischial tuberosity. In the adjacent figure, the thumb is slightly displaced laterally with respect to the sites of origin of these muscles on the ischial tuberosity.

ATTACHMENTS

- The long head of biceps femoris arises from the ischial tuberosity by a tendon shared with semitendinosus. This common site of origin lies medial to that of semimembranosus.
- The short head of biceps femoris arises from the groove of the linea aspera and from its lateral lip.

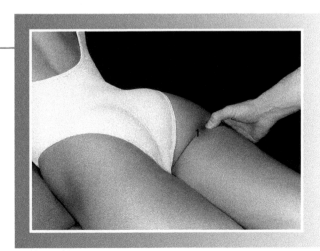

10
The knee

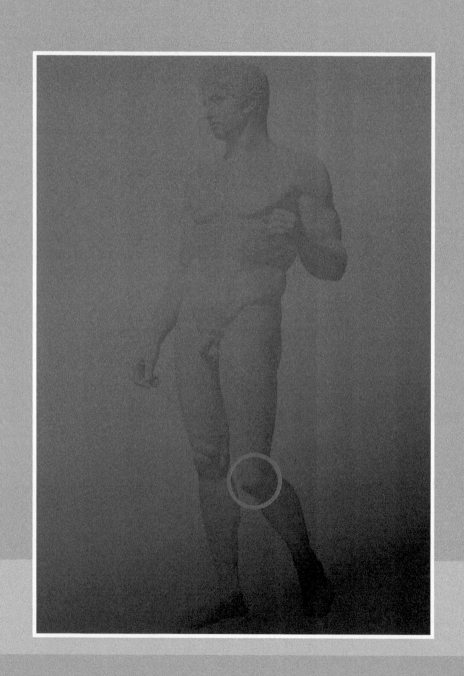

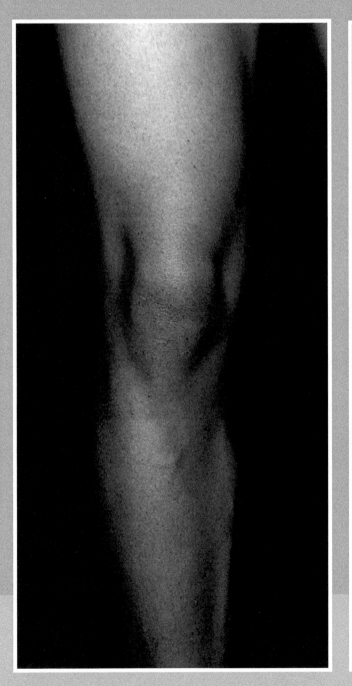
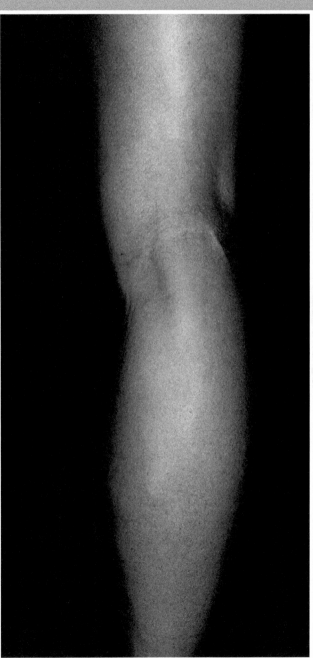

OSTEOLOGY

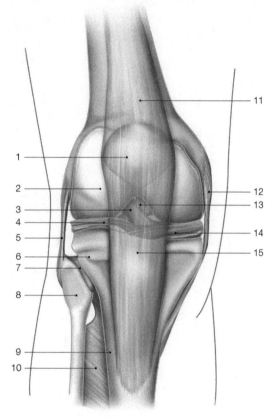

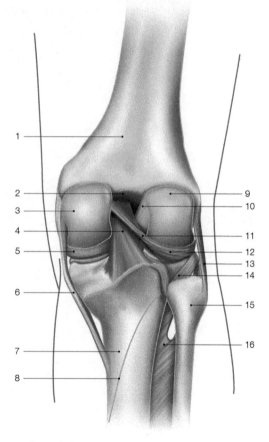

Osteology and arthrology of the knee (anterior view)

1. Patella
2. Patellar articular surface
3. Anterior cruciate ligament
4. Lateral meniscus
5. Fibular collateral ligament
6. Gerdy's tubercle
7. Anterior ligament of fibular head
8. Fibular head
9. Tibia
10. Interosseous membrane of thigh
11. Quadriceps tendon
12. Tibial collateral ligament
13. Posterior cruciate ligament
14. Medial meniscus
15. Patellar ligament

Osteology and arthrology of the knee (posterior view)

1. Femur
2. Intercondylar fossa
3. Medial femoral condyle
4. Posterior cruciate ligament
5. Medial meniscus
6. Tibial collateral ligament
7. Tibia
8. Soleal line
9. Lateral tibial condyle
10. Anterior cruciate ligament
11. Meniscofemoral ligament
12. Lateral meniscus
13. Fibular collateral ligament
14. Posterior ligament of fibular head
15. Fibular head
16. Interosseous membrane

THE ANTERIOR COMPARTMENT

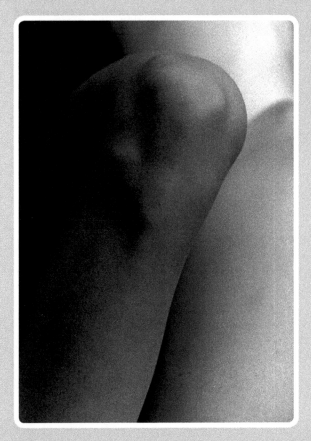

Fig. 10.3 Frontal view: knee flexed

The bony structures accessible to palpation are:

- The suprapatellar fossa (Fig. 10.4)
- The patella
  - the base (Fig. 10.5)
  - the anterior surface (Fig. 10.6)
  - the apex (Fig. 10.7)
  - the borders (Fig. 10.8)
  - the lateral approach to the posterior articular surface (Fig. 10.9)
  - the medial approach to the posterior articular surface (Fig. 10.10)
- The femur
  - the articular surfaces of the condyles (Fig. 10.13)
  - the oblique grooves on the condylar articular surfaces (Figs. 10.14 and 10.15)
- The tibia
  - the tibial plateau and the femorotibial space (Figs. 10.12 and 10.13)
  - the tibial tuberosity (Fig. 10.11).

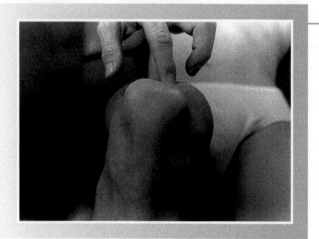

Fig. 10.4 The suprapatellar fossa

MA: This triangular fossa lies proximal to the femoral trochlea on the anterior surface of the distal end of the femur and accommodates the superior part of the patella during knee extension.

Flex the subject's knee maximally to be able to best palpate the fossa starting from the easily located base of the patella (see Fig. 10.5).

Fig. 10.5 The patellar base

MA: It is triangular in shape with a wide anterior base and an apex located posteriorly and is felt under the fingers as a sloping surface.

ATTACHMENTS

The quadriceps tendon is inserted into its anterior half, and the joint capsule is inserted posteriorly near its articular surface.

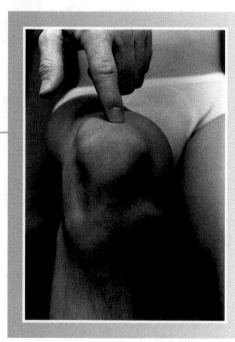

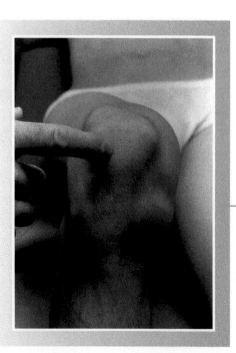

Fig. 10.6 The anterior aspect of the patella

MA: It is convex and pitted with numerous vascular openings and has an uneven surface with vertical ridges and depressions formed by the movement of the quadriceps tendon.

CLINICAL NOTE

In cases of recurrent dislocation (a condition seen in adolescents with genu valgum) the patella can be found on the lateral surface of the knee or astride the lateral border of the femoral trochlea.

Fig. 10.7 The patellar apex

MA: The apex points toward the distal extremity of the lower limb and receives the insertion of the patellar ligament. You can approach it with the knee flexed or extended.

CLINICAL NOTE

It can be the seat of an enthesopathy on the deep plane of the patellar tendon at its insertion.

Patellar tendinitis

It is more usually associated with the practice of certain sports: ball games played on hard courts (basketball, handball, etc.). The patellar apex becomes painful on palpation with pressure.

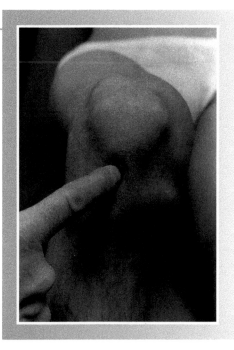

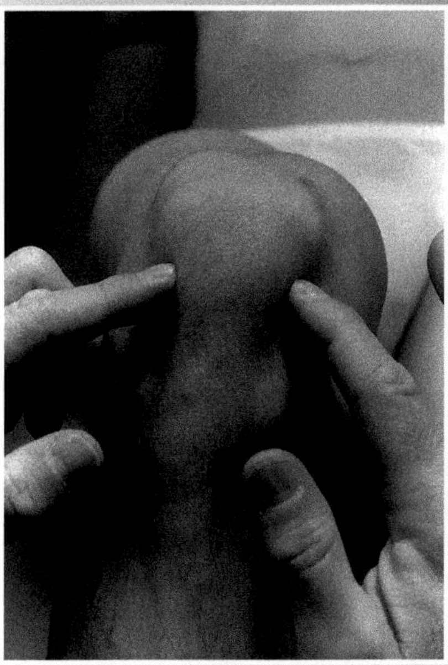

Fig. 10.8 The borders of the patella

MA: Its two borders run proximodistally and lateromedially with reference to the median axis of the patella. They are readily accessible to palpation.

ATTACHMENTS

These borders (more exactly the junctions of their margins and the base of the patella) provide attachment to the medial and lateral patellar retinacula, respectively.

CLINICAL NOTE

Cases of lateral dislocation of the patella can also be associated with an osteochondral fracture of the medial border of the patella, which can be detected on palpation. If on palpation you get the sensation of a "sensitive" cord running along the patella, you must think of a synovial fold or plica.

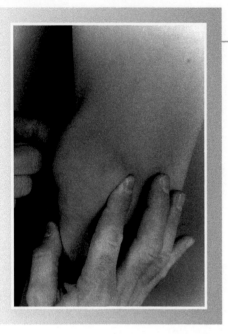

Fig. 10.9 The lateral approach to the lateral articular surface of the patella

MA: Only the most lateral part of this surface is accessible. Hyperextend the subject's knee with the quadriceps kept perfectly relaxed and you can feel it by simply displacing the patella laterally.

CLINICAL NOTE

Caution: This method of approach must be banned in cases of recurrent dislocation of the patella.

Fig. 10.10 The medial approach to the medial articular surface of the patella

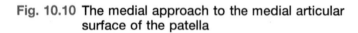

MA: Hyperextend the subject's knee with the quadriceps kept perfectly relaxed and you get access to it simply by displacing the patella medially.

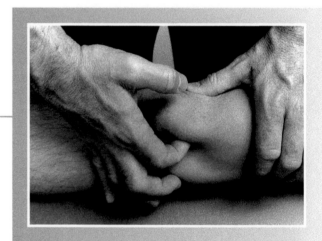

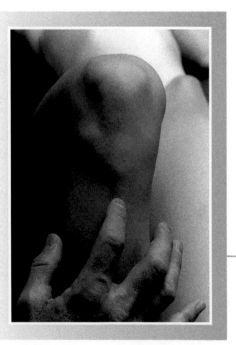

Fig. 10.11 The tibial tuberosity

MA: It is a triangular surface with its apex located distally, and it separates the tibial medial and lateral condyles anteriorly.

It is the site of insertion of the patellar ligament, which is a mixed structure made up superficially of active fibers from the quadriceps and passive fibers from the apex of the patella.

Fig. 10.12 The tibial plateau

MA: With the subject's knee flexed at 90°, put your thumbs on either side of the patellar ligament in the tibiofemoral joint space. Then simply move your thumbs distally to reach the nonarticular border of the plateau and keep palpating this border up to its point of contact with the femur.

Note: This approach also allows you to contact the tibiofemoral joint space.

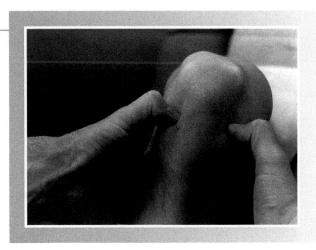

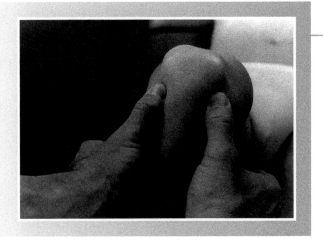

Fig. 10.13 The articular surfaces of the femoral condyles

MA: With the subject's knee flexed at 90°, put your thumbs on either side of the patellar ligament in the tibiofemoral joint space. Then simply move your thumbs upward to reach these surfaces.

If you have any difficulty, flex the knee even more and it will make access much easier.

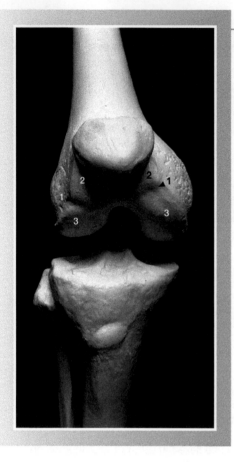

Fig. 10.14 Visualization of the oblique grooves

MA: These two grooves, cut into the cartilage-lined articular surface of the distal end of the femur, divide it into two parts:

- the articular surfaces lying anterior and proximal to these grooves belong to the femoral trochlea;
- the articular surfaces lying posterior and distal to these grooves are called the tibial condylar articular surfaces.

1. The oblique grooves separating the condylar and trochlear surfaces
2. The femoral trochlea, on which moves the posterior articular surface of the patella
3. The femoral condylar articular surfaces, which move on the menisci of the tibial plateau

Fig. 10.15 Approach to the oblique grooves

MA: For this approach the ideal position is with the knee slightly flexed beyond 90°. Then simply run your fingers along the articular surface between the patella and the condylar articular surfaces themselves in order to feel the two gutters or depressions that are the oblique grooves.

Note: The lateral oblique groove is most often the much easier one to feel with your fingers because it is more prominent.

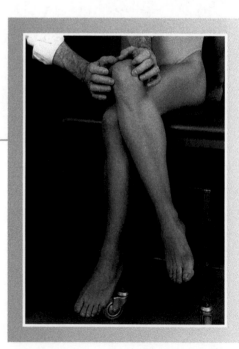

THE MEDIAL COMPARTMENT

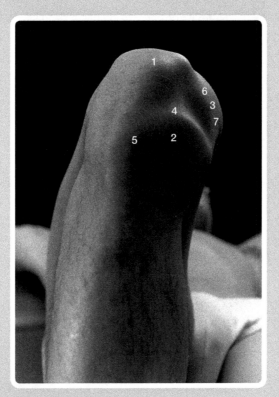

Fig. 10.16 Anteromedial view, with knee flexed

1. Patella
2. Medial tibial condyle
3. Medial femoral condyle
4. Tibial articular surface for the femur
5. Tibial tuberosity
6. Medial border of the femoral trochlea
7. Medial oblique groove

The bony structures accessible to palpation include:
- The femur
  - the medial epicondyle (Figs. 10.17 and 10.18)
  - the medial border of the trochlea (Figs. 10.19 and 10.20)
  - the femoral trochlea (Fig. 10.20)
  - the adductor tubercle (Fig. 10.21)
- The tibia
  - the medial tibial plateau (Fig. 10.22)
  - the inferior border of the medial tibial condyle (Fig. 10.23)
  - the superior part of the medial tibial border, which is the crucial structure for the localization of the anserine muscles (Fig. 10.24).

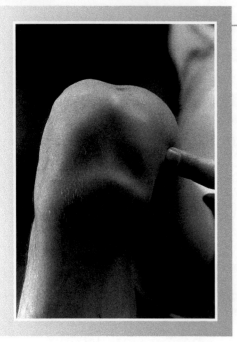

Fig. 10.17 The medial femoral epicondyle: anterior view

MA: It is a subcutaneous structure directly accessible to palpation, and it represents the most prominent bony projection on the rough aspect of the medial femoral condyle.

Note: Its posterior slope has a depression for the insertion of the tibial collateral ligament of the knee.

Fig. 10.18 The medial femoral epicondyle: medial view

MA: This medial view of the medial femoral epicondyle allows this structure to be visualized and localized more precisely.

ATTACHMENTS

Posterior to the medial epicondyle lie the following structures:
- a depression for the insertion of the tibial collateral ligament;
- the adductor tubercle, which lies at the medial end of the distal bifurcation of the linea aspera and receives the insertion of adductor magnus.

Distal and posterior to this tubercle there is a depression from which arises the medial head of gastrocnemius.

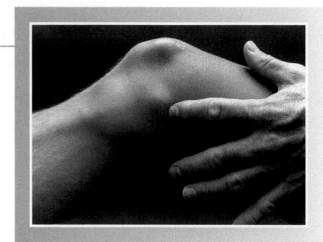

Fig. 10.19 The medial border of the femoral trochlea

MA: This border is the lateral boundary of the femoral trochlea and of the articular surface of the medial condyle.

With the subject's knee maximally flexed, there is easy access to this structure.

The medial oblique groove

It is the distal border of the rough medial aspect of the medial femoral condyle along its distal extremity. It is deeper posteriorly than anteriorly.

MA: Flex the subject's knee in order to free it from the adjacent musculotendinous structures.

Note: Do not forget that, when the knee is flexed, a large part of the distal articular surface of the femur lies in front of you.

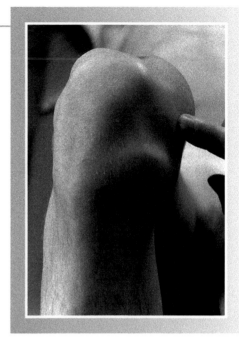

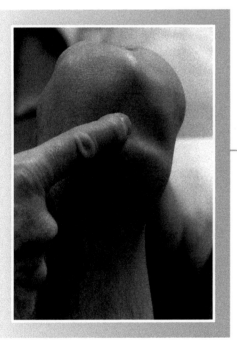

Fig. 10.20 The medial articular surface of the femoral trochlea

MA: Using your thumb and index finger, locate the medial edge of the tibiofemoral joint space. From this landmark run along the joint space, which your fingers will feel as a smooth surface bounded by the medial border of the medial trochlear surface.

Fig. 10.21 The adductor tubercle

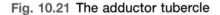

MA: This structure is not easy to locate per se, but you can find it by first locating the tendon of the vertical bundle of adductor magnus.

Then you need only follow this tendon to its insertion, where you will feel a projection, which is the adductor tubercle.

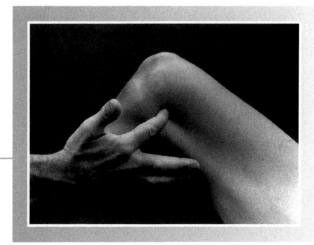

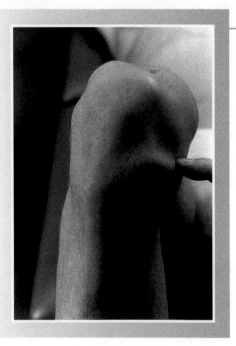

Fig. 10.22 The medial tibial plateau

MA: With the subject's knee flexed at 90° it is easy to locate this structure. Viewed from the front, the most medial part of the plateau is an important landmark to visualize, since it is from this site that you approach the tibial collateral ligament.

Note: Only the margin of the plateau is accessible to palpation, and not the plateau itself.

Fig. 10.23 The inferior border of the medial tibial condyle

MA: With the subject's knee flexed you need only locate the medial tibial condyle and follow it right to its proximal extremity. You will then easily "catch" this inferior border of the medial tibial condyle using the pads of one or two fingers.

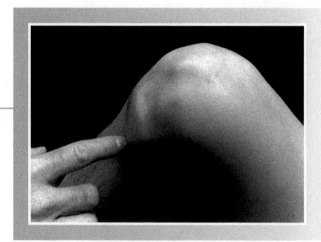

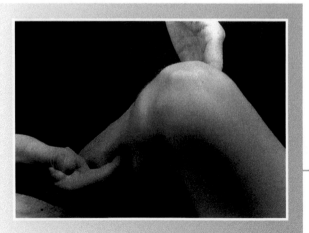

Fig. 10.24 The proximal part of the medial tibial border

MA: It is a notable bony structure where you can locate the three anserine muscles (semitendinosus, gracilis, and sartorius) at their site of insertion into the anteromedial aspect of the tibia close to its anterior border.

THE LATERAL COMPARTMENT

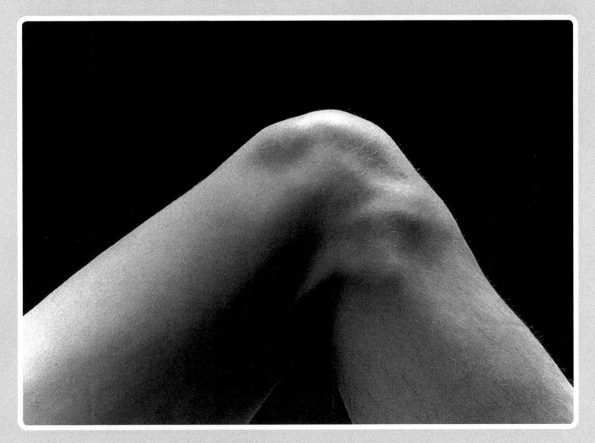

Fig. 10.25 Lateral view with the knee flexed

The bony structures accessible to palpation include:
- The femur
  - the lateral border of the suprapatellar fossa (Fig. 10.26)
  - the lateral border of the trochlea (Fig. 10.27)
  - the lateral epicondyle (Fig. 10.28)
  - the lateral articular surface of the trochlea (Figs. 10.29 and 10.30)
- The tibia
  - the lateral tibial plateau (Fig. 10.31)
  - Gerdy's tubercle (Figs. 10.32 and 10.33)
  - the lateral oblique crest (Fig. 10.30)
  - the medial oblique crest
- The fibula
  - the head (Fig. 10.35)
  - the neck (Fig. 10.36).

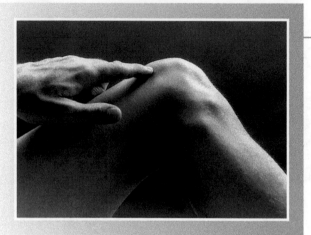

Fig. 10.26 The lateral border of the suprapatellar fossa of the femur

MA: It is more prominent than the medial border, the more so as the knee is brought progressively into full flexion.

Fig. 10.27 The lateral border of the lateral articular surface of the femoral trochlea

MA: It extends very far laterally in keeping with the markedly off-center displacement of the patella when the knee is flexed.

Note: As a result, the femoral trochlea becomes more uncovered medially than laterally when the knee is flexed.

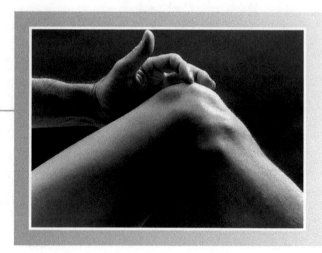

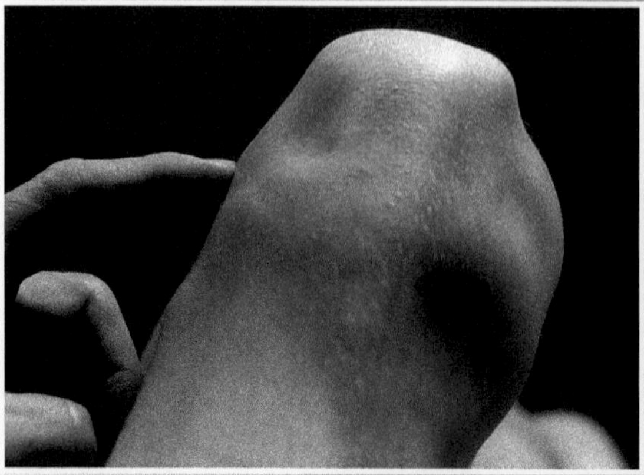

Fig. 10.28 The lateral femoral epicondyle

MA: It is less prominent than the medial epicondyle and lies on the middle portion of the lateral aspect of the condyle.

If you have any difficulty finding it, tighten the fibular collateral ligament by causing the lateral tibiofemoral joint space to gap as a result of flexing the subject's knee.

The lateral epicondyle is the femoral site of attachment of the above-mentioned ligament.

ATTACHMENTS

• Distal and posterior to the lateral epicondyle there is a groove for the origin of the popliteus tendon.
• Proximal and posterior to the epicondyle there is another groove providing origin for the lateral head of gastrocnemius.
• Running between these two grooves there is a crest to which is attached the fibular collateral ligament.

Fig. 10.29 The lateral border of the lateral lip of the femoral trochlea

MA: This margin limits the femoral trochlea laterally and also the tibial articular surface of the lateral condyle.

When the knee is fully flexed this structure is easily accessible.

The popliteal groove

It is the distal boundary of the rough lateral surface of the lateral condyle along its inferior margin. It is much deeper posteriorly than anteriorly.

MA: Flex the subject's knee in order to free it from the adjacent musculotendinous structures.

Note: Do not forget that, when the knee is flexed, the distal extremity of the femur is in front of you.

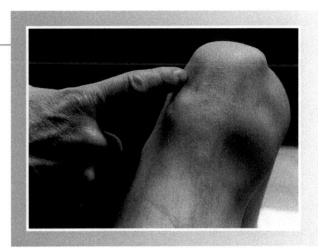

ATTACHMENTS

The capsule of the knee joint and the popliteus tendon are attached to this groove.

> **CLINICAL NOTE**
>
> The popliteus arises from this groove, where it is painful on palpation when its tendon is inflamed.

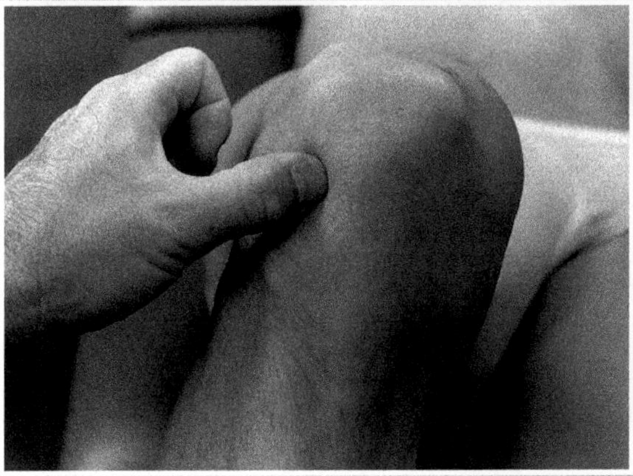

Fig. 10.30 The lateral lip of the femoral trochlea

MA: With your thumb, locate the lateral tibiofemoral joint space. Starting from this landmark, proceed along the articular surface, which will feel smooth under your fingers. This articular surface is bounded medially by the patellar ligament and the lateral border of the patella, and laterally by the lateral border of the femoral trochlea.

> **CLINICAL NOTE**
>
> In cases of recurrent partial or complete dislocation of the patella, this lip can be painful on palpation. It can also be painful after any overload of the articular surface resulting from intense overuse of the knee, however brief.

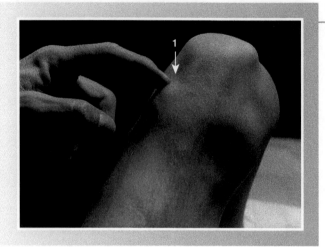

Fig. 10.31 The lateral tibial plateau

MA: When the knee is flexed at 90°, this structure can easily be found. Viewed from the front, its most lateral part is important to visualize because it provides the site of approach to the fibular collateral ligament at the level of the knee joint space.

Note: The margin of the tibial plateau is accessible to palpation, but not the plateau itself.

1. Space of the lateral tibiofemoral joint

CLINICAL NOTE

Meniscal cyst

It presents as an easily palpable firm nodule located in the anterolateral part of the space of the tibiofemoral joint.

Fig. 10.32 Gerdy's tubercle: lateral view

MA: It is the most prominent projection on the lateral tibial condyle. With the subject's knee flexed at 90°, you can investigate it just distal to the lateral tibial plateau and lateral to the tibial tuberosity.

1. Gerdy's tubercle
2. Lateral tibial epicondyle
3. Fibular head

ATTACHMENTS

The iliotibial tract is inserted into the tubercle.

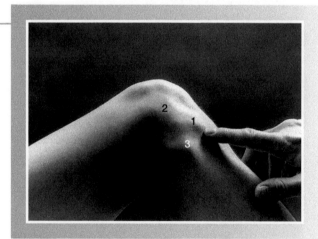

CLINICAL NOTE

Iliotibial syndrome is the result of the continual rubbing of the iliotibial tract over the lateral tibial epicondyle (2), which becomes painful on palpation, particularly if the practitioner extends the subject's knee while still applying pressure to the epicondyle. Pain is usually felt when the knee is flexed at 30° to 40°.

Fig. 10.33 Gerdy's tubercle

MA: The additional anterior view provides a more precise visualization and location of this tubercle. A further bony landmark is the fibular head, which is a bony structure lying posterior and distal to the tubercle.

ATTACHMENT

The iliotibial tract of the tensor fasciae latae.

> **CLINICAL NOTE**
>
> A varus force applied to an extended knee can lead to distal rupture of the iliotibial tract and an avulsion fracture of the tubercle. Palpation of the latter structure will be painful.

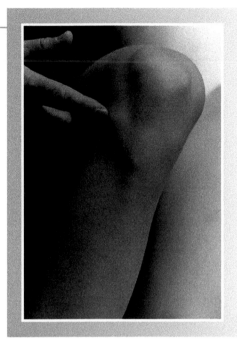

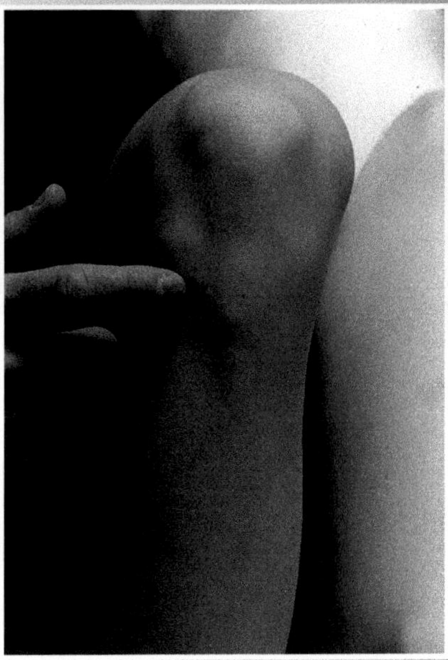

Fig. 10.34 The oblique line of the tibia: anterior view

MA: It is in effect a bony ridge running between Gerdy's tubercle and the lateral border of the tibial tuberosity. Its course is oblique superoinferiorly and posteroanteriorly, and it is directly accessible under the skin.

ATTACHMENTS

Proximal and medial to the oblique line:
- the iliotibial tract lying more medially
- the lateral patellar retinaculum

Distal to the oblique line and from posterior to anterior:
- biceps femoris
- fibularis longus
- extensor digitorum longus
- anterior tibialis

> **CLINICAL NOTE**
>
> All the above-mentioned attachment sites can be painful on palpation. You must perform your clinical palpation procedure according to which muscles are involved.

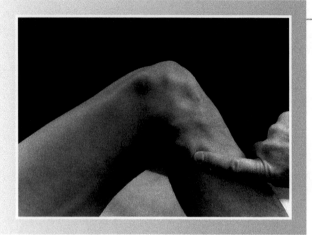

Fig. 10.35 The fibular head: lateral view

MA: There is an easy access to the fibular head, which you can bring out more prominently by first medially rotating the subject's knee.

Note: The styloid process is a bony projection arising posteriorly from the articular surface of the fibular head.

ATTACHMENTS

Laterally and from proximal to distal:
- the fibular collateral ligament
- biceps femoris
- fibularis longus

> **CLINICAL NOTE**
>
> All these above-mentioned insertion sites can be painful on palpation, and you must perform your clinical palpation according to which muscles are involved.

Fig. 10.36 The fibular neck: anterior view

MA: This structure lies between the proximal end of the fibula and its shaft and is notable insofar as the common fibular nerve curves around it before entering the leg.

> **CLINICAL NOTE**
>
> The common fibular nerve can be injured by compression due to an ill-fitting plaster cast. Some surgical procedures can cause injury to the nerve, as can lying on one's back for prolonged periods of time with a blanket that passively and "heavily" keeps the foot in plantar flexion.

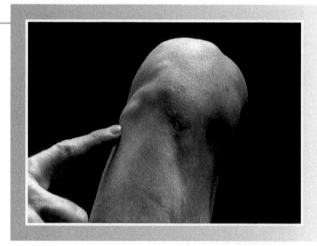

ARTHROLOGY

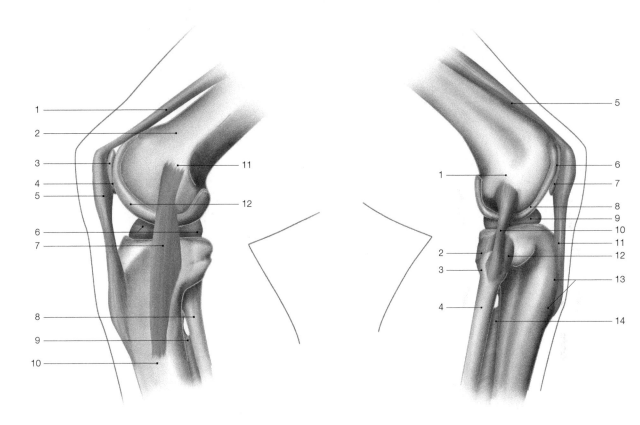

Osteology and arthrology of the knee (medial view)

1. Quadriceps tendon
2. Femur
3. Patella
4. Femoropatellar joint
5. Patellar ligament
6. Medial ligament
7. Tibial collateral ligament
8. Fibula
9. Interosseous membrane
10. Tibia (medial aspect)
11. Medial epicondyle
12. Medial femoral epicondyle

Osteology and arthrology of the knee (lateral view)

1. Lateral epicondyle
2. Posterior ligament of fibular head
3. Fibular head
4. Fibula
5. Quadriceps tendon
6. Femoral trochlea
7. Patella
8. Lateral femoral condyle
9. Lateral meniscus
10. Fibular collateral ligament
11. Patellar ligament
12. Anterior ligament of fibular head
13. Tibial tuberosity
14. Interosseous membrane

THE LIGAMENTS

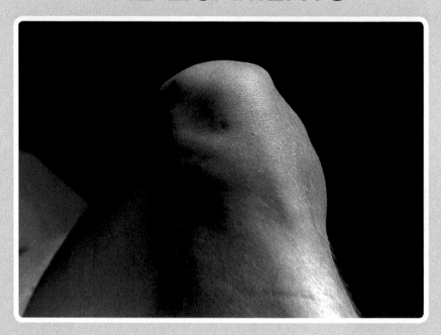

Fig. 10.37 **Anterior view of the knee**

The ligamentous structures accessible to palpation include:

- the fibular collateral ligament: visualization and stretching procedure (Figs. 10.38 and 10.39)
- the lateral patellar retinaculum: stretching procedure (Figs. 10.40–10.42)
- the tibial collateral ligament: visualization and stretching procedure (Figs. 10.43–10.46)
- the medial patellar retinaculum: visualization and stretching procedure (Figs. 10.47–10.49)
- the infrapatellar fat pad: visualization and approach (Fig. 10.50)

Fig. 10.38 Visualization of the fibular collateral ligament

MA: This ligament (1) runs from the lateral femoral epicondyle to the anterolateral part of the fibular head anterior to its apex.

ATTACHMENTS

- This ligament comprises two bundles (an anatomical peculiarity):
  - a superficial bundle separated from the biceps tendon by a synovial bursa;
  - a deep bundle, which is adherent to the capsule and is related to the popliteus tendon and its synovial bursa. The latter separates it from the lateral meniscus.

> **CLINICAL NOTE**
>
> A varus force applied to the knee, whether medially rotated or not, can cause either a mild sprain of this ligament, i.e., simple overstretching, or a more severe sprain with its disinsertion or avulsion of the bone at its insertion site.

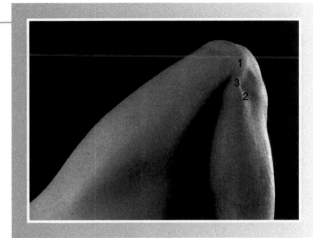

1. Origin from the femoral epicondyle
2. Insertion into the femoral head
3. Body of the ligament

Fig. 10.39 The fibular collateral ligament: stretching procedure

MA: In order to locate this ligament under the best conditions, it is preferable to stretch it. Once located, it is easy to investigate in all positions of the knee.

Have the subject adopt a posture as indicated in the adjacent figure. With one of your hands placed on the medial aspect of the knee, apply some pressure mediolaterally to open up the lateral part of the joint space and stretch the ligament as a result. Place your other hand opposite the joint space between the fibular head and the lateral femoral epicondyle.

Note: Your fingers will feel the ligament as a solid cylindrical cord of variable thickness depending on the individual. Those with genu varum will obviously have a stronger and thicker ligament because it is constantly under tension.

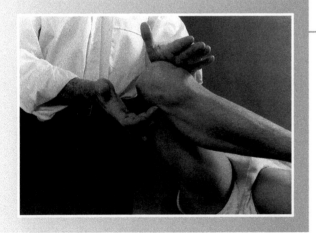

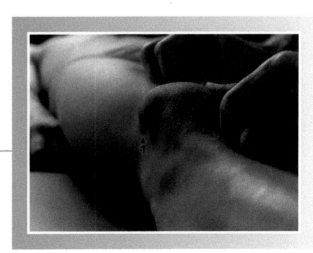

Fig. 10.40 Visualization of the lateral patellar retinaculum

MA: When the knee is fully extended, the quadriceps femoris is relaxed. You can push the patella laterally and as a result stretch this ligament (adjacent figure, 1), or you can push the patella medially with the same result. Then approach the lateral patellar retinaculum in a plane perpendicular to its course.

1. Lateral patellar retinaculum

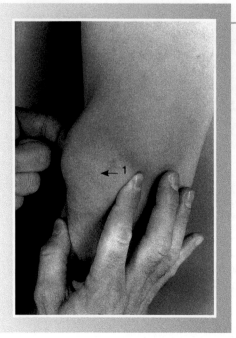

Fig. 10.41 Palpation of the lateral patellar retinaculum

MA: In this maneuver, pushing the patella mediolaterally (1) brings the retinaculum, as displayed in Figure 10.40, into a plane close to the midsagittal plane. As a reinforcement of the capsule it is felt under your fingers as a fibrous band.

1. Lateral displacement of the patella

CLINICAL NOTE

First case

The lateral patellar retinaculum can be painful because of tendinitis of the extensor apparatus of the knee, following intensive practice of such sports as cycling or running.

Second case

In the event of recurrent partial or (even more so) complete dislocation of the patella, the medial patellar retinaculum will be painful.

Fig. 10.42 Visualization of the concurrent stretching procedure for the lateral and medial patellar retinacula

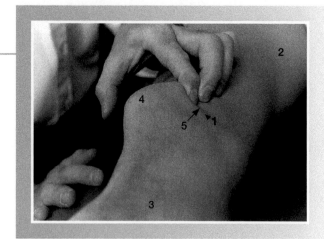

MA: Lateral traction exerted on the patella allows the medial patellar retinaculum to stand out (1) and the lateral patellar retinaculum (not shown in the adjacent figure) to be stretched simultaneously.

Note: During the procedure the medial patellar retinaculum is made to stretch in a plane that gets progressively closer to the midsagittal plane, whereas the lateral patellar retinaculum is made to stretch in a progressively more horizontal plane. The adjacent figure provides an inferomedial view.

1. Lateral traction exerted on the patella
2. Thigh
3. Leg
4. Patella
5. Visualization of the stretched medial patellar retinaculum

---

CLINICAL NOTE

In cases of complete chronic lateral dislocation of the patella, the medial patellar retinaculum is painful on palpation, and the subject shows signs of apprehension when the practitioner's hands approach his knee.

Fig. 10.43 Visualization of the tibial collateral ligament

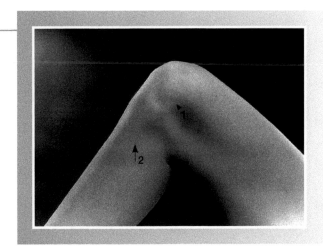

MA: This ligament (1) stretches from the apex of the medial femoral epicondyle, and also from a depression lying just posterior to the epicondyle, to the proximal part of the medial tibial border and its adjacent anteromedial aspect.

1. Proximal attachment of the ligament to the medial femoral condyle
2. Distal attachment of the ligament to the medial tibial border

ATTACHMENTS

• This ligament consists of a superficial and a deep bundle. The superficial bundle is attached proximally to the lateral femoral epicondyle, runs an oblique course anteromedially and is inserted into the medial tibial border deep to the tendons of the pes anserinus and to the intervening anserine bursa.
• The anatomic peculiarity of the deep bundle is the fact that it is shorter than the superior bundle. It is made up of two bundles of fibers, i.e., a meniscofemoral bundle and a meniscotibial bundle.

Fig. 10.44 The tibial collateral ligament: stretching procedure

MA: Two steps are used to stretch this ligament optimally.

First, with the subject's knee flexed at 90°, laterally rotate the leg to stretch the ligament.

Second, place your hand on his knee and push it medially while keeping his foot immobile on the table. The joint space will gap medially, and the ligament will be stretched even more.

Note: The same hand, whose fingers face the joint space, will feel the ligament as a rather flat fibrous band.

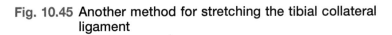

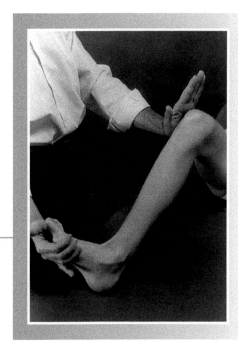

Fig. 10.45 Another method for stretching the tibial collateral ligament

MA: With the subject's heel resting on the table, grasp the medial border of her foot in the palm of your hand so as to rotate the leg laterally.

Then use your other hand, positioned flat on the lateral part of her knee, to push his knee medially so as to open up the joint space and stretch the ligament as a result.

Note: The ligament stands out at the level of the joint space (see Fig. 10.46).

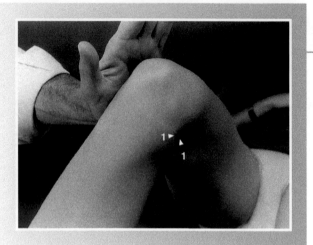

Fig. 10.46 Another method for stretching the tibial collateral ligament, similar to the previous one, but shown in close-up

MA: This figure is a close-up anteromedial view of the knee that demonstrates very clearly the stretching of the ligament.

Note: The ligament stands out at the level of the joint space.

> **CLINICAL NOTE**
>
> A knee injury caused by forced valgus displacement, with or without concomitant forced lateral rotation, results in overstretching of the ligament with possible avulsion of its proximal attachment. It is the classic mechanism underlying a sprain. This injury can be part of a more extensive injury that may include damage to the anterior cruciate ligament and the medial meniscus.

Fig. 10.47 Visualization of the transverse fibers of the medial patellar retinaculum with knee extended: medial view

MA: The knee is fully extended and the quadriceps relaxed. Either push the patella laterally so as to stretch the retinaculum, or push it medially with the same result.

Palpate the medial patellar retinaculum in the same way in both cases, using a transverse approach.

1. Medial patellar retinaculum

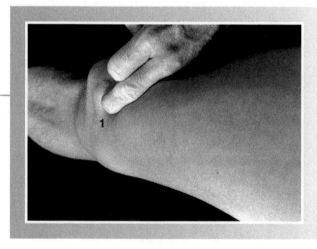

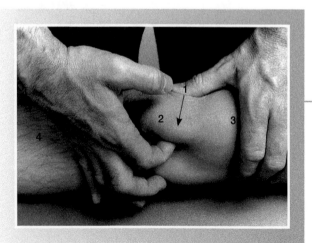

Fig. 10.48 Palpation of the medial patellar retinaculum

MA: This maneuver induces a partial medial dislocation of the patella and results in a stretching of the retinaculum in a plane that gets progressively closer to the midsagittal plane. The retinaculum reinforces the capsule and is felt under the fingers as a fibrous band.

1. Medial displacement of the patella
2. Patella
3. Quadriceps
4. Leg

Fig. 10.49 **Method for stretching the transverse fibers of the medial patellar retinaculum by pulling the patella laterally**

MA: This procedure, similar to that described in Figure 10.42, stretches the structure you are after in a plane that progressively approaches the horizontal plane. As a reinforcement of the capsule, it is felt by your fingers as a fibrous band.

1. Medial patellar retinaculum
2. Thigh
3. Leg
4. Patella

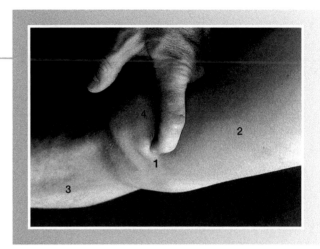

Fig. 10.50 **Visualization of the infrapatellar fat pad**

MA: There is a fat pad lying between the patellar ligament and the posterior nonarticular part of the patella and overlying the anterior intercondylar area of the tibial plateau. Laterally this fat pad extends halfway between the medial and lateral borders of the patella, forming a series of folds of fat. It is easily visible and becomes more prominent if the subject is asked to extend her knee, as shown in the adjacent figure.

Another method of approach: with the subject supine, the practitioner places his hand between her popliteal fossa and the table and asks her to flatten his hand. The fat pad will appear on both sides of the patella and of each patellar ligament.

Note: It is more prominent in women than in men.

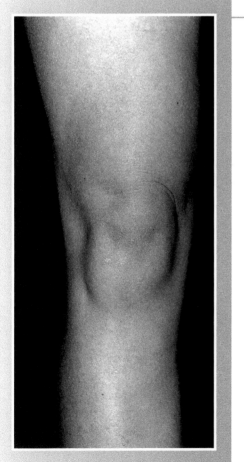

> **CLINICAL NOTE**
>
> **The infrapatellar fat pad syndrome (Hoffa's disease)**
>
> In this condition the fat pad can become swollen and painful on palpation.
>
> - During a knee operation the drainage tubes pass through the fat pad, which can remain painful for a very long time.

NERVES AND BLOOD VESSELS

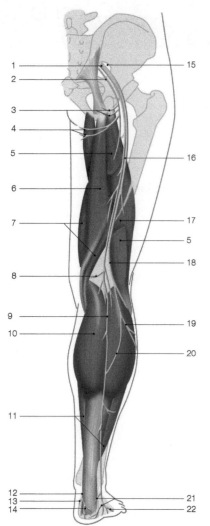

Sciatic nerve and posterior femoral cutaneous nerve

1. Sciatic nerve
2. Posterior femoral cutaneous nerve
3. Inferior clunial nerves
4. Perineal branches
5. Long head of biceps femoris
6. Semitendinosus
7. Semimembranosus
8. Articular branch
9. Sural nerve
10. Medial head of gastrocnemius
11. Soleus
12. Tibial nerve
13. Medial and lateral plantar nerves
14. Medial calcaneal branches
15. Greater sciatic notch
16. Common fibular branch of the sciatic nerve
17. Short head of biceps femoris
18. Common fibular nerve
19. Lateral sural cutaneous nerve
20. Sural communicating nerve
21. Lateral calcaneal branches
22. Lateral dorsal cutaneous nerve

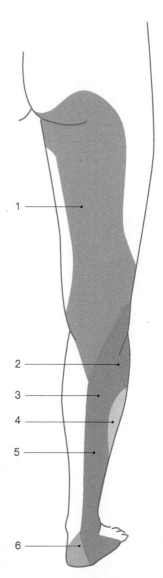

Sciatic nerve and posterior femoral cutaneous nerve

1. Posterior femoral cutaneous nerve

Sciatic nerve:
2. Common fibular nerve via the lateral sural cutaneous nerve
3. Medial sural cutaneous nerve
4. Superficial fibular nerve
5. Sural nerve
6. Tibial nerve via the medial calcaneal branches

THE MAIN NERVES AND BLOOD VESSELS

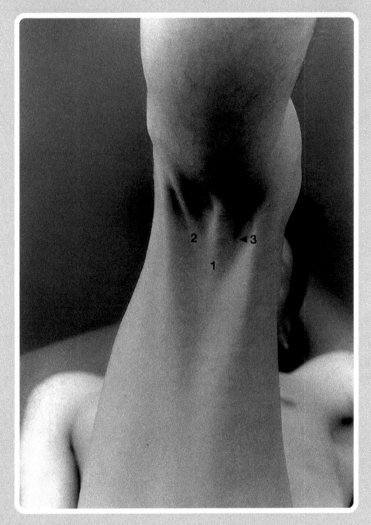

Fig. 10.51 Posterior view of the popliteal fossa: subject supine with hip and knee flexed

1. Tibial nerve (Figs. 10.52–10.56)
2. Common fibular nerve (Figs. 10.52–10.55, and 10.57–10.60)
3. Popliteal artery (Figs. 10.54, 10.55, 10.58, and 10.61–10.64)

Note: The arrow indicates the notable landmarks for an optimal approach to the popliteal artery.

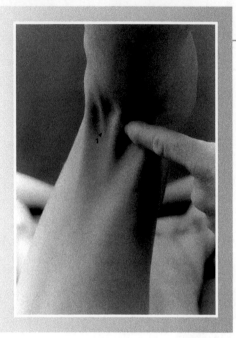

Fig. 10.52 Close-up of the tibial nerve: subject supine with hip and knee flexed

MA: The index finger points to the tibial nerve.

1. Common fibular nerve

Fig. 10.53 Display of the tibial, common fibular, and lateral sural cutaneous nerves

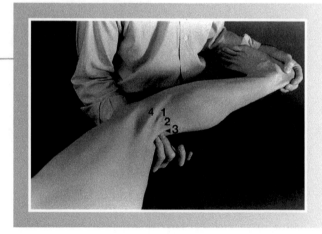

MA: With the subject lying on one side, the practitioner flexes her hip beyond 90°, flexes her knee slightly and also dorsiflexes her ankle. In the figure his index finger points to the structures being looked for.

Captions for Figures 10.53 and 10.54

1. Common fibular nerve
2. Lateral sural cutaneous nerve
3. Tibial nerve
4. Biceps femoris tendon

Fig. 10.54 Close-up of the popliteal fossa: visualization of the nerves mentioned above

MA: The same display technique is used as shown in Fig. 10.53: the subject lies on her side, her ankle is passively dorsiflexed to the maximum, her knee is slightly flexed and her hip is progressively flexed more or less maximally.

If this procedure fails to bring out the nerve in the middle of the popliteal fossa, you must then ask the subject to flex her trunk while simultaneously flexing her head and her neck.

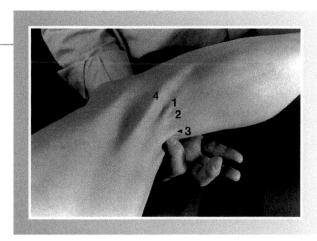

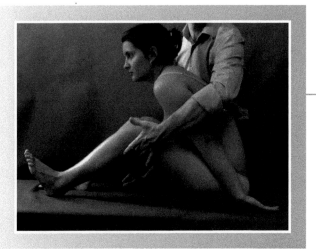

Fig. 10.55 Palpation of the tibial nerve and of the common fibular nerve in the popliteal fossa: initial phase

MA: The subject is seated on the examining table with three joints of her lower limb flexed (foot dorsiflexed, knee flexed, and hip flexed), and her trunk slightly flexed. Place your hand in her left popliteal fossa while standing on the opposite side.

Note: The subject's knee needs to be flexed adequately according to the shape of her body in order to stretch optimally the nerve you wish to palpate.

Fig. 10.56 Palpation of the tibial nerve: stretching procedure

MA: From the initial position shown in the previous figure, flex the subject's trunk and head until your fingers can feel in the middle of the popliteal fossa a solid cylindrical cord the size of a little finger.

Note: Since female subjects are generally more flexible than their male counterparts, occasionally you may well have to resort to submaximal flexion of head and trunk while calibrating the appropriate degree of knee flexion.

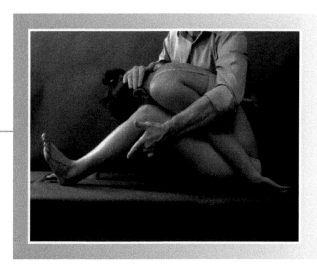

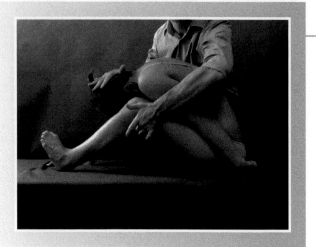

Fig. 10.57 Palpation of the common fibular nerve: stretching procedure

MA: Starting from the position where the tibial nerve is already stretched (described in Fig. 10.56), you need only ask the subject to invert and plantar-flex her foot until you can feel under your fingers a solid cylindrical cord (finer than the tibial nerve). You can palpate it in the lateral part of the popliteal fossa along the medial border of the biceps femoris. It continues its course in the proximolateral part of the knee as it wraps itself around the fibular head.

Note: As for the tibial nerve, in women the knee is extended to a greater degree than in men.

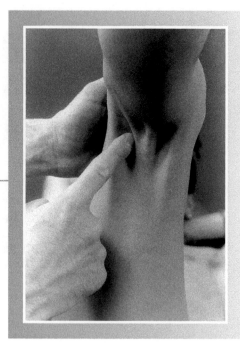

Fig. 10.58 Posterior view of the popliteal fossa: the subject lying supine with hip and knee flexed.

MA: The index finger points to the common fibular nerve.

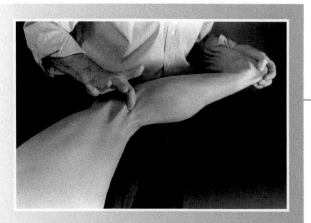

Fig. 10.59 Display of the common fibular nerve

MA: The subject lies on her side. The mode of display is similar to that described for the nerves in the popliteal fossa (Fig. 10.55). The index finger points to the structure you are after.

Fig. 10.60 Display of the lateral sural cutaneous nerve

MA: The subject lies on her side. The method of display is the same as that described for the common fibular nerve (Fig. 10.53).

The index finger points to the structure you are looking for.

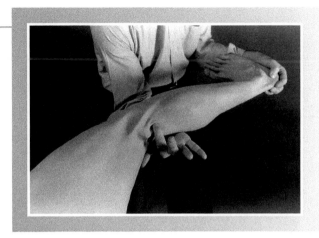

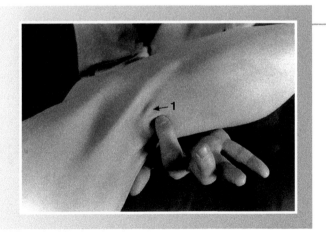

Fig. 10.61 Close-up of the popliteal fossa

MA: For the method of display, see Figure 10.53. The index finger shows the lateral sural cutaneous nerve. Lateral to it lies the common fibular nerve (1) as it runs toward the fibular neck.

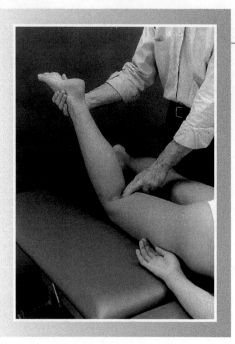

Fig. 10.62 Taking the popliteal arterial pulse in the popliteal fossa: stage 1

MA: Extend the subject's knee more or less maximally to allow you to place the pads of two or three fingers in the superomedial part of the popliteal fossa on top of the semimembranosus tendon.

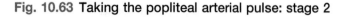

Fig. 10.63 Taking the popliteal arterial pulse: stage 2

MA: Flex the subject's knee progressively and move your palpating finger pads toward the central part of the popliteal fossa, seeking the popliteal pulse, which you can feel close to the tibial nerve.

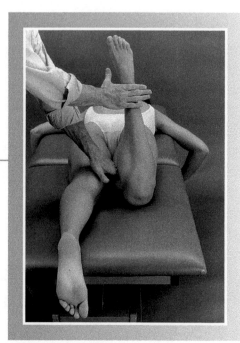

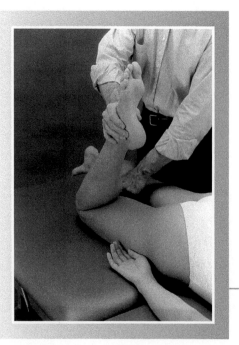

Fig. 10.64 Taking the popliteal arterial pulse: stage 3

MA: Keep the subject's knee more or less maximally flexed to relax optimally the posterior fibrous structures of the knee. This will facilitate your access to the popliteal artery, which you can feel medial to the tibial nerve.

11
The leg

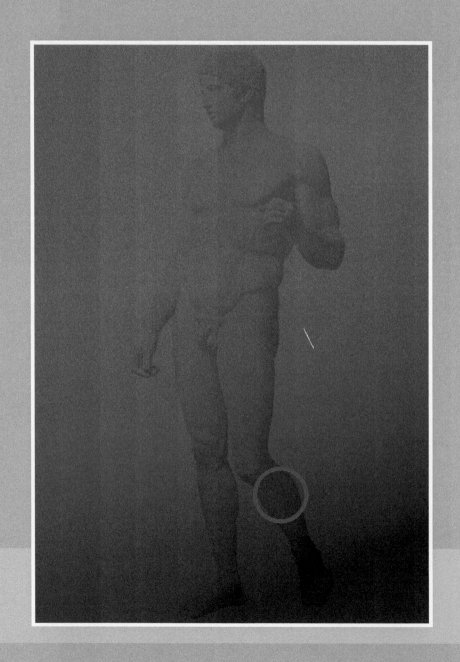

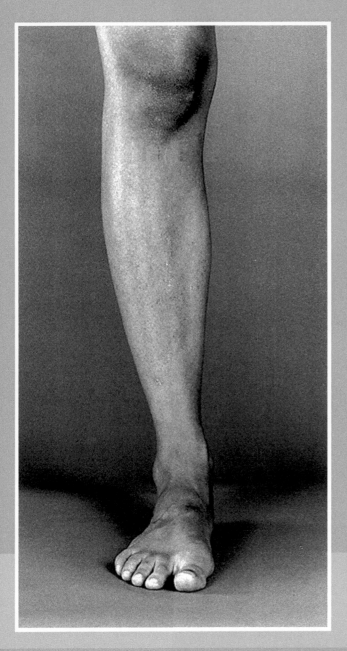
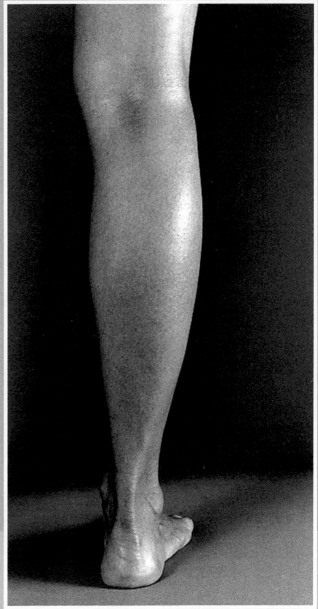

OSTEOLOGY

Attachments of the anterior muscles of the leg

1. Rectus femoris
2. Lateral patellar retinaculum
3. Iliotibial tract
4. Aponeurosis of biceps femoris
5. Fibularis longus
6. Biceps femoris
7. Extensor digitorum longus
8. Extensor hallucis longus
9. Fibularis tertius
10. Adductor magnus
11. Medial patellar retinaculum
12. Semimembranosus
13. Patellar ligament
14. Gracilis
15. Sartorius
16. Semitendinosus
17. Interosseous membrane
18. Tibialis anterior

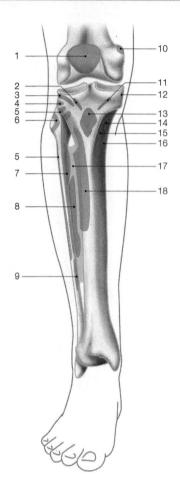

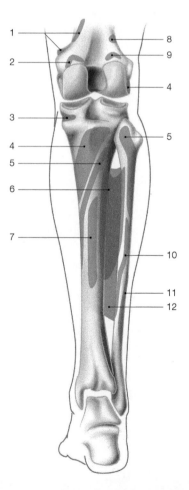

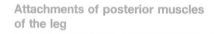

Attachments of posterior muscles of the leg

1. Adductor magnus
2. Medial head of gastrocnemius
3. Semimembranosus
4. Popliteus
5. Soleus
6. Tibialis posterior
7. Flexor digitorum longus
8. Plantaris
9. Lateral head of gastrocnemius
10. Fibularis brevis
11. Flexor hallucis longus
12. Interosseous membrane

THE BONES OF THE LEG

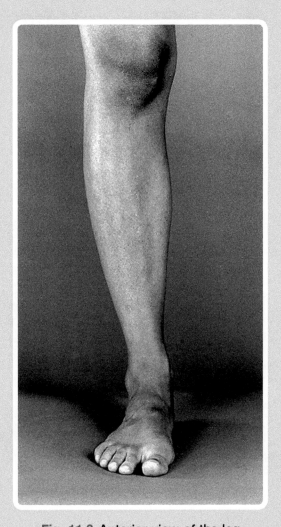

Fig. 11.3 Anterior view of the leg

The bony structures accessible to palpation are:
- The tibia:
  – the anterior border (Fig. 11.4)
  – the medial border (Fig. 11.5)
  – the medial aspect (Fig. 11.6)
  – the posterior aspect (Fig. 11.7)
- The fibula:
  – the lateral aspect (Fig. 11.8).

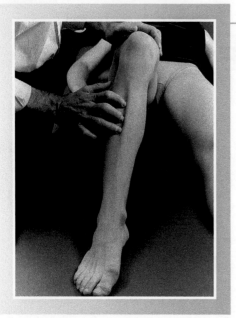

Fig. 11.4 The anterior tibial border

MA: It extends from the tibial tuberosity down to the medial malleolus. In its proximal three quarters it has the shape of a crest, known as the tibial crest (the shin). In its distal quarter it veers medially toward the medial malleolus and becomes blunt. As it lies directly under the skin, the anterior border is accessible in its entirety and is quite easy to investigate.

Fig. 11.5 The medial tibial border

MA: It stretches from the medial tibial condyle to the medial malleolus and limits the medial aspect of the tibial shaft. It is also accessible to investigation in its entirety.

> **CLINICAL NOTE**
>
> A fatigue fracture presents as a very distinct spot, acutely painful on palpation and more likely to lie in the distal third of the medial border, whereas periosteal pain is felt over a large area in its middle third. Pain on palpation of this structure can reveal the presence of a periostitis or of a fatigue fracture.

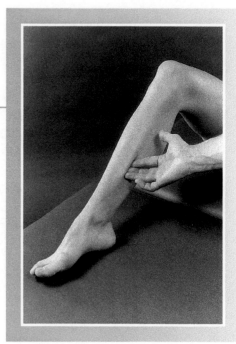

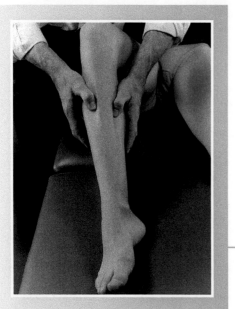

Fig. 11.6 The medial aspect of the tibia

MA: It is flat and smooth and lies directly under the skin along its entire length. Its proximal part near the tuberosity receives the insertion of the anserine muscles. As it lies between the anterior border and the medial border, it is entirely accessible to investigation.

Fig. 11.7 The posterior aspect of the tibia

MA: It is partially accessible to examination posterior to the medial tibial border and particularly at the proximal and distal ends of the shaft.

In the adjacent figure the subject's leg is laterally rotated to allow adequate palpation of this surface very close to its proximal extremity and posterior to its medial tibial border. You must take care to have the subject's posterior thigh muscles in a thoroughly relaxed state.

ATTACHMENTS

- Popliteus is inserted into the soleal line and its upper lip.
- Soleus is inserted into the soleal line.
- Tibialis posterior arises laterally and flexor digitorum longus medially from the lower lip of the soleal line.
- Distal to the soleal line there is a vertical ridge separating the insertion of flexor digitorum longus medial to it from that of tibialis posterior lateral to it.

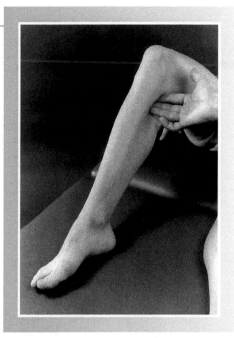

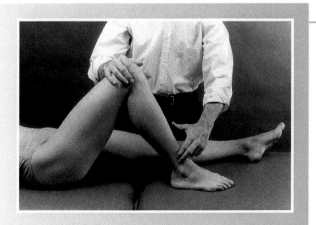

Fig. 11.8 The lateral aspect of the fibula

MA: It is directly accessible in its distal part. Its distal end bears an oblique ridge that runs superoinferiorly and anteroposteriorly and divides into two parts:

- an anterior triangular part lying directly under the skin and easily accessible to palpation;
- a posterior part, on which slide the tendons of fibularis brevis and fibularis longus.

CLINICAL NOTE

A fatigue fracture can be detected by applying palpation with pressure at the junction of the proximal two thirds and of the distal third of the fibula. From this point, move your fingers proximally and distally in search of the precise location of the fracture.

ATTACHMENTS

The superiorly convex lateral aspect forms along its intermediate part a longitudinal groove that gives origin to fibularis longus and fibularis brevis.

THE JOINTS OF THE LEG

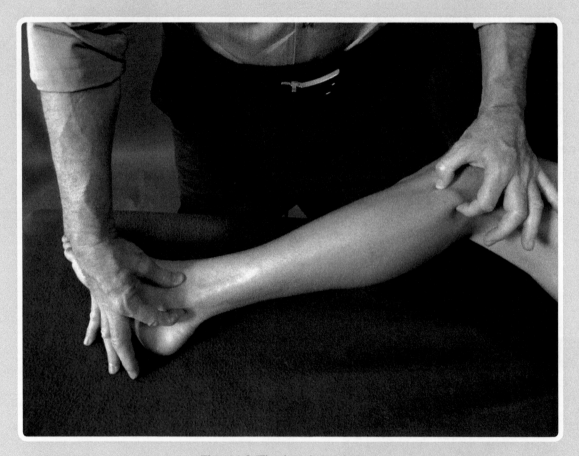

Fig. 11.9 The leg: lateral view

The notable articular structures of the leg are the proximal and distal tibiofibular joints (Fig. 11.10).

ARTHROLOGY

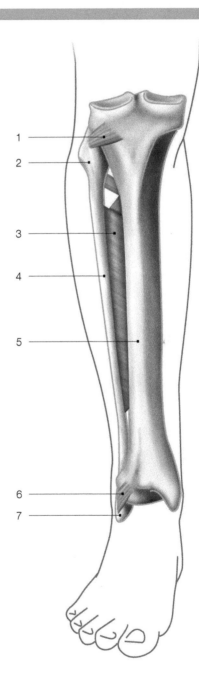

Arthrology of the leg

1. Anterior ligament of the fibular head
2. Fibular head
3. Interosseous membrane
4. Fibula
5. Tibia
6. Anterior tibiofibular ligament
7. Lateral malleolus

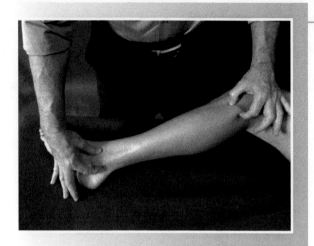

Fig. 11.10 The proximal and distal tibiofibular joints

MA: The proximal tibiofibular joint is a plane synovial joint uniting the tibia to the fibula. It is maintained by a capsule and two ligaments, one anterior and the other posterior.

> **CLINICAL NOTE**
>
> This joint can be the seat of a complete dislocation (a rare occurrence), of a subluxation (with misalignment of the fibular head relative to the tibia), of hypermobility, and even of a microtraumatic arthropathy. Pain is the major clinical sign. Palpation and mobilization of the fibular head are the key clinical approaches.

MA: The distal tibiofibular joint is a syndesmosis that unites the distal tibial and fibular epiphyses. It is maintained by three ligaments: anterior, posterior, and interosseous. The interosseous ligament unites the two articular surfaces, whose distinguishing feature is the absence of articular cartilage.

MYOLOGY

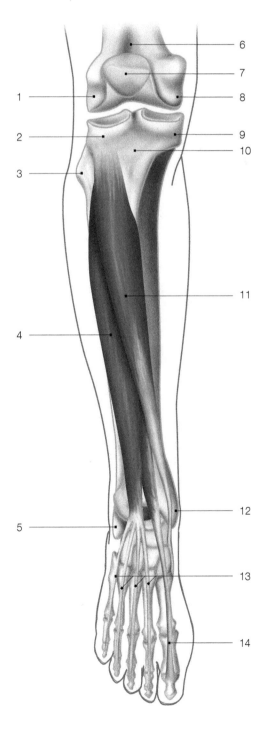

Muscles of the leg (anterior compartment)

1. Lateral epicondyle
2. Lateral tibial condyle
3. Fibular head
4. Extensor digitorum longus
5. Lateral malleolus
6. Femur
7. Patella
8. Medial epicondyle
9. Medial tibial condyle
10. Tibial tuberosity
11. Tibialis anterior
12. Medial malleolus
13. Tendons of extensor digitorum longus
14. Tendon of extensor hallucis longus

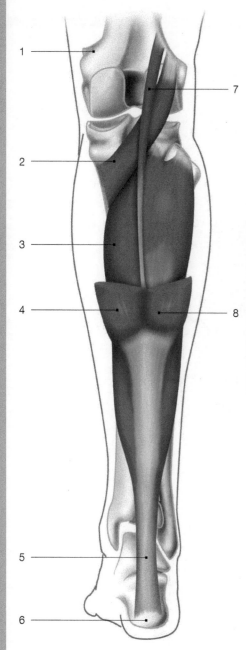

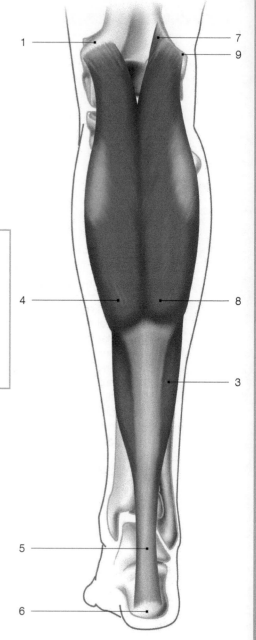

Triceps surae (posterior view after removal of gastrocnemius)

1. Medial femoral epicondyle
2. Popliteus
3. Soleus
4. Medial head of gastrocnemius
5. Calcaneal tendon (Achilles tendon)
6. Calcaneus
7. Plantaris
8. Lateral head of gastrocnemius
9. Lateral femoral epicondyle

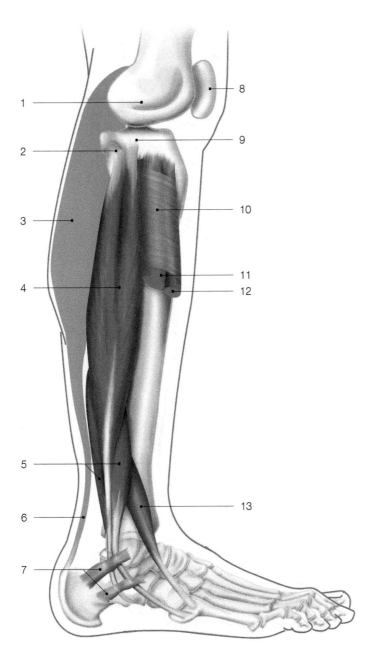

Muscles of the thigh (lateral compartment)

1. Femur
2. Fibular head
3. Triceps surae
4. Fibularis longus
5. Fibularis brevis
6. Calcaneal tendon
7. Superior and inferior fibular retinacula
8. Patella
9. Lateral tibial condyle
10. The deep fascia of leg (crural fascia)
11. Extensor digitorum longus
12. Tibialis anterior
13. Fibularis tertius

Deep muscles of the leg (posterior compartment)

1. Medial tibial condyle
2. Soleal line
3. Flexor digitorum longus
4. Medial malleolus
5. Tendon of insertion of tibialis posterior
6. Tendon of flexor hallucis longus
7. Fibular head
8. Tibialis posterior
9. Flexor hallucis longus
10. Calcaneal tuberosity
11. Lateral malleolus
12. Tendon of flexor digitorum longus

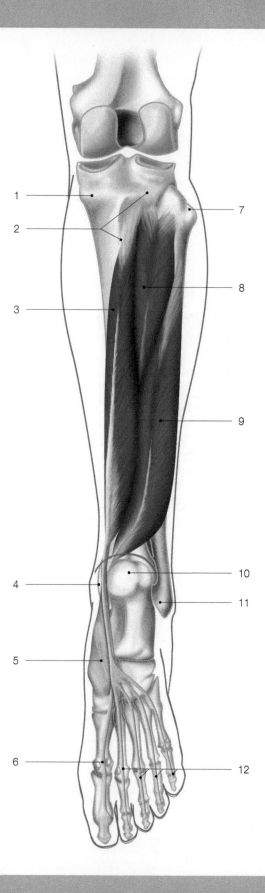

ANTERIOR GROUP OF LEG MUSCLES

It consists of the following four muscles:
- Tibialis anterior (Figs. 11.12–11.15)
- Extensor hallucis longus (Figs. 11.16–11.20)
- Extensor digitorum longus (Figs. 11.21 and 11.22)
- Fibularis tertius (Fig. 11.23).

Note: Extensor digitorum brevis also helps to extend the toes, but it is an intrinsic muscle of the foot, unlike the other three extensor muscles. It will be dealt with in Figs. 12.124, 12.140, 12.141, 12.143, and 12.144.

ACTIONS

- Tibialis anterior adducts, supinates, and dorsiflexes the foot on the leg.
- Extensor digitorum longus abducts, pronates, and dorsiflexes the foot on the leg and extends the toes.
- Extensor hallucis longus extends the big toe and helps in dorsiflexing the foot.
- Fibularis tertius dorsiflexes and everts the foot.

INNERVATIONS

- Tibialis anterior: deep fibular nerve + common fibular nerve (L4, L5, S1)
- Extensor digitorum longus: deep fibular nerve (L4, L5, S1)
- Extensor hallucis longus: deep fibular nerve (L4, L5, S1)
- Fibularis tertius: superficial fibular nerve (L5, S1)

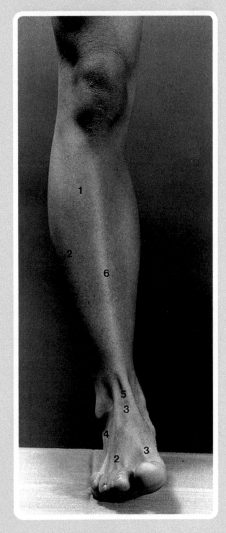

Fig. 11.11 Anterior view of the leg
1. Tibialis anterior
2. Extensor digitorum longus
3. Extensor hallucis longus
4. Fibularis tertius
5. Inferior extensor retinaculum
6. Anterior tibial border

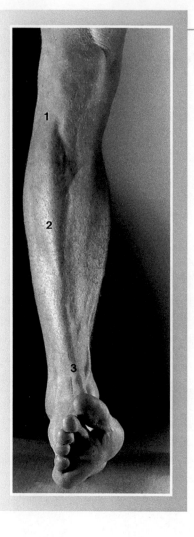

Fig. 11.12 Anterior view of tibialis anterior

1. Origin
2. Body
3. Distal tendon

Fig. 11.13 The distal part of the tibialis anterior tendon

MA: First adduct, supinate, and dorsiflex the subject's foot and then place the pads of your fingers on the medial border of his foot in order to resist his movements and thus bring out this tendon. It is the most medial of the anterior tendons of the instep, and it lies just anterior to the medial malleolus (1) and to the navicular.

ATTACHMENTS

In the adjacent figure the pads of two of the practitioner's fingers lie opposite the tendon near its distal insertion into the anteroinferior part of the medial aspect of the medial cuneiform (2). This insertion extends farther distally as a tendinous slip that inserts into a tubercle on the inferomedial part of the base of the first metatarsal.

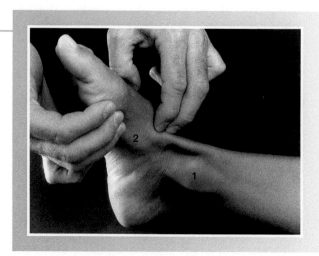

Fig. 11.14 Tibialis anterior in the leg

MA: This tendon (1) lies laterally alongside the tibial crest (the anterior tibial border) and is continuous proximally with the body of the muscle (2), which stays lateral to the crest and medial to extensor digitorum longus.

To bring out this muscle, ask the subject to perform the same movements as described in Fig. 11.13.

Note: As seen in the figure, it is a simple task to bring out this muscle.

1. Tendon of tibialis anterior
2. Body of tibialis anterior

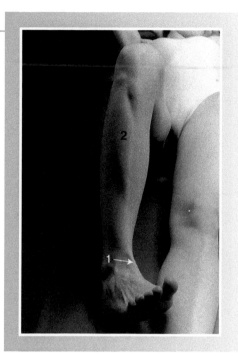

CLINICAL NOTE

Compartment syndrome

This is due to an increase in intramuscular pressure within a leg compartment, resulting in ischemia of the tissues and pain. All three leg compartments can be affected.

Acute anterior compartment syndrome

This can follow an injury complicated or not by a fracture and treated by a plaster cast that is too tight or by a supporting splint.

Apart from trauma it can follow any utilization of the muscles of the compartment so intense that the subject is forced to stop his effort.

On palpation the compartment feels very tender and very swollen. On testing it is painful, and its muscles are deficient. The dermatome of the deep fibular nerve reveals sensory disturbances. In a very short time (a few hours) paralysis sets in and sensory disturbances get worse in the dermatome.

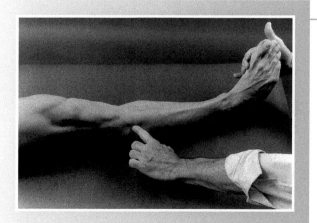

Fig. 11.15 The origin of tibialis anterior

MA: Ask the subject to place his foot in the same position as that shown in Figure 11.13, since this series of foot movements is specific for the visualization of this muscle. At the same time resist his movements by placing your fingers on the medial border of his foot in order to get a good feel of this muscle as it "tightens up" under your fingers.

ATTACHMENTS

It arises from Gerdy's tubercle, the oblique line, and the proximal two thirds of the anterolateral aspect of the tibia.

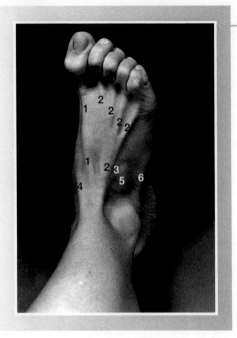

Fig. 11.16 The extensor apparatus of the toes

1. Extensor hallucis longus
2. Extensor digitorum longus
3. Fibularis tertius
4. Tibialis anterior
5. Extensor digitorum brevis
6. Fibularis brevis

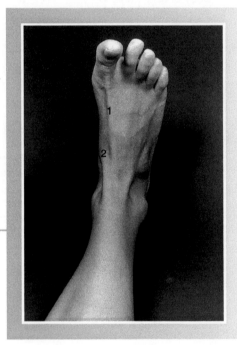

Fig. 11.17 Anterior view of the ankle

1. Extensor hallucis longus
2. Tibialis anterior

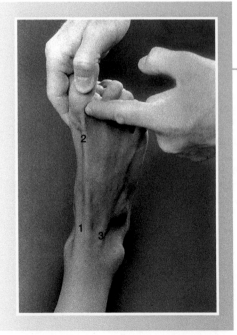

Fig. 11.18 The tendon of extensor hallucis longus near its insertion

MA: Ask the subject to extend his entire big toe and meanwhile resist this movement by placing your thumb flat on the dorsum of the distal phalanx of the big toe, causing the latter to go into plantar flexion.

The practitioner's index finger shows the tendon near its insertions into the base of the dorsal aspect of the distal phalanx of the big toe and into the sides of the base of the proximal phalanx of the big toe.

ATTACHMENTS

This muscle arises from the middle part of the medial aspect of the fibula anterior to the interosseous membrane and is inserted by two lateral tendinous slips into the base of the proximal phalanx and into the distal phalanx of the big toe.

CAPTION OF FIGURES 18, 19, 20

1. Tibialis anterior
2. Extensor hallucis longus
3. Extensor digitorum longus

Fig. 11.19 The tendon of extensor hallucis longus at the level of the instep

MA: The same set of movements has been performed by subject and practitioner as in Figure 11.18. The practitioner's index finger now points to the tendon as it crosses the instep.

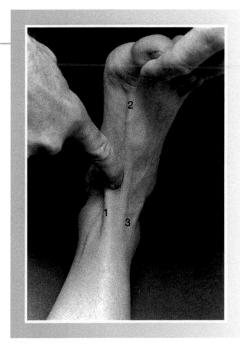

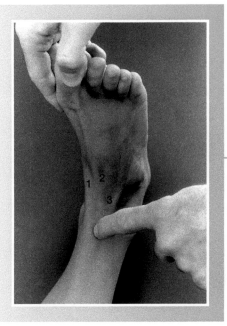

Fig. 11.20 The body of extensor hallucis longus in the distal part of the leg

MA: After ascending deep to the two extensor retinacula, the tendon joins the body of the muscle as it lies between tibialis anterior on its medial side and extensor digitorum longus on its lateral side.

Fig. 11.21 The tendons of extensor digitorum longus in the dorsum of the foot

MA: Place your distal hand as shown in the adjacent figure in order to resist the subject's extension of his toes.

Then you must run your fingers along the tendons for the four toes from their distal ends to the instep. In the adjacent figure, the common tendon is approached at the level of the instep.

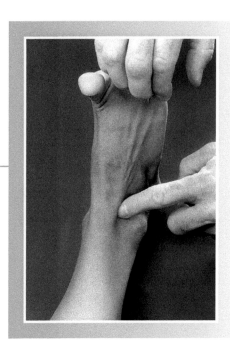

ATTACHMENTS

- This muscle arises from the lateral tibial condyle, lateral to that of tibialis anterior and from the proximal two thirds of the medial aspect of the fibula along its anterior border.
- The tendons for the four toes split along the dorsal surfaces of the proximal phalanges before inserting into the bases of the middle and distal phalanges.

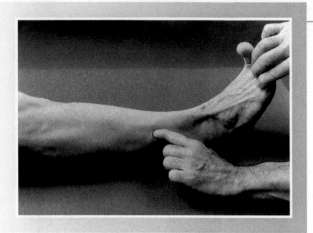

Fig. 11.22 Extensor digitorum longus in the leg

MA: Before it becomes tendinous, the body of the muscle courses along the full length of the leg between fibularis longus and fibularis brevis on its lateral side and tibialis anterior on its medial side.

Carefully locate these last two muscles by taking advantage of their actions and you will be better able to find the muscle you are looking for.

Moreover, it is useful to ask the subject to keep his foot actively dorsiflexed, abducted and "pronated" in order for you to appreciate even better the contraction of this muscle at this level.

Fig. 11.23 Fibularis tertius

MA: This muscle, when present, appears as a tendon on the lateral border of the tendon of extensor digitorum longus for the fifth toe.

To bring out this tendon, simply ask the subject to evert his foot with or without any resistance on your part.

ATTACHMENTS

- The tendon runs toward the dorsal surface of the base of the fifth metatarsal, where it is inserted.
- It arises from the distal third of the medial aspect of the fibula.

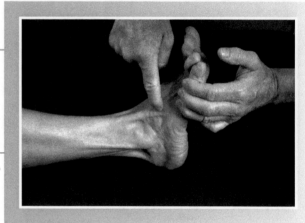

THE LATERAL GROUP OF MUSCLES

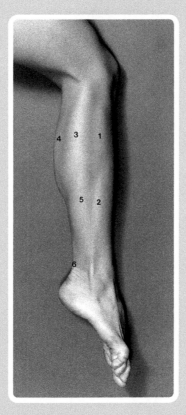

Fig. 11.24 Lateral view of the leg

1. Fibularis longus
2. Fibularis brevis
3. Lateral head of gastrocnemius
4. Medial head of gastrocnemius
5. Soleus
6. Calcaneal tendon

This group consists of two muscles:

- Fibularis longus (Figs. 11.25–11.28, 11.33, and 11.34)
- Fibularis brevis (Figs. 11.29–11.32).

ACTIONS

- Fibularis longus:
  - It abducts, pronates, and plantar-flexes the foot.
  - It lowers the first metatarsal by displacing it laterally and thus unifies the entire metatarsus.
  - It stabilizes the foot laterally in the coronal plane, acting synergistically with fibularis brevis.

- Fibularis brevis:
  - It pronates and abducts the foot.
  - It stabilizes the foot laterally in the coronal plane.

INNERVATIONS

- Fibularis longus: superficial fibular nerve (L4, L5, S1)
- Fibularis brevis: superficial fibular nerve (L4, L5, S1)

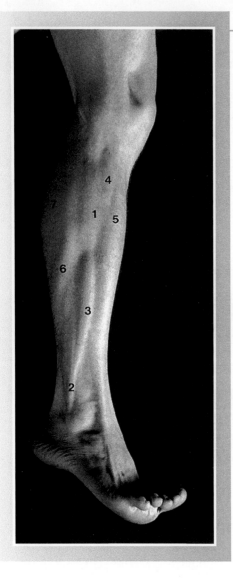

Fig. 11.25 Fibularis longus and related muscles

1. Fibularis longus
2. Tendon of fibularis longus
3. Fibularis brevis
4. Extensor digitorum longus
5. Tibialis anterior
6. Soleus
7. Lateral head of gastrocnemius

Fig. 11.26 The tendon of fibularis longus on the lateral border of the foot

MA: Ask the subject to abduct his foot already plantar-flexed, a movement that the practitioner can oppose.

After being reflected at the level of the lateral malleolus, the tendon lies flat on the lateral aspect of the calcaneus and passes deep to the fibular trochlea before entering the groove for its tendon on the cuboid on the lateral border of the foot.

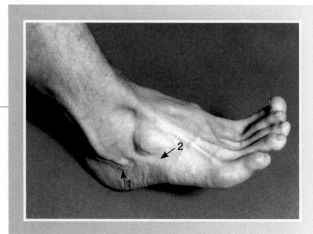

1. Tendon of fibularis longus
2. Tendon of fibularis brevis

Fig. 11.27 The tendon of fibularis longus in the leg

MA: Ask the subject to perform the same actions as described in Fig. 11.26. At this level the tendon courses along half of the lateral aspect of the leg. It lies flat on the body of fibularis brevis, which extends beyond its margins anteriorly and posteriorly.

ATTACHMENTS

- It arises from the lateral tibial condyle lateral to the origin of the extensor digitorum longus, from the anterolateral aspect of the fibular head, and from the proximal third of the lateral aspect of the fibular shaft.
- It is inserted into the posterolateral tuberosity of the first metatarsal, sending more often than not tendinous slips to the medial aspect of the cuneiform or to the second metatarsal and also to the first dorsal interosseus.

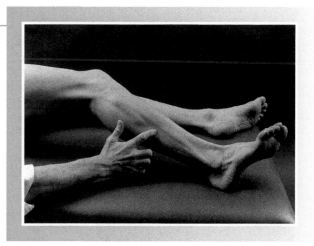

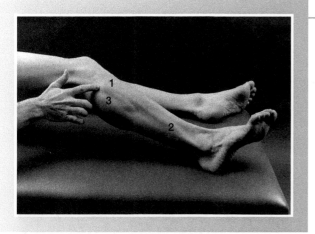

Fig. 11.28 The body of fibularis longus

MA: Ask the subject to abduct and plantar-flex his foot (as shown in Fig. 11.27), and the body of the muscle will stand out on the proximal part of the lateral aspect of the leg between extensor digitorum longus anteriorly and soleus posteriorly, as indicated by the practitioner's index finger.

CLINICAL NOTE

A tear can occur, though rarely, in this muscle. Targeted palpation of its body, when painful, can reveal such a tear, and the diagnosis can be confirmed by the presence of a notch in the muscle indicating a tear in its fibers. Clinical testing of this muscle (requiring inversion of the foot) will show pain and reduced muscular activity.

1. Extensor digitorum longus
2. Fibularis brevis
3. Soleus

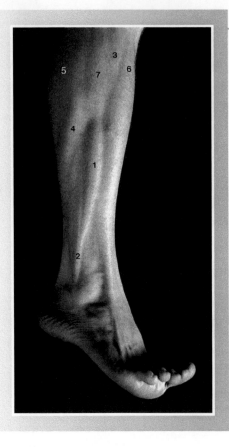

Fig. 11.29 Fibularis brevis and related muscles

1. Fibularis brevis
2. Tendon of fibularis longus
3. Extensor digitorum longus
4. Soleus
5. Lateral head of gastrocnemius
6. Tibialis anterior
7. Fibularis longus

Fig. 11.30 The tendon of fibularis brevis in its most distal course on the lateral border of the foot

MA: Abducting the subject's foot, with or without any opposition, is enough to bring out this tendon. You must then follow its course along the lateral border of the foot to its insertion into the tuberosity of the fifth metatarsal.

Note: To improve the visualization of its passage on the lateral aspect of the calcaneus dorsal to the fibular trochlea, please see Figs. 12.12–12.19.

1. Fibularis longus
2. Tendon of fibularis longus
3. Fibularis brevis

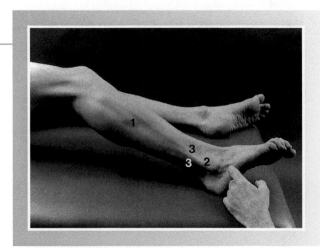

Fig. 11.31 Fibularis brevis in the leg

MA: Ask the subject to perform the same movement as shown in Figure 11.30. The body of the muscle will stand out anterior to the fibularis longus tendon. Having the subject perform a series of contractions and relaxations will help you to get a better view of the location of the relaxed muscle.

ATTACHMENTS

The muscle arises from the distal two thirds of the lateral aspect of the fibula and is inserted into the tuberosity of the fifth metatarsal.

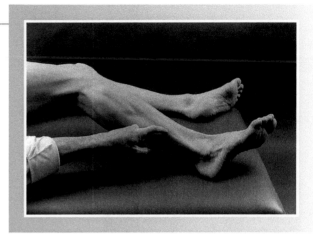

> **CLINICAL NOTE**
>
> A tear in the muscle can always occur, particularly during sports activities. Targeted palpation of the body of the muscle, if painful, indicates the presence of a tear and can also reveal a notch in the muscle consistent with a tear in the muscle fibers. Testing of this muscle (abduction of the foot against resistance) will be painful and show reduced muscular function.
>
> Stretching the muscle by abducting the foot will induce or exacerbate the pain.

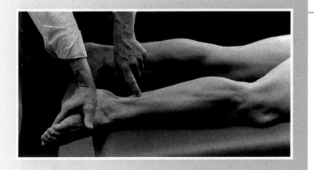

Fig. 11.32 Fibularis brevis in the leg: another view

MA: The subject performs the same movement as shown in Fig. 11.31. You can also ask him to plantar-flex his foot to bring out the contraction of the muscle even better.

You can also feel the body of the muscle posterior to the tendon of fibularis longus, depending on the physiques of the subjects examined.

Global approach

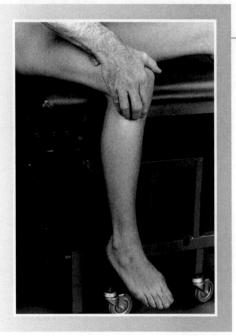

Fig. 11.33 Global location of tibialis anterior, extensor digitorum longus, and fibularis longus

MA: The subject sits on the edge of the table with or without his legs crossed, and his foot hangs down in a normally relaxed state. (The subject can also lie down on his back with his trunk raised so that he has visual control of his foot movements.)

Using your thumb and your fingers, place your hand on the superolateral part of the leg between the fibular head and the tibial tuberosity.

Fig. 11.34 Global location of muscles as described above: close-up

MA: To be more precise, place your fifth and fourth fingers flat on the anterior part of the fibular head, and your third and second fingers on the lateral border of the tibial tuberosity, just distal to the tibial oblique line and Gerdy's tubercle. When your global contact is in place, your fifth finger faces fibularis longus, your fourth finger faces extensor digitorum longus, and your third and second fingers face tibialis anterior.

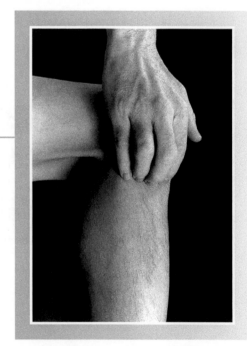

Fig. 11.35 Locating the proximal part of tibialis anterior

MA: From the starting point described in Figures 11.33 and 11.34, proceed by asking the subject to adduct, supinate, and dorsiflex his foot.

You will feel the muscle contracting under your fingers, and more precisely under your second and third fingers.

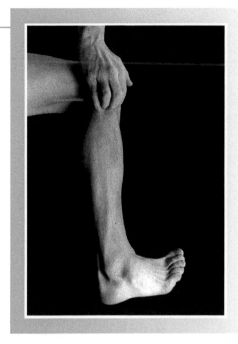

Fig. 11.36 Locating the proximal part of extensor digitorum longus

MA: From the starting point described in Figures 11.33 and 11.34, ask the subject to abduct, pronate, and dorsiflex his foot.

You will feel the muscle contracting under your fingers – more precisely, under your fourth finger.

Note: This muscle is not necessarily clearly felt at this level. It can be covered by a well-developed tibialis anterior or fibularis longus or even by both these muscles.

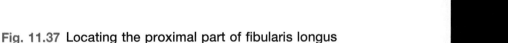

Fig. 11.37 Locating the proximal part of fibularis longus

MA: From the starting point already described, proceed by asking the subject to perform abduction, pronation, and plantar flexion of his foot, which are precisely the actions of fibularis longus.

As the muscle tightens it will be felt under your fingers and more precisely under your fourth and fifth fingers.

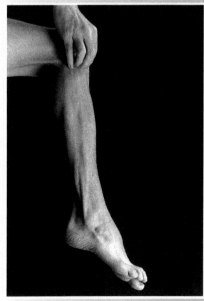

THE POSTERIOR MUSCLE GROUP

The **superficial plane** of this group comprises:

- triceps surae (Fig. 11.39), which consists of:
  - medial head of gastrocnemius (Figs. 11.40–11.42)
  - lateral head of gastrocnemius (Figs. 11.40, 11.43, and 11.44)
  - soleus (Figs. 11.45–11.49)
- plantaris (Figs. 11.44 and 11.51).

The **deep plane** of this group comprises:

- tibialis posterior (Figs. 11.52–11.55)
- flexor digitorum longus (Figs. 11.56–11.59)
- flexor hallucis longus (Figs. 11.60–11.64)
- popliteus (Figs. 11.65 and 11.66).

ACTIONS

- Triceps surae and plantaris:
  - They plantar-flex the ankle.
  - Both heads of gastrocnemius are weak participants in knee flexion and are mobilized much less during plantar flexion of the foot when the knee is flexed.
  - Plantaris takes part in the same actions as the gastrocnemius. (It is, however, often absent, and its action is of secondary importance anyway.)
- Tibialis posterior:
  - It adducts and supinates the foot.
  - It also helps to plantar-flex the foot.
- Flexor digitorum longus:
  - It flexes the distal phalanx on the middle phalanx, the middle phalanx on the proximal phalanx, and the proximal phalanx on the corresponding metatarsal; it acts only on the last four toes.
  - It helps in plantar flexion of the ankle.
- Flexor hallucis longus:
  - It flexes the distal phalanx on the proximal phalanx and the proximal phalanx on the first metatarsal.
- Popliteus:
  - It medially rotates the leg.

INNERVATIONS

- Triceps surae: tibial nerve (L5, S1, S2)
- Plantaris: tibial nerve (L5, S1, S2)
- Tibialis posterior: tibial nerve (L5, S1)
- Flexor digitorum longus: tibial nerve (L5, S1, S2)
- Flexor hallucis longus: tibial nerve (L5, S1, S2)
- Popliteus: tibial nerve (L4, L5, S1)

Plantaris: distally its tendon blends with that of triceps surae, but it can remain separate.

Note: For teaching purposes the gastrocnemius, soleus, and plantaris will be dealt with in this order and separately.

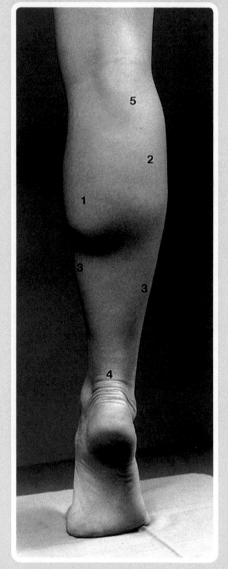

Fig. 11.38 Posterior view of the leg

1. Medial head of gastrocnemius
2. Lateral head of gastrocnemius
3. Soleus
4. Calcaneal tendon (Fig. 11.50)
5. Plantaris

The superficial plane

Fig. 11.39 Triceps surae and related muscles

1. Medial head of gastrocnemius (Figs. 11.40–11.42)
2. Lateral head of gastrocnemius (Figs. 11.40, 11.43, and 11.44)
3. Soleus (Figs. 11.45–11.49)
4. Calcaneal tendon (Fig. 11.50)
5. Fibularis longus
6. Tendon of fibularis longus
7. Fibularis brevis
8. Lateral malleolus
9. Posterior aspect of calcaneus
10. Fibular head
11. Tendon of biceps femoris

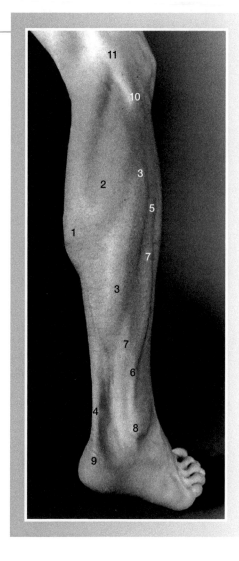

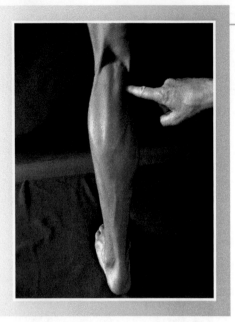

Fig. 11.40 Visualization of the two heads of gastrocnemius

MA: Triceps surae and particularly gastrocnemius can become highly developed as a result of certain sporting activities, like cycling.

> **CLINICAL NOTE**
>
> A third head of gastrocnemius can lead to compression of the tibial artery.
>
> **Posterior compartment syndrome**
>
> After an injury, a fracture treated by splinting or an overly tight cast can be complicated by this syndrome.
>
> Apart from injury, it can also follow utilization of the muscles of this compartment so intense that it forces the subject to stop his effort.
>
> On palpation the compartment is very tender and very swollen. Testing elicits pain and reveals muscular insufficiency. The dermatome of the tibial nerve is the seat of sensory disturbances. In a short time (a few hours) paralysis sets in and the sensory disturbances get worse.

Fig. 11.41 Medial head of gastrocnemius (1) in the leg

MA: Place your forearm on the sole of the subject's foot and use it to induce him to perform a series of plantar flexions of his ankle while you hold his calcaneus in the palm of your distal hand and prevent him from flexing his knee. These two sets of movements performed by the subject are produced by gastrocnemius. Look for the muscle itself on the posteromedial part of his leg superficial to the soleus.

Note: The body of the medial head of gastrocnemius extends farther distally than that of the lateral head.

> **CLINICAL NOTE**
>
> Partial or total disinsertion of this muscle can occur exactly where the practitioner's thumb is positioned in the adjacent figure (at the musculotendinous junction). When seen early, the notch in the muscle can be felt under the practitioner's fingers, and it is painful for the subject. When seen later, the calf will be swollen and tight, requiring careful handling on examination. The method of approach described in Figure 11.40 will make the pain worse. The diagnosis can be confirmed by stretching the subject's triceps surae, achieved by dorsiflexion of his foot with the knee extended.

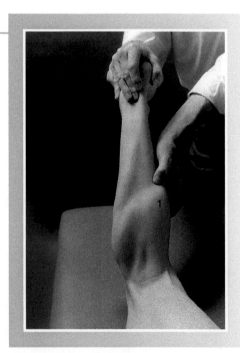

Fig. 11.42 Medial head of gastrocnemius (1) at the knee

MA: The method of tightening the muscle is the same as that described in Fig. 11.41.

> ### CLINICAL NOTE
>
> The body of this muscle (1) can be overstretched and even torn. When seen early, the latter condition can be diagnosed by the presence of a notch felt under the practitioner's fingers; when seen later, the edema present will make examination more difficult. In the clinical history the subject will describe a feeling of "a dagger thrust into" his calf or more simply a feeling of receiving a blow.

ATTACHMENTS

- The muscle arises from many structures, i.e., from the posteromedial corner of the knee (which is a reinforcement of the capsule posterior to the medial femoral condyle), from the adductor tubercle, from the adjacent part of the capsule, and from the popliteal surface of the femur. It is thus accessible in the medial part of the popliteal fossa, since it forms its inferomedial border.
- It is inserted with soleus and the lateral head of gastrocnemius on the posterior aspect of the calcaneus via the calcaneal tendon.

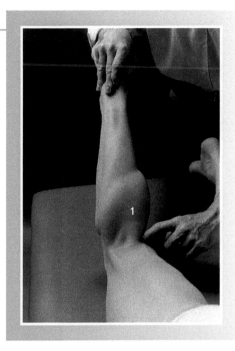

Fig. 11.43 Lateral head of gastrocnemius (1) in the leg

MA: Here again use your distal hand, which cradles the heel, and your forearm, which lies flat on the sole of the subject's foot, to resist simultaneously his attempt to plantar-flex his ankle and flex his knee. These combined muscular actions bring out the muscle you are after.

It is always useful to have the subject go through a contraction-relaxation series so that you can better feel the muscle as it contracts.

> ### CLINICAL NOTE
>
> There can also be partial or total disinsertion of this muscle exactly where the practitioner has placed his index finger and his middle finger as shown in the adjacent figure, i.e., at the musculotendinous junction. The subject feels pain under the practitioner's palpating fingers. When seen later, the calf will be swollen and tight, making examination more difficult.

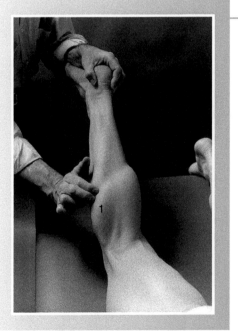

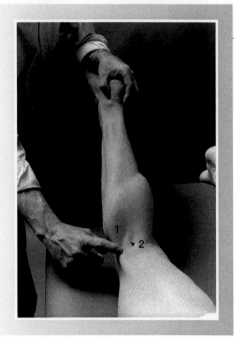

Fig. 11.44 Lateral head of gastrocnemius (1) at the knee and plantaris (2)

MA: The method for tightening these muscles is the same as that described in Fig. 11.43.

The proximal part of the lateral head of gastrocnemius represents an important region in the field of palpatory anatomy, since it forms the inferolateral border of the popliteal fossa. Its proximal end is bordered medially by plantaris (2), lying in a deeper plane.

Note: The body of popliteus, lying in the superoposterior part of the knee, can be approached indirectly through the fleshy medial and lateral bodies of the heads of gastrocnemius (palpation not shown). Caution is essential with deep palpation of this area because of the presence of the tibial nerve.

> **CLINICAL NOTE**
>
> The body of this muscle (1) can also be affected by some muscular lesions (overstretching, tears), but much less frequently than the body of the medial head.

ATTACHMENTS

- Like the medial head, the lateral head of gastrocnemius arises from the corresponding retrocondylar posterolateral reinforcement of the knee capsule, from the lateral femoral epicondyle and from the vicinity of the capsule and of the popliteal surface.
- It is inserted with soleus and the medial head of gastrocnemius into the posterior aspect of the calcaneus via the calcaneal tendon.
- Popliteus arises from the popliteal groove distal to the lateral femoral epicondyle and is inserted into the tibia proximal to the soleal line.

Fig. 11.45 Soleus

MA: Visualization of soleus: its fibular head in its entirety

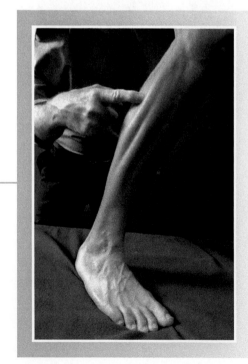

Fig. 11.46 Soleus: fibular head in its distal part

MA: The most distal part of the fibular head of soleus lies superficial to fibularis brevis (2) and posterior to the tendon of fibularis longus (3). With the palm of your distal hand, cradle the subject's heel and place your forearm flat on the sole of his foot in order to resist his plantar flexion. The technique of repeated contractions and relaxations is ideal to bring out the muscle. Look for it along the fibula between the posteriorly located lateral head of gastrocnemius (1) and the anteriorly located fibularis brevis and fibularis longus.

ATTACHMENTS

The fibular head of soleus is the part of the body of the muscle arising from the fibula, i.e., the posterior aspect of its head and the proximal quarter of its shaft. It is more extensive on the lateral aspect of the leg than is its medial head on the medial aspect.

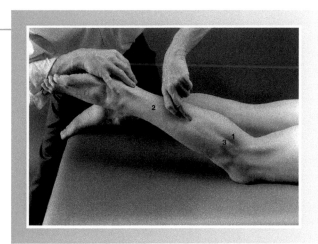

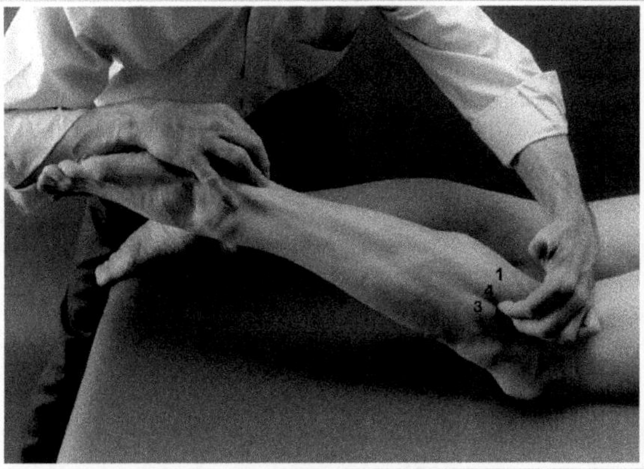

Fig. 11.47 Soleus: its fibular head in its proximal part

MA: The middle and proximal parts of its fibular head (4) lie posterior to fibularis longus (3) and anterior to the lateral head of gastrocnemius (1).

ATTACHMENTS

The two tendinous heads arising from the tibia and the fibula fuse into a single aponeurosis that gives rise to the muscle fibers on its posterior and anterior surfaces. As this tendinous aponeurosis is thus embedded inside the muscle, it is called the intramuscular fascia. The tendinous aponeurosis of soleus blends with the two heads of gastrocnemius before inserting into the posterior aspect of the calcaneus via the calcaneal tendon.

Fig. 11.48 Soleus: the tibial head

MA: Take hold of the calcaneus in the palm of your hand while placing your forearm flat on the sole of the subject's foot in order to resist his plantar flexion of the ankle.

The technique of repeated contractions and relaxations is ideal for bringing out the body of the muscle. Look for it along the medial border of the tibia down to its middle third and anterior to the medial head of gastrocnemius.

ATTACHMENTS

The tibial head is part of the body of the muscle, arising from the lower lip of the inferomedial half of the soleal line and from the middle third of the medial tibial border. It extends much less over the medial surface of the leg than does the fibular head on the lateral surface of the leg.

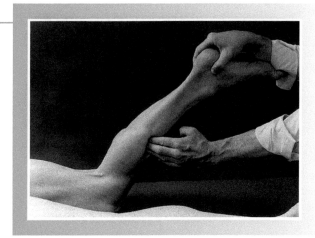

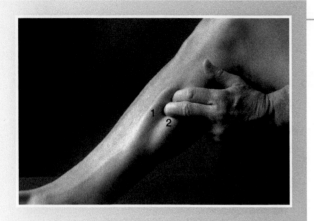

Fig. 11.49 Soleus: another view

MA: Visualization of the tibial head of soleus in its full length

1. Tibial head of soleus
2. Medial head of gastrocnemius

Fig. 11.50 Calcaneal tendon

MA: With the subject's heel held in the palm of your hand and your forearm resting flat on the sole of his foot, you can vary the degree of tension in the tendon. You can tighten the tendon in two ways:

- by exerting pressure on the sole of his foot so as to dorsiflex the foot and thus pull on the tendon;
- by using the technique of repeated contractions and relaxations of the tendon produced by plantar flexion of the foot.

Note: Once the tendon is located, you can also gain access to it in a relaxed state and on its three surfaces (posterior, anterior, and lateral). It is the bulkiest tendon in the body.

> **CLINICAL NOTE**
> Please see Figs. 12.128–12.129.

ATTACHMENTS

The calcaneal tendon is formed by the union of the gastrocnemius and soleus muscles and is inserted into the distal half of the posterior aspect of the calcaneus.

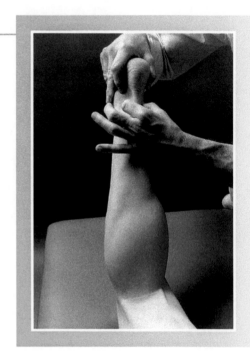

Fig. 11.51 Plantaris in the popliteal fossa

MA: This muscle lies anterior to the lateral head of the gastrocnemius and runs along its medial border. It is often absent and not easily accessible except in its proximal part in the popliteal fossa.

With the palm of your distal hand holding the subject's heel and your forearm pressed against the sole of his foot, you can prevent him simultaneously from plantar-flexing his foot and flexing his knee.

How you will feel the contraction of this muscle depends on the subject's build. You can feel it (1) in the popliteal fossa medial to the lateral head of gastrocnemius.

Note: The label (1) indicates more the course of the muscle than the muscle itself, which lies deep.

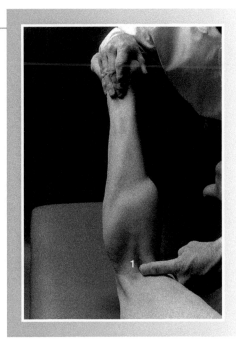

CLINICAL NOTE

This muscle can become disinserted or can be torn. Clinical testing of it is similar to that described for gastrocnemius.

ATTACHMENTS

- It arises from the lateral tibial condyle proximal and medial to the lateral head of gastrocnemius.
- It is inserted medial to the calcaneal tendon on the posterior aspect of the calcaneus.

The deep plane

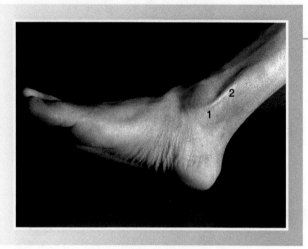

Fig. 11.52 Tibialis posterior and related muscles (medial view)

1. Tendon of tibialis posterior
2. Body of tibialis posterior

MA: Note: Refer to Figure 11.56 to observe the relations of this muscle with the other two tendons of the medial retromalleolar groove, which also belong to the deep muscular plane of the leg:

• flexor digitorum longus;
• flexor hallucis longus.

Fig. 11.53 The tendon of tibialis posterior between the tuberosity of the navicular and the medial malleolus

MA: With your distal hand guide and/or resist the subject's adduction of his foot, which has already been plantar-flexed. You will feel the tendon between the two structures mentioned above. In some cases, it is helpful to locate first the tuberosity of the navicular (see Figs. 12.37, 12.38 and 12.83).

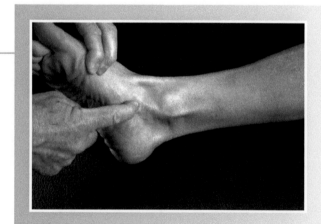

CLINICAL NOTE

The tendon can rupture at this level, and the rupture can be felt under your fingers as a notch along the course of the tendon. Obesity linked with a pes planus valgus is a predisposing factor among joggers, mainly because of the hyperpronation of their feet.

Fig. 11.54 The tendon of tibialis posterior at the ankle

MA: With your distal hand, guide and/or oppose the subject's adduction of his foot, which is already in the position of plantar flexion. You can see the tendon lying posterior to the medial malleolus and you can feel it under your fingers as a very "hard" cylindrical cord.

CLINICAL NOTE
At this level the tendon can be affected by two conditions: tenosynovitis or anterior dislocation of the tendon over the medial malleolus.

ATTACHMENTS

- The tibialis posterior arises from:
  – the proximal two thirds of the posterior aspect of the tibia lateral to the vertical ridge that separates it from flexor digitorum longus;
  – the proximal two thirds of the medial aspect of the fibula posterior to its interosseous border.
- It is inserted into all the tarsal bones, except the talus, and into all the metatarsal bones except the first and the fifth.

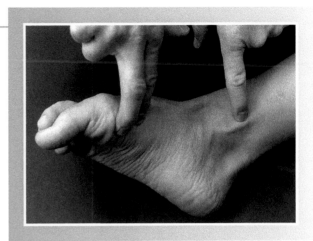

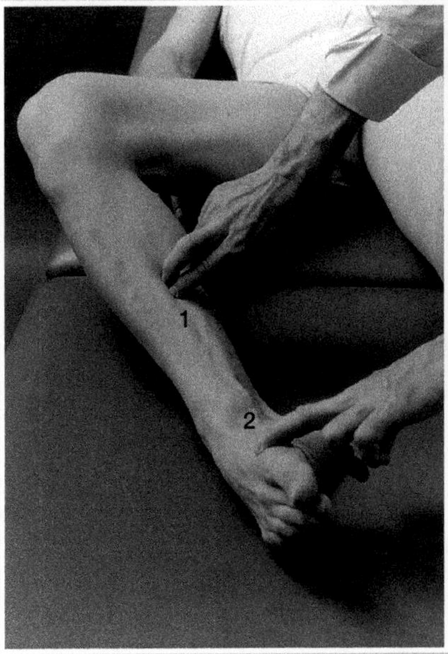

Fig. 11.55 The tendon and body of tibialis posterior

MA: The subject's leg rests on its lateral surface. To feel properly the muscle contracting, you simply have to move your finger pads along the medial tibial border (1). It is easier to feel if you use the technique of repeated contractions and relaxations. Start with the subject's foot in plantar flexion and ask him to adduct his foot repeatedly against resistance. The body of the muscle, which terminates in the tendon of tibialis posterior (2), courses anterior to flexor digitorum longus until it reaches the arcade formed at the distal tibial origin of the latter muscle, about 10 cm (4 inches) proximal to the medial malleolus. After passing under the arcade, the body of tibialis posterior comes to lie medial to that of flexor digitorum longus. At this level it is not directly accessible to palpation, since it is covered by triceps surae.

CLINICAL NOTE
If the muscle is torn, palpation will reveal a tender area in the soft tissues near the medial tibial border. During testing of the muscle (inversion of the plantar-flexed foot against resistance), the pain gets worse and is also associated with muscle weakness. Likewise, stretching the muscle by performing movements opposite to those used during testing will also cause pain.

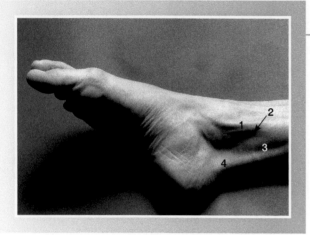

Fig. 11.56 Flexor digitorum longus and related muscles (medial view)

1. Tibialis posterior
2. Flexor digitorum longus
3. Flexor hallucis longus
4. Calcaneal tendon

Fig. 11.57 The tendons of flexor digitorum longus in the sole of the foot

MA: Your distal hand guides and/or gently resists a succession of rapid flexions of his toes with the ankle in the neutral position. Place your other hand flat on the sole of the subject's foot while holding its lateral border in your palm. Your contact is wide enough to allow you to feel the contraction of the muscle. You cannot directly feel the tendons themselves under your fingers, as they are masked by those of flexor digitorum brevis.

Note: You can better feel the contraction of these two muscles under your fingers if the proximal phalanges of the subject's toes are already hyperextended.

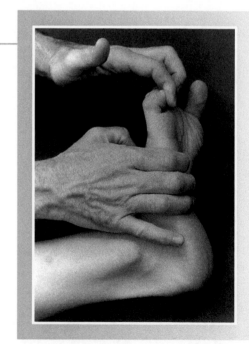

Fig. 11.58 Flexor digitorum longus in the medial retromalleolar groove

MA: The subject flexes his toes repeatedly in rapid succession, with his foot resting on its heel or on its lateral border.

You can feel the tendon close to the medial malleolus posterior to the tendon of tibialis posterior.

ATTACHMENTS

* The muscle arises from:
  – the medial part of the inferior lip of the soleal line of the tibia;
  – the middle third of the posterior aspect of the tibia medial to the vertical ridge that separates it from tibialis posterior.
* It is inserted into the bases of the distal phalanges of toes II–IV.

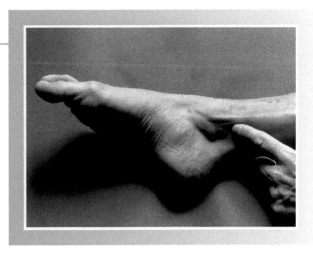

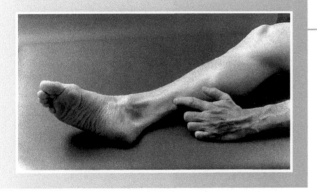

Fig. 11.59 The body of flexor digitorum longus in the distal third of the leg

MA: The subject's leg lies on its lateral border, and his ankle is relaxed. The practitioner's index finger shows the body of the muscle running posterior to tibialis posterior down to the arcade formed by its distal fibers arising from the tibia and located about 10 cm (4 inches) proximal to the medial malleolus. Beyond this arcade the body of the muscle comes to lie lateral to that of tibialis posterior and anterior to the medial or tibial head of soleus.

You can feel the contraction of the muscle better with the help of the technique of repeated contractions and relaxations, so ask the subject to flex his toes repeatedly in rapid succession.

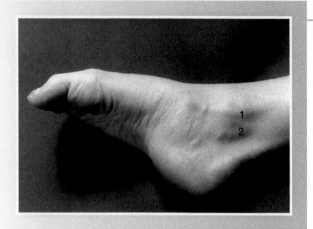

Fig. 11.60 Flexor hallucis longus

Note: Refer to Figure 11.56 in order to visualize the relations of this muscle with the other two tendons that cross the medial retromalleolar groove and also belong to the deep plane of the leg (tibialis posterior and flexor digitorum longus).

1. Tendon of tibialis posterior
2. Tendon of flexor hallucis longus as it passes posterior to the talus between the medial and lateral tubercles on its posterior surface

Fig. 11.61 Flexor hallucis longus in the sole of the foot

MA: First place the subject's ankle in the neutral position and have his leg resting on its heel or on its lateral border. Then proceed using your distal hand, guiding and/or opposing his repeated rapid flexions of his big toe.

Place your other hand on the plantar aspect of his first metatarsal, using a wide grip, the better to feel the contraction of the muscle. This method provides a better approach to the tendon, which is felt somewhat like a cord under your fingers.

Note: You will feel this tendinous structure much better if you first hyperextend the proximal phalanx of his big toe. You can leave the distal phalanx unopposed so that you can better feel the tendon.

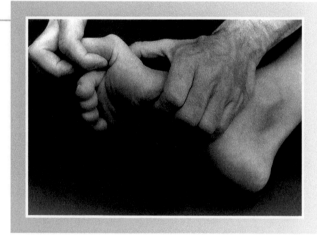

Fig. 11.62 Flexor hallucis longus in its retrotalar course

MA: First place the subject's ankle in the neutral position, with his leg resting on its posterolateral surface. Then proceed using your distal hand to guide and/or oppose his repeated rapid flexions of his big toe.

You will feel the muscle between the posteromedial and posterolateral tubercles of the talus and posterior to the tendon of flexor digitorum longus.

ATTACHMENTS

- It arises from the distal three quarters of the posterior aspect of the fibula.
- It is inserted into the base of the distal phalanx of the big toe after passing between the two sesamoid bones of the metatarsophalangeal joint.

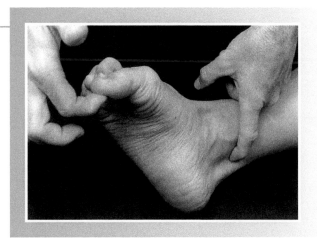

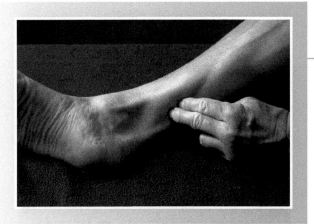

Fig. 11.63 Flexor hallucis longus: medial approach

MA: This figure simply allows you to better visualize the body of the muscle (indicated by the practitioner's two fingers), as it runs posterior to flexor digitorum longus and along the medial border of the calcaneal tendon.

If you ask the subject to perform repeated rapid flexions of his big toe, you can better feel the contraction of the muscle in the medial retromalleolar groove between the medial malleolus and the calcaneal tendon.

Fig. 11.64 Lateral approach to flexor hallucis longus

MA: The body of the muscle is also palpable from the lateral border of the calcaneal tendon.

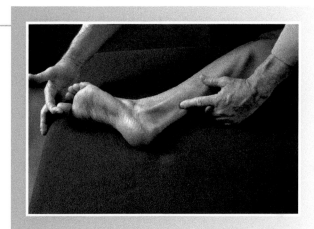

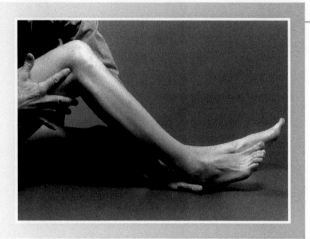

Fig. 11.65 The tendon of popliteus

MA: With one hand resist the subject as he flexes his knee and place your other hand posterior to the fibular collateral ligament.

You will feel the tendon you are seeking just posterior to the ligament mentioned above. Your ability to feel this tendon is not guaranteed in every subject. It can be "interfered with" by contraction of the lateral head of gastrocnemius.

Fig. 11.66 Origin of popliteus

MA: You can also feel its tendinous origin in the popliteal groove of the lateral femoral condyle.

The popliteal groove of the lateral femoral condyle

Distally it borders the lateral aspect of the lateral condyle, which feels rough to the touch and provides its inferior limit. The groove is much deeper posteriorly than anteriorly.

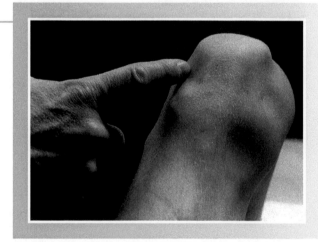

12

The ankle and the foot

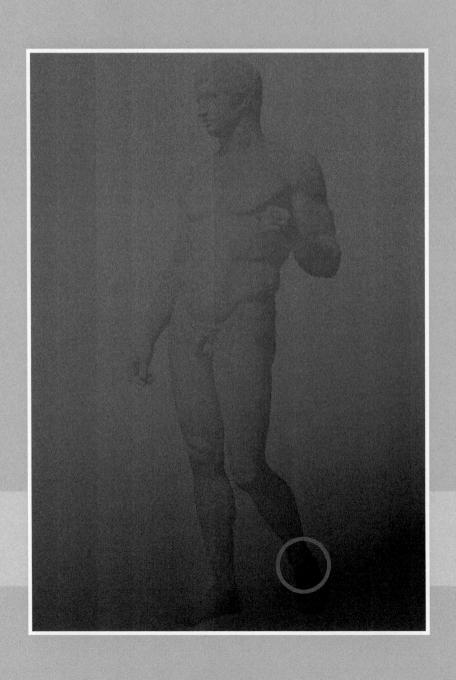

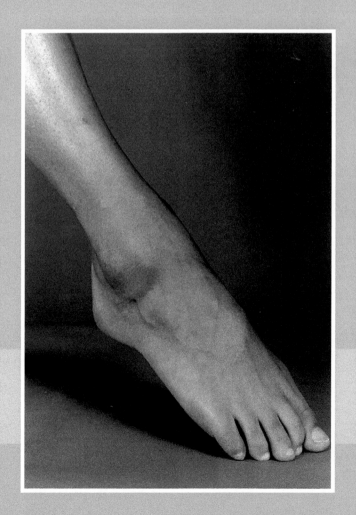 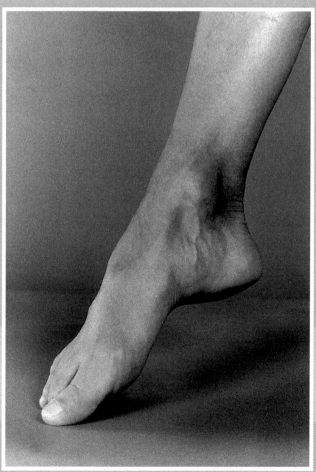

OSTEOLOGY

Bones of the foot (lateral view)

1. Posterior talofibular ligament
2. Posterior talocalcaneal ligament
3. Calcaneofibular ligament
4. Tubercle for insertion of calcaneofibular ligament
5. Calcaneal tendon
6. Abductor digiti minimi
7. Inferior fibular retinaculum
8. Fibular trochlea
9. Anterior tibiofibular ligament
10. Plantar calcaneocuboid ligament
11. Extensor digitorum brevis and extensor hallucis brevis
12. Dorsal calcaneocuboid ligament
13. Fibularis brevis
14. Dorsal cuboideonavicular ligament
15. Cuboid bone
16. Dorsal cuneocuboid ligament
17. Fibularis tertius
18. Fifth metatarsal
19. Articular surface of fibular malleolus
20. Interosseous talocalcaneal ligament
21. Dorsal intercuneiform ligaments
22. Bifurcate ligament
23. Navicular bone
24. Dorsal cuneonavicular ligaments
25. Medial cuneiform bone
26. Intermediate cuneiform bone
27. Lateral cuneiform bone

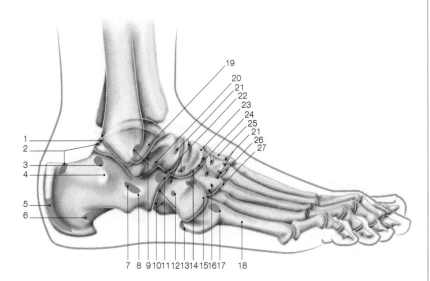

Bones of the foot (medial view)

1. Tibialis anterior
2. Navicular bone
3. Plantar calcaneonavicular ligament
4. Tibionavicular ligament
5. Anterior tibiotalar ligament
6. Medial talocalcaneal ligament
7. First metatarsus
8. Medial cuneiform bone
9. Tibialis posterior
10. Plantar calcaneocuboid ligament
11. Tibiocalcaneal ligament
12. Quadratus plantae
13. Abductor hallucis
14. Plantar aponeurosis
15. Calcaneal tendon
16. Posterior talocalcaneal ligament
17. Posterior tibiotalar ligament
18. Articular surface of tibial malleolus

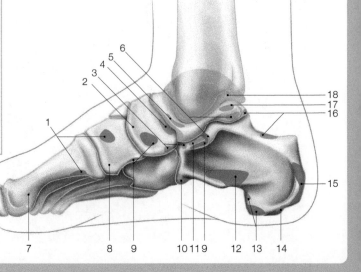

Bones of the foot (plantar view)

1. Calcaneal tendon
2. Plantar aponeurosis
3. Abductor hallucis
4. Quadratus plantae
5. Tibialis posterior
6. Plantar calcaneonavicular ligament
7. Flexor hallucis brevis
8. Tibialis anterior
9. Fibularis longus
10. Adductor hallucis
11. Dorsal interossei
12. Sesamoid bones
13. Flexor digitorum brevis
14. Flexor hallucis longus
15. Abductor digiti minimi
16. Long plantar ligament
17. Plantar calcaneocuboid ligament
18. Opponens digiti minimi
19. Fibularis brevis
20. Flexor digiti minimi brevis
21. Flexor digitorum longus

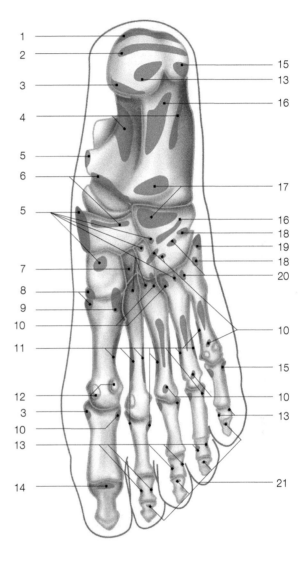

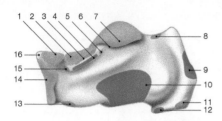

Calcaneus (medial view)

1. Anterior talar articular surface
2. Middle talar articular surface
3. Tibiocalcaneal ligament
4. Tibialis posterior
5. Medial talocalcaneal ligament
6. Interosseous talocalcaneal ligament
7. Posterior talar articular surface
8. Posterior talocalcaneal ligament
9. Calcaneal tendon
10. Quadratus plantae
11. Plantar aponeurosis
12. Abductor hallucis
13. Plantar calcaneocuboid ligament
14. Articular surface for the cuboid bone
15. Plantar calcaneonavicular ligament
16. Rostral process

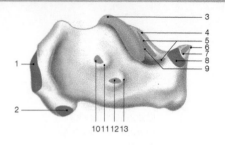

Calcaneus (lateral view)

1. Calcaneal tendon
2. Abductor digiti minimi
3. Posterior talar articular surface
4. Middle talar articular surface
5. Interosseous talocalcaneal ligament
6. Rostral process
7. Bifurcate ligament
8. Extensor digitorum brevis and extensor hallucis brevis
9. Calcaneal sulcus
10. Calcaneofibular ligament
11. Tubercle for insertion of calcaneofibular ligament
12. Inferior fibular retinaculum
13. Fibular trochlea

Calcaneus (plantar view)

1. Abductor hallucis
2. Medial tubercle of calcaneal tuberosity
3. Quadratus plantae
4. Sustentaculum tali
5. Tibialis posterior
6. Plantar calcaneonavicular ligament
7. Articular surface for the cuboid bone
8. Plantar aponeurosis
9. Flexor digitorum brevis
10. Abductor digiti minimi
11. Lateral tubercle of calcaneal tuberosity
12. Long plantar ligament
13. Plantar calcaneocuboid ligament
14. Anterior tubercle

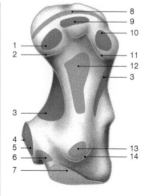

Calcaneus (dorsal view)

1. Extensor digitorum brevis and extensor hallucis brevis
2. Bifurcate ligament
3. Rostral process
4. Calcaneal tuberosity
5. Posterior talar articular surface
6. Sustentaculum tali
7. Interosseous talocalcaneal ligament
8. Calcaneal sulcus
9. Middle talar articular surface
10. Anterior talar articular surface

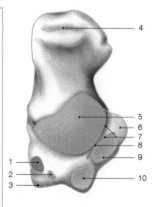

THE LATERAL BORDER

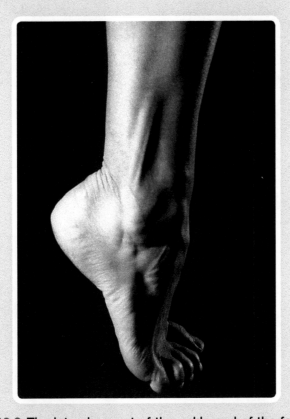

Fig. 12.3 The lateral aspect of the ankle and of the foot

The bony structures accessible to palpation include:

- The fifth metatarsal bone:
  - the head (Fig. 12.4)
  - the lateral border of its shaft (Fig. 12.5)
  - the plantar border of its shaft (Fig. 12.6)
  - the base of the fifth metatarsal and the other bones on the lateral border of the foot: they can be located using a global approach on the lateral border of the foot (Fig. 12.7)
  - the tuberosity of the fifth metatarsal (Fig. 12.8)
- The cuboid:
  - the lateral border (Fig. 12.9)
  - the dorsal aspect (Fig. 12.10)
  - the plantar aspect (Fig. 12.11)
- The calcaneus:
  - the lateral aspect (Fig. 12.12)
  - the rostral process (Fig. 12.13)
  - the articular surface for the cuboid (Fig. 12.14)
  - the sinus tarsi (Fig. 12.15)
  - the fibular trochlea (Fig. 12.16)
  - the tubercle for the insertion of the calcaneofibular ligament (Fig. 12.17)
  - the posterior part of the lateral aspect (Fig. 12.18)
  - the dorsal surface: the lateral part of the posterior segment (Fig. 12.19)
- The talus:
  - the lateral aspect of the neck (Fig. 12.20)
  - the lateral process (Fig. 12.21)
- The lateral malleolus:
  - the anterior border (Fig. 12.22)
  - the apex (Fig. 12.23)
  - the posterior border (Fig. 12.24).

The fifth metatarsal

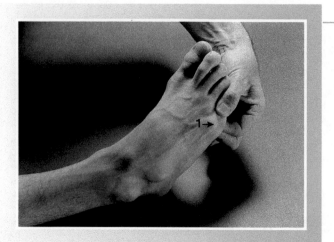

Fig. 12.4 The head of the fifth metatarsal

MA: You need only plantar-flex the fifth toe to bring out the head (1) of the fifth metatarsal on the dorsal aspect of the lateral border of the foot. This procedure also allows you to locate the metatarsophalangeal joint.

Fig. 12.5 The lateral aspect of the body of the fifth metatarsal

MA: As it lies directly under the skin, you can easily run your fingers over it. It lies just dorsal to abductor digiti minimi.

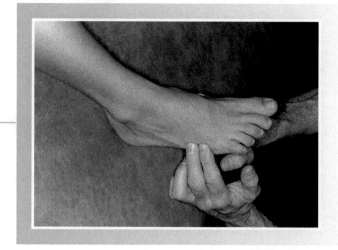

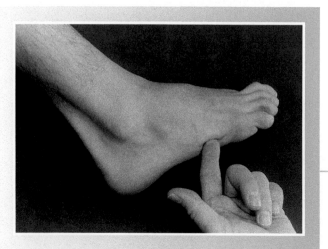

Fig. 12.6 The plantar border of the fifth metatarsal

MA: Your index finger will feel this border as a well-defined curve with a plantar concavity. In the adjacent figure the practitioner's index finger pushes aside abductor digiti minimi in order to gain contact with the bony structure being looked for.

Fig. 12.7 "Global" location of the bones on the lateral border

MA: With the subject's foot in a normally relaxed state and resting on a table or on your knee, position your proximal hand on his instep in a grip that gently closes over the lateral border of his foot, while placing the lateral border of your little finger against his lateral malleolus.

Your little finger is now in contact with the dorsal and lateral aspects of the talar neck, the floor of the sinus tarsi, and the anterior superolateral angle (rostral process) of the calcaneus. Your ring finger lies opposite the cuboid and your middle finger rests on top of the base of the fifth metatarsal.

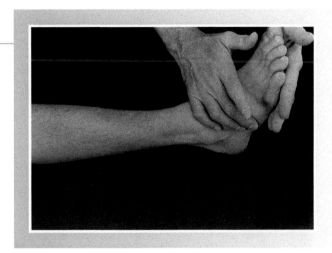

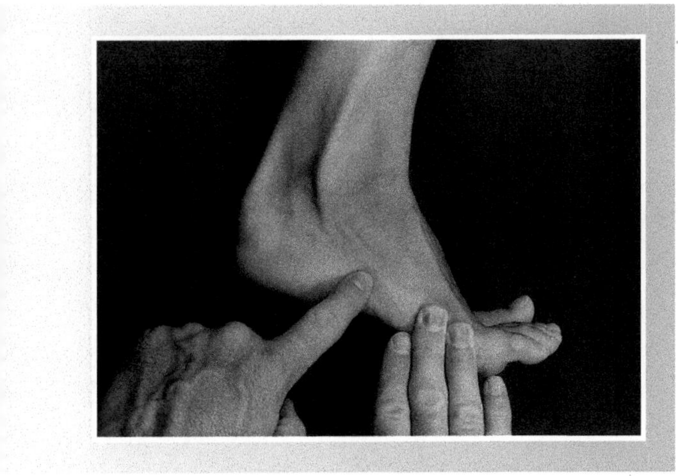

Fig. 12.8 The tuberosity of the fifth metatarsal

MA: With its posterior extremity articulating with the cuboid, the fifth metatarsal has a distinctive feature, i.e., a prominent tuberosity, which projects posteriorly, inferiorly, and laterally beyond its base. It is the bony structure you are after, and it gives attachment to the tendon of fibularis brevis. This bony projection extends posteriorly to cover partially the lateral border of the cuboid.

> **CLINICAL NOTE**
>
> This structure can be the seat of an avulsion fracture caused by pulling on the fibularis brevis as the foot is twisted into inversion and plantar flexion.

The cuboid

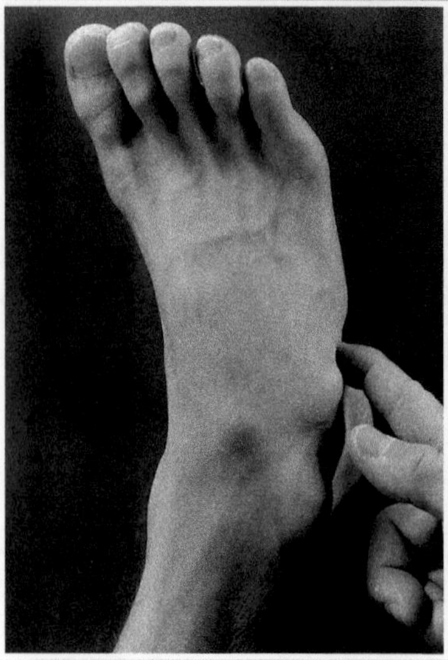

Fig. 12.9 The lateral border of the cuboid

MA: The cuboid is the bony structure next to the tuberosity of the fifth metatarsal in the hindfoot. Once you locate the tuberosity, you simply need to let your fingers glide into the adjacent depression lying proximal to it on the lateral border of the foot, and you will reach a ridge-like border, which is the structure you are looking for.

Note: The tendon of fibularis brevis runs along this border and can impede palpation of it, unless the muscle is in a relaxed state.

> **CLINICAL NOTE**
>
> The cuboid can be partially dislocated, in which case passive movements of pronation and supination of the forefoot will be painful. Use palpation with pressure to elicit pain at the level of the four joint spaces connecting the cuboid with the other five bones that surround it (calcaneus, navicular, lateral cuneiform, metatarsals IV and V).

Fig. 12.10 The dorsal aspect of the cuboid

MA: Two notable bony structures will help you to locate this aspect of the cuboid:
• the tuberosity of the fifth metatarsal, already located (Fig. 12.8);
• the rostral process of the calcaneus (Fig. 12.13).

These two bony structures are the anterior and posterior limits of the structure you are after, which must therefore lie between them.

Starting from the lateral border of the cuboid already located by your thumb (see Fig. 12.9), you need only move it slightly toward the dorsal aspect of the foot to make contact with the bony structure you are interested in.

Note: It is a rough subcutaneous surface that slopes distally and laterally and is easy to investigate. The tendon of fibularis brevis runs along its lateral border and extensor digitorum brevis covers it partially.

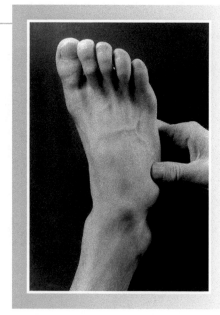

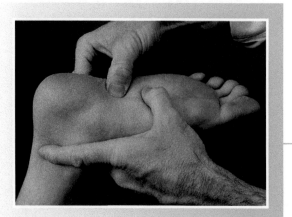

Fig. 12.11 The plantar aspect of the cuboid

MA: Once you have located the tuberosity of the fifth metatarsal and the rostral process of the calcaneus, you need only put your thumb between these two structures and move it round the lateral border of the foot, and therefore the lateral border of the cuboid, in order to reach its plantar surface.

The calcaneus

Fig. 12.12 The lateral aspect of the calcaneus

MA: First adduct and slightly supinate the subject's forefoot so as to bring out the anterior articular surface of the calcaneus and "uncover" it partially.

Then place your thumb on this surface and your index finger on the posterior aspect of the calcaneus in order to appreciate fully the size of this bone relative to the other bones of the foot.

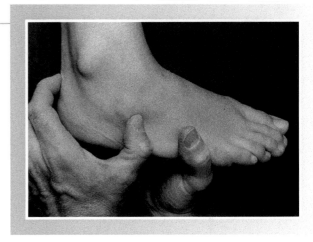

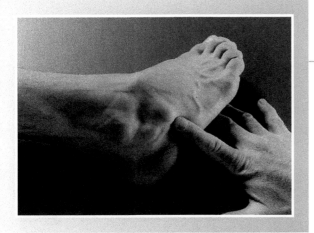

Fig. 12.13 The rostral process of the calcaneus

MA: This process corresponds to the anterior superolateral angle of the calcaneus and is the posterior limit of the lateral part of the calcaneocuboid joint space. It is easily accessible if the forefoot is already supinated. It can be very prominent in some subjects, as is the case shown in this figure.

Note: Locating this structure is of interest, since it allows you to determine clearly the size of the calcaneus, which is bound to vary from subject to subject.

Fig. 12.14 The plantar aspect of the calcaneal anterior articular surface for the cuboid

MA: To uncover the dorsal anterolateral aspect of this articular facet it most often suffices to ask the subject to adduct and supinate his already slightly flexed forefoot.

If this is not good enough, you can carry out this maneuver without his participation, i.e., immobilize his calcaneus with one hand and, with the other, adduct, supinate, and slightly plantar-flex his forefoot.

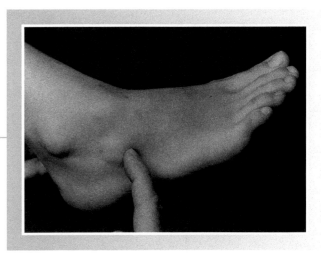

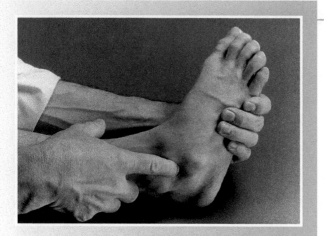

Fig. 12.15 The tarsal sinus

Reminder: The tarsal sinus is formed by the interlocking of the calcaneus and the talus. It is a sulcus that progressively widens, mediolaterally and posteroanteriorly. Its "floor" is the calcaneus and its "'roof" is the talus or, more accurately, the sulcus tali. The superimposition of these two sulci forms the canal called the tarsal sinus. Thus the sinus itself is not accessible, but its floor is, precisely at the point where it emerges onto the dorsal surface of the anterior segment of the calcaneus.

Note: The posterior part of the tarsal sinus is filled by the two bundles of the interosseous talocalcaneal ligament.

MA: With the subject's foot in the neutral position, first place your index finger on the anterior border of the lateral malleolus and then move it slightly toward the sole of the foot. The pad of your finger will feel the structure you are looking for as a depression. Extensor digitorum brevis can be a hindrance as you try to approach this structure. Therefore, make sure that it is relaxed or pushed aside. The tendon of extensor digitorum longus and the lateral part of the talar neck lie on its medial side.

Fig. 12.16 The fibular trochlea

MA: This bony projection lies about one finger-breadth distal to the lateral malleolus. The fibular trochlea separates the groove for fibularis longus (which underlies it) from the groove for fibularis brevis (which overlies it).

Note: The trochlea may be absent.

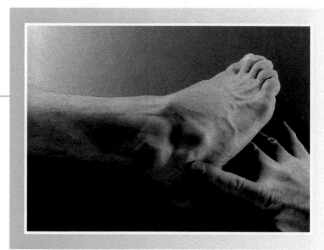

Fig. 12.17 The tubercle for the insertion of the calcaneofibular ligament

MA: This tubercle is not always well defined. It gives attachment to the calcaneofibular ligament (1) (previously known as the calcaneoperoneal or as the middle bundle of the lateral collateral ligament of the ankle). When the foot is in the neutral position, the tubercle lies about one finger-breadth dorsal and posterior to the fibular trochlea (2) and one finger-breadth plantar to the lateral part of the space of the talocalcaneal joint.

Note: The tubercle may not always be present. In its absence the calcaneofibular ligament is inserted directly into the lateral aspect of the calcaneus.

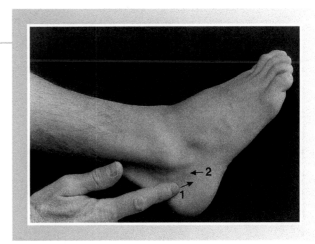

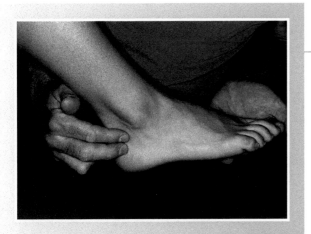

Fig. 12.18 The posterior part of the lateral aspect of the calcaneus

MA: It feels flat and rough under your fingers and extends over most of the directly subcutaneous lateral aspect of the calcaneus. In the adjacent figure, the practitioner's contact is placed slightly behind it to allow the best possible view of the bony structure of interest.

CLINICAL NOTE

Pain felt on palpation of the posteroinferior part of the lateral aspect of the calcaneus must raise the possibility of calcaneal apophysitis (Sever's disease), usually encountered in children.

Fig. 12.19 The superolateral part of the posterior segment (the dome) of the calcaneus

MA: In the adjacent figure the practitioner's index finger rests on the bony structure mentioned above in Fig. 12.18 and lies posterior to the talus and lateral to the calcaneal tendon.

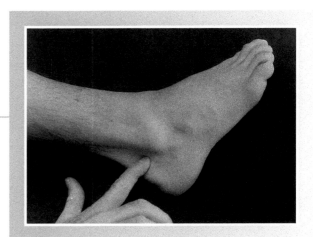

The talus

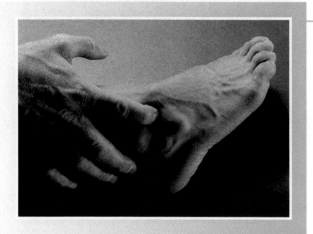

Fig. 12.20 The lateral aspect of the talar neck

MA: Start by putting the subject's foot in the neutral position and placing your index finger on the anterior border of the lateral malleolus. Then move your index finger slightly anteromedially, and it will face the structure you are looking for. Now you need only tilt his forefoot slightly into supination to make this lateral aspect even more accessible.

Fig. 12.21 The lateral process of the talus (1)

MA: Invert the subject's foot in order to free up the lateral process from the lateral malleolus and you will be able to feel it.

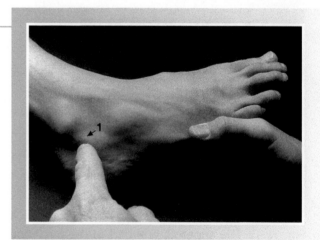

> **CLINICAL NOTE**
>
> This process can be fractured by injuries sustained in the practice of certain winter sports (skiing, snowboarding, etc.). A fracture can also occur in the absence of any injury. Pain on palpation with pressure will raise this possibility.

ATTACHMENTS

This process, to which is attached the lateral talocalcaneal ligament, lies just dorsal to the lateral part of the talocalcaneal joint space.

The lateral malleolus

Fig. 12.22 The anterior border of the lateral malleolus

MA: To its "highest" or proximal part is attached the anterior tibiofibular ligament, and to its "lowest" or distal part are attached the anterior talofibular ligament and the calcaneofibular ligament.

CLINICAL NOTE

In case of a sprain or a pull of the anterior talofibular ligament, this border will be painful on palpation with pressure. You must also consider a possible fracture with avulsion of part of this border when palpation with pressure elicits an exquisite pain.

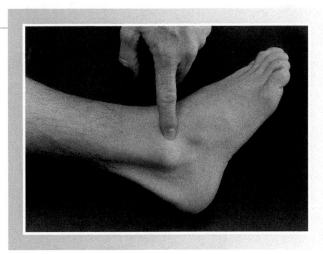

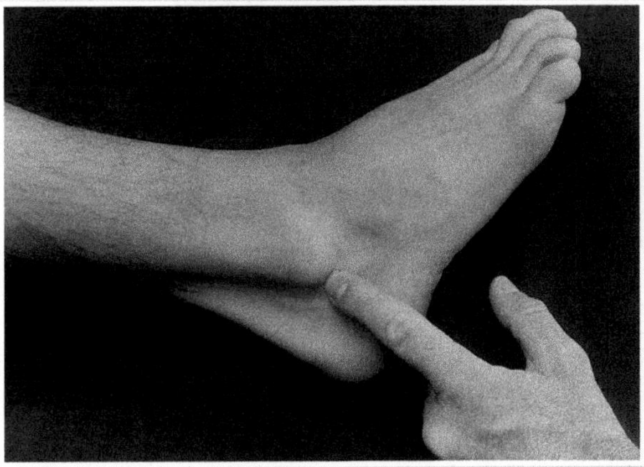

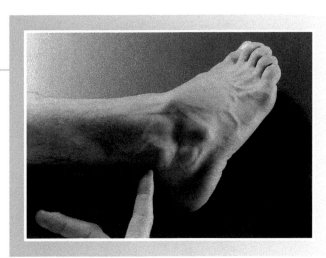

Fig. 12.23 The apex of the lateral malleolus

MA: The distinctive feature of this apex is the presence, just anterior to its highest point, of a notch to which is attached one part of the calcaneofibular ligament, while the other part is inserted into the most distal part of the anterior fibular border. It is thus an important landmark for locating the fibular insertions of the ligament.

CLINICAL NOTE

If the calcaneofibular ligament is sprained it will be painful on palpation with pressure.

Fig. 12.24 The posterior border of the lateral malleolus

MA: Simply ensure that fibularis longus and fibularis brevis are in a relaxed state or pushed aside in order to avoid any hindrance to your approach from these tendons, which lie posterior to this border.

Note: This border gives attachment to the posterior tibiofibular ligament and also to the posterior talofibular ligament.

CLINICAL NOTE

If palpation with pressure is painful, you must consider the possibility of a lesion involving the ligamentous structures inserted here (refer to Fig. 12.23).

THE MEDIAL BORDER

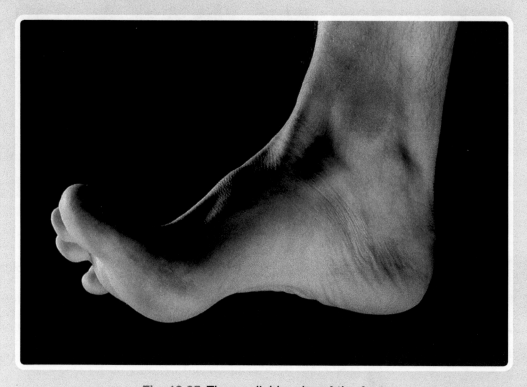

Fig. 12.25 The medial border of the foot

The bony structures accessible to palpation are:
- The first metatarsal:
  - the phalanges of big toe and head of the first metatarsal; dorsal approach (Fig. 12.26)
  - the head: plantar approach (Fig. 12.27)
  - the body (Figs. 12.28–12.31)
  - "global" approach to the bones of the medial border of the foot (Fig. 12.32)
  - the posteromedial tuberosity (Fig. 12.33)
  - the posterolateral tuberosity (Fig. 12.34)
- The medial cuneiform:
  - the medial aspect: locating it with the help of tibialis anterior (Fig. 12.35)
  - the dorsal aspect (Fig. 12.36)
- The navicular:
  - its tuberosity: "direct" approach (Fig. 12.37)
  - its tuberosity: locating it with the help of tibialis posterior (Fig. 12.38)
- The talus:
  - the ligament-related or middle portion of the talar head (Fig. 12.39)
  - the neck (Fig. 12.40–12.41)
  - the posteromedial tubercle (Fig. 12.42)
  - the posterolateral tubercle (Fig. 12.43)
- The calcaneus:
  - sustentaculum tali (Fig. 12.44)
  - calcaneal sulcus (Fig. 12.45)
- The medial malleolus:
  - anterior border (Fig. 12.46)
  - inferior extremity (Fig. 12.47)
  - posterior border (Fig. 12.48).

The first metatarsal

Fig. 12.26 The phalanges of the big toe and the head of the first metatarsal: dorsal approach

MA: The phalanges are easy to examine, with the reminder that each toe has three phalanges, except for the big toe with only two.

By meticulous palpation you can identify the medial, lateral, plantar, and dorsal aspects of the shaft of each phalanx.

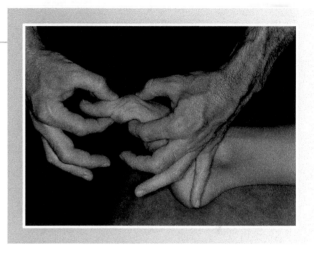

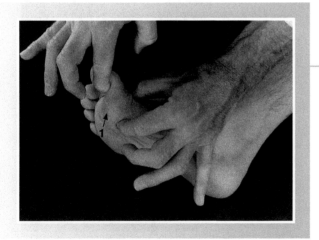

Fig. 12.27 The head and sesamoid bones of the first metatarsal: plantar approach

MA: Place the pad of the index finger of your distal hand on the plantar aspect of the proximal phalanx so as to extend it, and you will feel the plantar aspect of the base of this phalanx, the plantar articular surface of the head of the first metatarsal, and the two sesamoid bones.

Note: The distal extremity or head of each metatarsal bears a convex articular surface more extensive on its plantar (1) than on its dorsal aspect. The grip shown here allows you to free this articular surface adequately.

Fig. 12.28 The medial aspect of the first metatarsal

MA: It lies in the medial part of the foot. It is directly under the skin and has the distinction of lying in the dorsal half of the medial border of the foot, whereas the plantar half of this border contains only soft tissues.

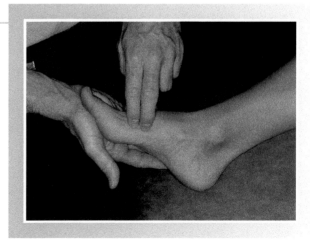

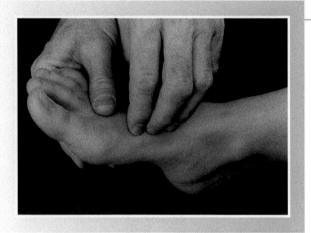

Fig. 12.29 The dorsal aspect of the first metatarsal

MA: The shaft of every metatarsal is like a triangular prism. Its dorsal aspect is narrow overall but much wider posteriorly than anteriorly.

Note: A distinctive anatomical feature of each metatarsal is the sloping nature of both the medial and the lateral borders of its dorsal aspect.

Fig. 12.30 The lateral aspect of the first metatarsal

MA: The lateral aspects of all the metatarsals respectively combine with the medial aspects of the adjacent metatarsals to form a special space known as the intermetatarsal or interosseous space.

ATTACHMENTS

- All four dorsal interossei arise from the adjacent sides and dorsal aspects of the two metatarsals that demarcate the corresponding interosseous space.
- The three plantar interossei arise from the plantar aspects of the sides of the metatarsals facing the axis of the foot, which passes through the second toe, and also from the plantar borders and bases of these metatarsals.

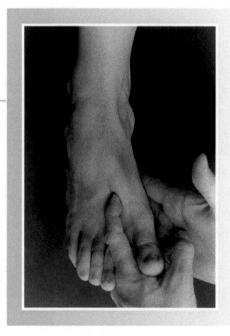

Fig. 12.31 The plantar border of the shaft of the first metatarsal

MA: You can see very clearly the plantar or inferior border of the shaft of the first metatarsal, which you can feel under your fingers as a concave structure.

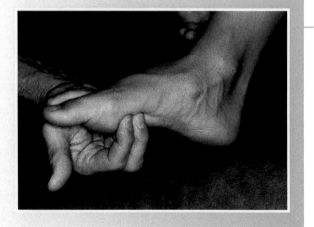

Fig. 12.32 "Global" approach to the bones on the medial border of the foot

MA: The subject's foot is normally relaxed and rests on the table or on the practitioner's knee.

The latter places his proximal hand on the subject's instep and closes it gently over the medial border of the foot, while keeping the ulnar border of his little finger on the anterior border of the medial malleolus.

In the case presented here:

- The practitioner's little finger faces the medial aspect of the talar neck.
- His ring finger faces the navicular.
- His middle finger faces the medial cuneiform.
- His index finger faces the base of the first metatarsal.

Note: This global approach to the bony structures of the medial border of the foot can be considered reliable in the majority of subjects, except, of course, for extreme cases.

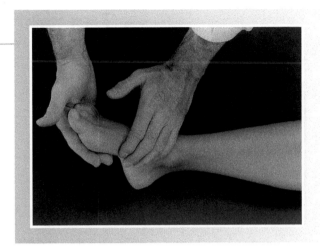

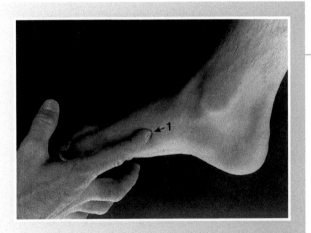

Fig. 12.33 The posteromedial tuberosity of the first metatarsal

MA: Slide your index finger between the body of abductor hallucis and the plantar border of the first metatarsal, which feels like a curved structure under your fingers. Follow the medial border of its shaft, and you will encounter the tuberosity on its base near the joint space.

ATTACHMENTS

The tuberosity receives the metatarsal insertion of tibialis anterior, while the medial part of the medial cuneiform (1) receives the other insertion.

Fig. 12.34 The posterolateral tuberosity of the first metatarsal

It is located on the plantar aspect, lateral and posterior to the posteromedial tuberosity and receives the main insertion of fibularis longus.

It is clear that this bony projection, buried as it is under the soft tissues, will be more easily felt after some muscle loss, as in the case of a subject bedridden for a long time. Otherwise you must apply a pressure strong enough to detect this structure.

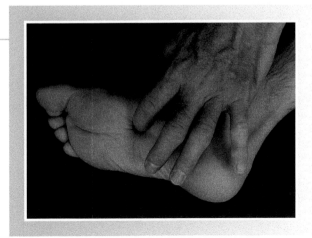

The medial cuneiform

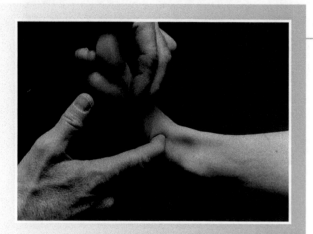

Fig. 12.35 The medial aspect of the medial cuneiform: location with the help of tibialis anterior

MA: An efficient way of localizing this aspect of the bone is to stretch tibialis anterior, which is inserted here. Just ask the subject to supinate and dorsiflex his foot with or without any resistance on your part.

Fig. 12.36 Lateral view of the dorsal border of the medial cuneiform

MA: The medial cuneiform lies on the medial border of the foot, between the navicular and the first metatarsal, and its dorsal (1) border is ridge-shaped, particularly posteriorly.

Note: This feature of the bone is shown in the adjacent picture, which provides a lateral view, chosen on purpose to highlight it.

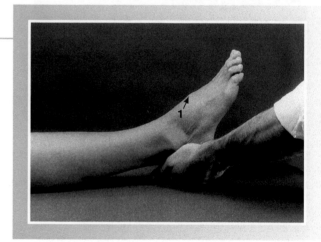

The navicular

Fig. 12.37 The tuberosity of the navicular: "direct approach"

MA: It is accessible posterior to the tendon of tibialis anterior. In many subjects it is clearly visible, as in the adjacent figure.

Note: There can be a supernumerary bone on top of this tuberosity (sometimes known as the "accessory navicular bone"), the result of a secondary center of ossification in the navicular. This supernumerary bone may not fuse at all with the navicular and remain quite mobile, or it may fuse with the navicular via a fibrous band while retaining a low level of mobility.

ATTACHMENTS

This tuberosity juts out on the plantar part of the medial aspect of the navicular (1) and is the site of insertion for tibialis posterior.

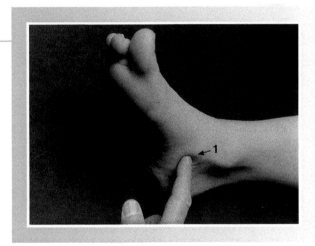

> **CLINICAL NOTE**
>
> When this supernumerary bone is present, the appropriate shoe must be worn. If the shoe is too narrow, it will irritate the zone of contact, producing a pain that will likely become permanent. Pain is also felt in cases of tibialis posterior tendinitis.
>
> **Note:** The navicular itself can be fractured (fatigue fracture). Pain felt mostly on its dorsal aspect during palpation with pressure should raise this possibility.

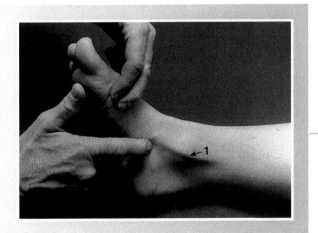

Fig. 12.38 The tuberosity of the navicular: location using tibialis posterior

MA: Stretching tibialis posterior (1) is an efficient way of locating this tuberosity when it is less prominent.

First plantar-flex the subject's foot and then simply ask him to adduct it.

Starting from the medial malleolus, follow the tibialis posterior tendon until you reach the tuberosity you are after.

The talus

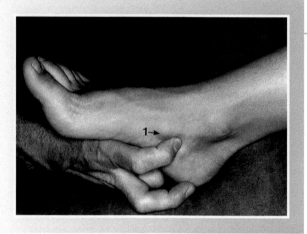

Fig. 12.39 The ligament-related or middle portion of the talar head

MA: As indicated by its name, this part of the bone is related to the plantar calcaneonavicular ligament.

It lies posterior to the anterosuperior region of the talar head, which articulates with the navicular.

Just place your fingers posterior to the tuberosity of the navicular (1) on the medioplantar border of the foot and you will be able to feel it as a smooth surface under your fingers.

Note: Depending on the subject, it is sometimes useful to keep the forefoot abducted and pronated, the better to feel this structure under your fingers on the medioplantar aspect of the foot between the navicular tuberosity and the sustentaculum tali.

Fig. 12.40 The medial part of the talar neck

MA: The medial part of the talar neck (1) is examined mainly between the tendon of tibialis anterior (2) laterally and that of tibialis posterior medially (3).

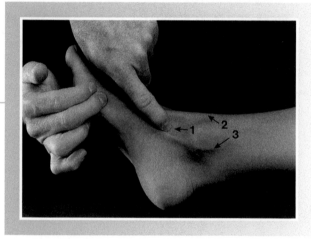

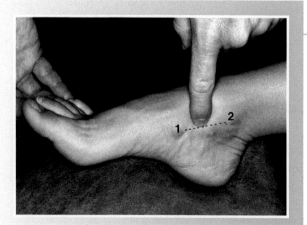

Fig. 12.41 The medial part of the talar neck: second approach

MA: In addition to its location using the tibialis tendons, as shown in the previous figure, you can also locate this structure using an imaginary line stretching from the navicular tuberosity (1) to the medial malleolus (2).

If you move your finger from the midpoint of this line toward the malleolus (2), it will face the talar neck, which is felt as a rough surface under your fingers. If you move your finger from the midpoint of this line toward the plantar surface of the foot, it will face the ligament-related portion of the talar head, which has a smooth texture on palpation.

Note: A rough ridge, felt sometimes as a tubercle depending on the subject, separates these two parts of the talus: the ligament-related portion of the talar head and the talar neck.

Fig. 12.42 The posteromedial tubercle of the talus

MA: It is important to remember that this bony structure (1) belongs to the posterior aspect of the talus and that it gives insertion to the posterior tibiotalar or the deep bundle of the deltoid ligament.

From this bony structure the medial talocalcaneal ligament also runs toward the posterior border of the sustentaculum tali.

CLINICAL NOTE

During such sports as high jump, classical dance, and also soccer, the tubercle is crushed whenever the calcaneus hits the tibia (the posterolateral tubercle is also affected; see Fig. 12.43).

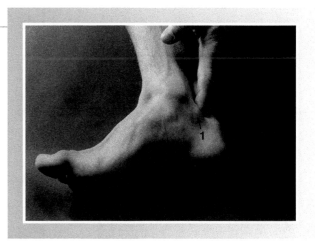

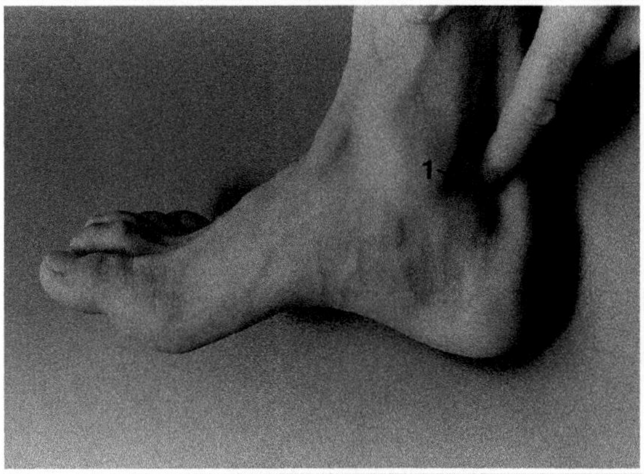

Fig. 12.43 The posterolateral tubercle of the talus

MA: This tubercle (1) also belongs to the posterior surface of the talus. You must first place your fingers flat on the medial part of the calcaneal tendon and then look for it at the level of the posterior border of the talus, where it is accessible.

Note: In most subjects it is not easily accessible, but it is an important bony structure because it is the site of attachment of the posterior talofibular ligament.

ATTACHMENTS

Attached to this tubercle are the posterior talofibular ligament and the posterior talocalcaneal ligament, which terminates on the posterodorsal surface of the calcaneus.

Between these two posteromedial and posterolateral tubercles there is a groove for the passage of the tendon of flexor hallucis longus.

CLINICAL NOTE

Supernumerary bone

An os trigonum can be present on top of the posterolateral tubercle. It can even fuse with the tubercle to give what is known as the trigonal process.

In the first case, the os trigonum can be mobilized by palpation.

In the second case, palpation will reveal on the top of the calcaneus a very prominent bony structure that has no mobility and can be fractured. Both passive and active plantar flexion of the foot will elicit pain.

The calcaneus

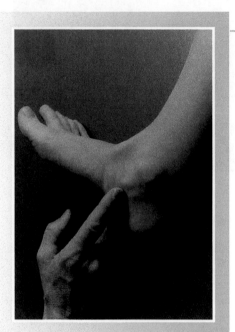

Fig. 12.44 The sustentaculum tali

MA: It lies a finger-breadth distal to the medial malleolus. You can also approach it on its inferior surface by gliding your contact from the calcaneus.

The superior part of the sustentaculum supports the middle talar articular surface of the calcaneus.

The space of the medial talocalcaneal joint is quite close, lying between the sustentaculum and the talus.

ATTACHMENTS

- From the anterior border of the sustentaculum the plantar calcaneonavicular ligament runs toward the middle part of the talar head before inserting into the navicular.
- From its posterior border the medial talocalcaneal ligament stretches toward the posteromedial tubercle of the talus.
- A groove runs dorsal to it and houses the tendon of flexor digitorum longus.
- Another groove running plantar to it houses the tendon of flexor hallucis longus.
- It also provides attachment to tibialis posterior.
- The tibiocalcaneal ligament is attached to the posterior part of the superficial bundle of the deltoid ligament.

Fig. 12.45 The calcaneal sulcus

MA: It runs in a dorsoplantar and proximodistal direction and occupies most of the medial surface of the calcaneus. It is bordered proximally and inferiorly by the medial process of the calcaneal tuberosity (1) and distally and superiorly by the sustentaculum tali (2), whose prominence varies with the subject.

Note: The calcaneal sulcus is "closed" medially by the flexor retinaculum, running from the medial malleolus to the medial aspect of the calcaneus. It allows the passage of tibialis posterior, flexor digitorum longus, and flexor hallucis longus. In this sulcus all the tendons are surrounded by synovial sheaths and accompany the tibial nerve and the posterior tibial artery.

> **CLINICAL NOTE**
>
> Any pain elicited by palpation with pressure on the medial aspect of the calcaneal tuberosity should suggest calcaneal apophysitis, which can occur in children.

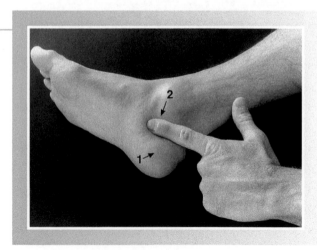

The medial malleolus

Fig. 12.46 The anterior border of the medial malleolus

MA: It is thick and rough and provides attachment to the superficial bundle of the deltoid ligament.

ATTACHMENTS

Also attached to this border is the capsule of the ankle joint (a hinge joint).

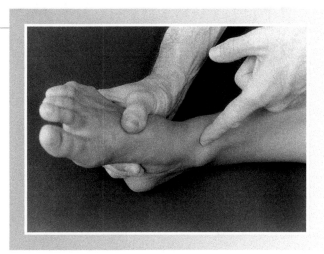

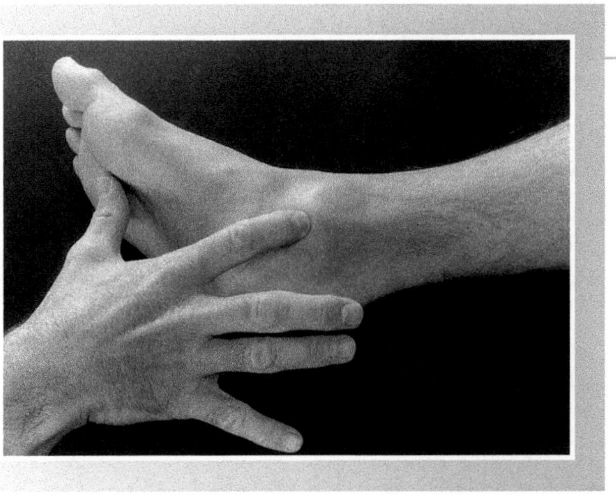

Fig. 12.47 The distal extremity of the medial malleolus

MA: It consists of two tubercles (one anterior and the other posterior) separated by a notch.

ATTACHMENTS

The notch gives attachment to the superficial and deep bundles of the medial collateral ligament or deltoid ligament of the ankle joint.

> **CLINICAL NOTE**
>
> A severe sprain of this ligament is extremely rare, but, on the other hand, the ligament can be pulled as a result of a traumatic eversion of the foot.

Fig. 12.48 The posterior border of the medial malleolus

MA: It contains an oblique groove running proximodistally and lateromedially. It is easily accessible to the investigator if the tendons in this area are kept in a relaxed state, i.e., that of tibialis posterior, which is the most anteriorly located, and that of flexor digitorum longus, which lies posterior to the former.

Note: In reality, these two tendons are retromalleolar and run inside their own individual osteofibrous sheaths.

ATTACHMENTS

Attached to this posterior border is the capsule of the ankle joint.

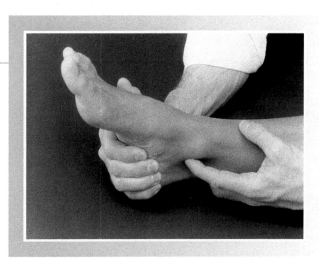

THE ANTERIOR ASPECT OF THE ANKLE AND THE DORSAL ASPECT OF THE FOOT

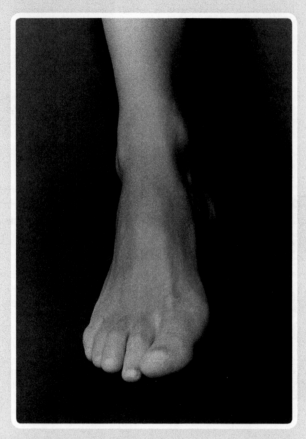

Fig. 12.49 Anterior view of the ankle and dorsal view of the foot

The notable structures accessible to palpation are:

- the dorsal aspects of the metatarsal heads (Fig. 12.50)
- the fifth metatarsal (Fig. 12.51)
- the fourth metatarsal (Fig. 12.52)
- the third metatarsal (Fig. 12.53)
- the second metatarsal (Fig. 12.54)
- the first metatarsal (Fig. 12.55)
- the talar neck (Fig. 12.56)
- the anterior border of the distal extremity of the tibia (Fig. 12.57)
- other methods of approach (Figs. 12.58–12.61).

Fig. 12.50 The metatarsal heads: dorsal view

MA: You need only use a global palmar grip for all the subject's toes in order to plantar-flex his foot enough to bring out the metatarsal heads. Obviously you can also use this method to bring out each metatarsal in succession.

> **CLINICAL NOTE**
>
> **Interdigital neuritis (commonly known as Morton's neuroma)**
>
> It occurs between the second and third or the third and fourth metatarsal heads. To elicit pain, just press together the two metatarsal heads involved so as to compress the affected nerve. This condition is most often due to the wearing of shoes that are too tight. It can also result from a fatigue fracture at the level of a metatarsal.

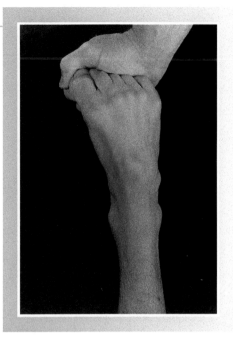

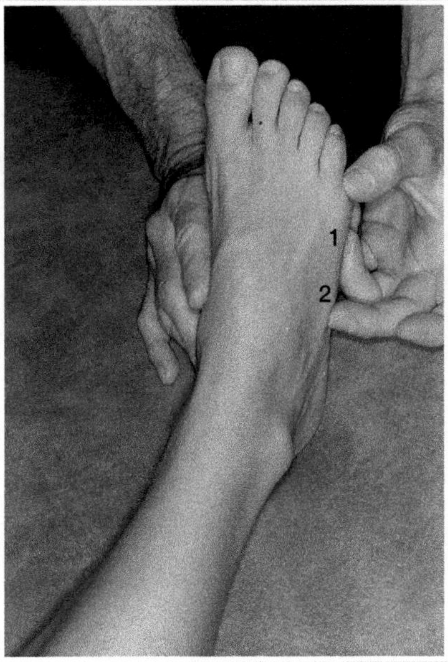

Fig. 12.51 The fifth metatarsal

MA: First locate its head and its base and then place your fingers facing the appropriate tarsometatarsal joint (Fig. 12.92). You are now able to grip the fifth metatarsal between your thumb and your index finger.

It is interesting to note the position and the size of this bone relative to the other metatarsals. Its base articulates posteriorly with the cuboid and medially with the fourth metatarsal. Its posterolateral surface bears a tuberosity or styloid process.

> **CLINICAL NOTE**
>
> The base of the fifth metatarsal can also be the seat of an insertional tendinitis or of an avulsion fracture of the tuberosity secondary to intense overuse of fibularis brevis.
>
> Distal (1) or proximal (2) fracture of its shaft: in both cases palpation with pressure elicits a sharp pain.

451

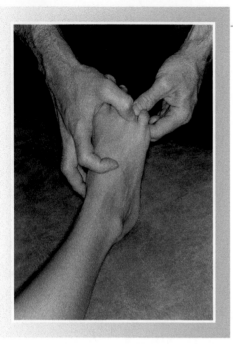

Fig. 12.52 The fourth metatarsal

MA: Locate its head and its base after locating the appropriate tarsometatarsal joint space.

> **CLINICAL NOTE**
>
> It can be the seat of a fatigue fracture, revealed by an exquisite pain felt on palpation of the dorsal and plantar aspects of its shaft, associated occasionally with a swelling related to the metatarsal.
>
> The pain gets worse when the subject is standing, walking, or standing on tiptoe.
>
> **Note:** This occurs typically with excessive walking but can occur under different circumstances.

Fig. 12.53 The third metatarsal

MA: Locate its head and base after locating the appropriate metatarsal joint space.

> **CLINICAL NOTE**
>
> It can be the seat of a fatigue fracture, revealed by an exquisite pain felt on palpation of its dorsal and plantar aspects. Regardless of whether the second, third, or fourth metatarsal is affected, the forefoot can be swollen. Excessive walking, running, and track sports can cause this injury.

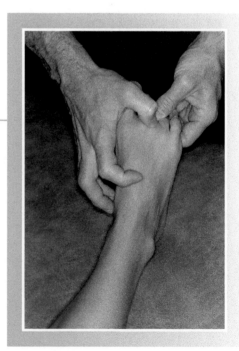

Fig. 12.54 The second metatarsal

MA: Locate its head and base after locating the appropriate tarsometatarsal joint space.

Note: It is the longest of all the metatarsals.

> **CLINICAL NOTE**
>
> It can be the seat of a fatigue fracture revealed by an exquisite pain on palpation of its dorsal and plantar aspects, occasionally coupled with a swelling related to the metatarsal.
>
> The pain gets worse when the subject is standing, walking, or standing on tiptoe.
>
> **Note:** It occurs typically with excessive walking but can also occur under different circumstances.

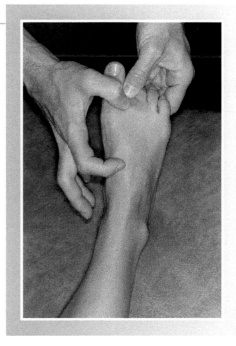

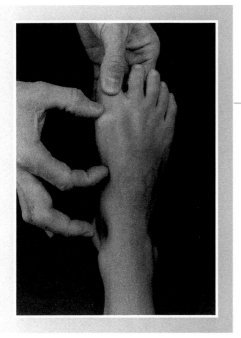

Fig. 12.55 The first metatarsal

MA: Locate its head and base after locating the appropriate tarsometatarsal joint space. It is the shortest and bulkiest of all the metatarsals.

> **CLINICAL NOTE**
>
> **Hallux valgus:** This is a more or less painful adducted big toe. In hyperalgesic states all movements of the big toe are painful. A bunion indicates a bursitis on the medial part of the head of the first metatarsal, which appears inflamed, red, and more or less painful on palpation. One of its causes is again the wearing of shoes that are too high and too narrow.

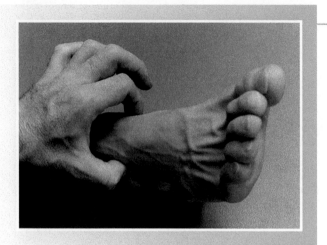

Fig. 12.56 The talar neck

MA: In the adjacent figure the practitioner is gripping the lateral and medial aspects of the talar head with his index finger lying on its medial aspect. These two parts of the neck have already been seen when the lateral and the medial borders of the foot were looked at, respectively.

The dorsal aspect of the talar neck lies between the practitioner's thumb and his index finger.

> **CLINICAL NOTE**
> It can be painful on palpation:
> - on its lateral aspect, after a sprain or a pull of the anterior talofibular ligament;
> - on its medial aspect, after a pull of the deltoid ligament.

Fig. 12.57 The anterior border of the inferior extremity of the distal tibial epiphysis

MA: Note: This is the border that fits snugly into the transverse groove on the dorsal aspect of the talar neck whenever the ankle is dorsiflexed.

> **CLINICAL NOTE**
> Pain, exacerbated by palpation with pressure applied distal to the anterior border of the distal tibial epiphysis, can result from injury to the capsule or to the extensor retinaculum.

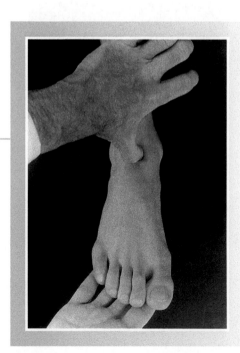

Other methods of approach

The palpatory approaches described below are meant to make it easier to learn the articular approaches relevant to this region.

Fig. 12.58 The dorsal aspect of the talar neck

MA: The practitioner's middle finger comes to rest on the dorsal aspect of the talar neck posterior to the navicular tuberosity.

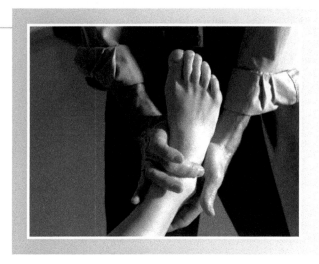

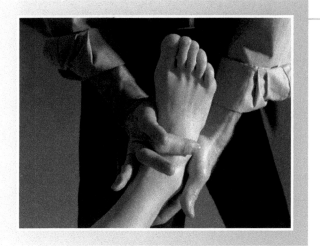

Fig. 12.59 The dorsal aspect of the navicular

MA: Its easily palpable tuberosity is a helpful landmark for the localization of the dorsal aspect of the bone you are interested in.

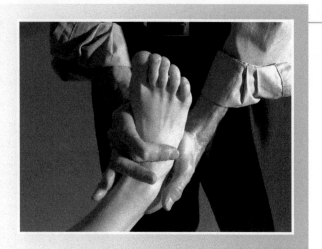

Fig. 12.60 **The dorsal aspects of the three cuneiforms**

MA: Starting from the dorsal aspect of the navicular the practitioner allows his middle finger to slide distally ahead of the navicular tuberosity and come to rest on the dorsal aspects of the three cuneiforms.

Fig. 12.61 **The dorsal aspect of the base of the first metatarsal**

MA: The practitioner usually approaches it by allowing his middle finger to slide distally from the dorsal aspects of the three cuneiforms to the dorsal aspect of the base of the first metatarsal.

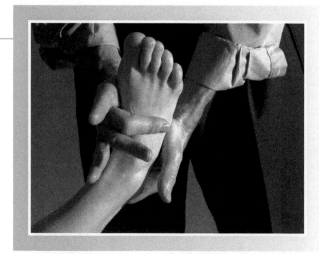

THE POSTERIOR ASPECT OF THE ANKLE AND OF THE FOOT

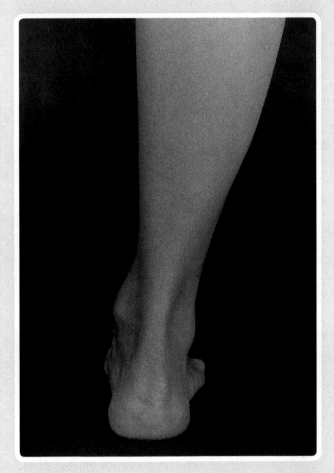

Fig. 12.62 Posterior view of the ankle and of the foot

The bony structures accessible to palpation are:

- the medial malleolus (Fig. 12.63)
- the sustentaculum tali (Fig. 12.64)
- the posterior aspect of the calcaneus (Fig. 12.65)
- the posterior segment of the dorsal aspect of the calcaneus (Fig. 12.66)
- the lateral malleolus (Fig. 12.67)
- the fibular trochlea (Fig. 12.68).

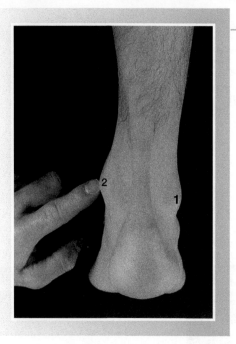

Fig. 12.63 The medial malleolus

MA: You previously located this structure, now indicated by your index finger, when you were looking for the medial border of the subject's foot (Fig. 12.32). This figure shows a different view meant to highlight the medial malleolus topographically with respect to the other anatomical structures in the region.

Note: This view underscores the "high" position of the medial malleolus (2) relative to that of the lateral malleolus (1).

1. Lateral malleolus
2. Medial malleolus

Fig. 12.64 The sustentaculum tali

MA: This structure, also indicated by the practitioner's index finger (2), was dealt with when the medial border of the foot was under investigation (Fig. 12.44). This posterior view confirms its topographical location with respect to the medial malleolus (1), i.e., about one finger-breadth distal to it.

1. Medial malleolus
2. Sustentaculum tali

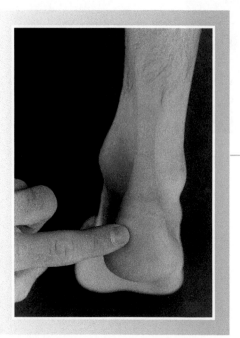

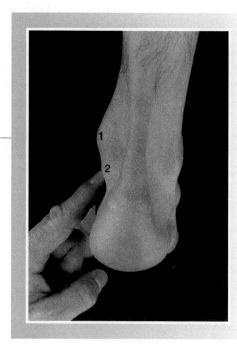

Fig. 12. 65 The posterior aspect of the calcaneus

MA: It is narrow and smooth superiorly and bulky and rough inferiorly. Your fingers will feel it overall as a triangle with a wide inferior base.

ATTACHMENTS

The calcaneal tendon is inserted into its inferior part.

> **CLINICAL NOTE**
>
> **Posterior calcaneal apophysitis (Sever's disease)**
>
> This is a disease occurring in children. Palpation with pressure elicits a pain that also extends along the posteromedial and/or the posterolateral border of the calcaneus.

Fig. 12.66 The posterior segment of the dorsal aspect of the calcaneus

MA: It is concave in the sagittal plane and convex in the horizontal plane. You can approach it on both sides of the calcaneal tendon.

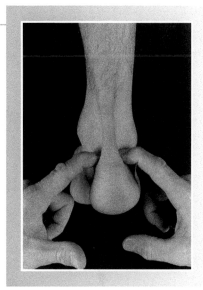

Fig. 12.67 The lateral malleolus and the lateral process of the talus

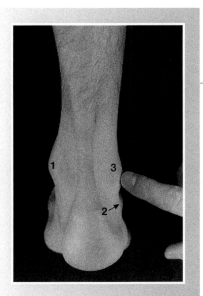

MA: The structure designated by the index finger has already been dealt with when the lateral border of the foot was under investigation. The different visual angle presented here underscores its "low" location relative to the medial malleolus (1) and its location relative to the fibular trochlea (2) (see Fig. 12.68).

1. Medial malleolus
2. Fibular trochlea or peroneal tubercle
3. Lateral malleolus

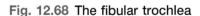

CLINICAL NOTE

The lateral process of the talus lying between the apex of the lateral malleolus and the fibular trochlea (2) can be fractured. "Invert" the calcaneus in order to bring out this process distal to the lateral malleolus. In case of a fracture, the pain elicited by palpation with pressure gets worse and becomes exquisite.

Fig. 12.68 The fibular trochlea

MA: This structure has already been dealt with when the lateral border of the foot was under investigation (Fig. 12.16). The visual angle presented here underscores its location with respect to the apex of the lateral malleolus (1), which lies about a finger-breadth proximal to it.

Note: It may be absent in some subjects.

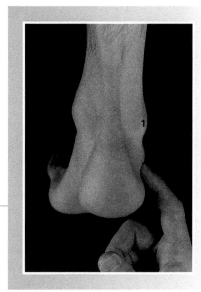

THE PLANTAR ASPECT

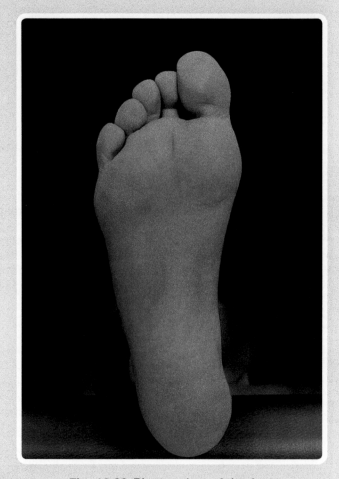

Fig. 12.69 Plantar view of the foot

The bony structures accessible to palpation are:
- the heads of the five metatarsals (plantar view) (Fig. 12.70)
- the plantar aspect of the cuboid (Fig. 12.71)
- the medial and sesamoid bones (Figs. 12.72 and 12.73)
- the posterolateral tuberosity of the first metatarsal (Fig. 12.74)
- the anterior calcaneal tubercle (Fig. 12.75)
- the posterior segment of the plantar surface of the calcaneus (calcaneal tuberosity) (Fig. 12.76)
- the medial process of the calcaneal tuberosity (Fig. 12.77)
- the lateral process of the calcaneal tuberosity (Figs. 12.76 and 12.78)
- other methods of approach (Figs. 12.79–12.85).

Fig. 12.70 The heads of the five metatarsals (plantar view)

MA: Each metatarsal is characterized by having its head covered by a convex articular surface that is peculiar in being much more extensive on its plantar side than on its dorsal side.

This specific feature for each metatarsal can be recognized on palpation as a large smooth convex surface (1) just proximal to the relevant metatarsophalangeal joint.

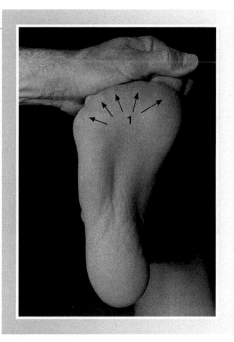

> ### CLINICAL NOTE
>
> #### Morton's neuroma
>
> This is a form of nerve pain on the plantar aspect of the forefoot. It is the result of irritation or compression of the plantar digital nerve in an intermetatarsal space. It is seen essentially in women wearing high-heeled shoes that are too narrow (a common occurrence among women), in conjunction with some morphologic abnormality of the foot, e.g., the flat foot and/or the convex forefoot.
>
> #### Avascular necrosis of the head of the second or third metatarsal
>
> This is a disease afflicting adolescents as a complication of osteochondritis of the metatarsal heads. Palpation elicits an exquisite pain between two metatarsal heads (mostly between those of the second and third metatarsals). On history taking, the subject mentions that pain is brought on by standing or walking.

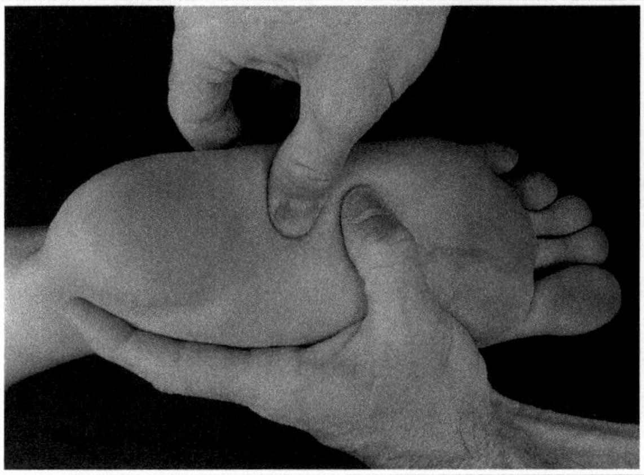

Fig. 12.71 The plantar aspect of the cuboid

MA: We have already dealt with this bone when studying the lateral border of the foot (Figs. 12.7–12.11). Once you have located the tuberosity of the fifth metatarsal and the rostral process of the calcaneus, simply place your thumb between these two structures, and then move it around the lateral border of the foot, and consequently around the lateral border of the cuboid, in order for your thumb to land on its plantar surface. The ridge on the cuboid (in the adjacent figure) can easily be felt, particularly in bedridden patients.

ATTACHMENTS

This surface of the bone bears a large number of attachments. In its middle part there is a ridge, which ends laterally with a tuberosity, and to which are attached the intrinsic muscles of the foot (opponens digiti minimi, flexor digiti minimi brevis, adductor hallucis) and one extrinsic muscle (tibialis posterior). Distal to the ridge there is a groove through which passes the tendon of fibularis longus.

> ### CLINICAL NOTE
>
> When palpation elicits an exquisite pain between two metatarsal heads (mostly between those of the second and third), the subject gives a clinical history of pain on standing or walking.

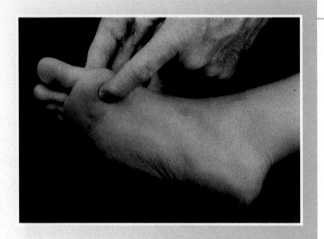

Fig. 12.72 The medial sesamoid bone

MA: You need only place the pad of one finger on the plantar aspect of the head of the first metatarsal and then rub it from side to side. With this method you can feel under your finger two "tubercles" separated by a depression.

In the adjacent figure the index finger is seen curving under the medial sesamoid bone.

ATTACHMENTS

The medial sesamoid is attached to the capsule and to the ligaments of the first metatarsophalangeal joint. It is embedded within the abductor muscles of the big toe and in the medial head of the flexor hallucis brevis.

> **CLINICAL NOTE**
>
> Excessive tenderness felt on palpation of the medial sesamoid suggests the possibility of a sesamoiditis and also of a fatigue fracture. Fracture of this sesamoid (usually both sesamoids are involved) causes:
>
> - exquisite pain on palpation with pressure,
> - pain when the big toe is passively dorsiflexed,
> - pain when the big toe is plantar-flexed against resistance.

Fig. 12.73 The lateral sesamoid bone

MA: Use the same method of approach as in Fig. 12.72. You need only move your index finger toward the lateral border of the foot to feel the lateral sesamoid under your finger just beyond the depression mentioned above.

ATTACHMENTS

Like the medial sesamoid, the lateral sesamoid is attached to the capsule and ligaments of the metatarsophalangeal joint of the big toe. It is embedded within the lateral head of flexor hallucis brevis and in the transverse and oblique heads of adductor hallucis.

Note: The tendon of flexor hallucis longus runs between these two sesamoids.

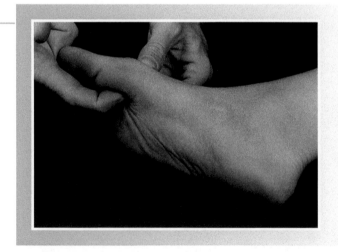

> **CLINICAL NOTE**
>
> Excessive tenderness felt on palpation of the lateral sesamoid raises the possibility of a sesamoiditis and also of a fatigue fracture.
>
> Fracture of this sesamoid (usually both sesamoids are involved) causes:
>
> - exquisite pain on palpation with pressure,
> - pain when the big toe is passively dorsiflexed,
> - pain when the big toe is plantar-flexed against resistance.

Fig. 12.74 The posterolateral tuberosity of the first metatarsal

MA: After locating the base of the first metatarsal, move your finger on the plantar aspect of the foot toward its lateral border (the adjacent figure indicates its location).

Note: Since this tuberosity lies deep in the tissues, it is advisable to apply an adequate amount of pressure on palpation so as to gain access to it. The use of the thumb may turn out to be a more efficient method of approach.

ATTACHMENTS

This tuberosity receives the insertion of fibularis longus.

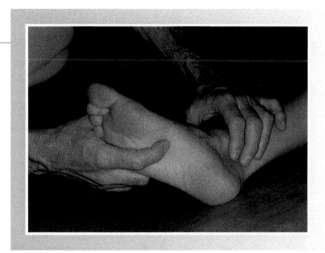

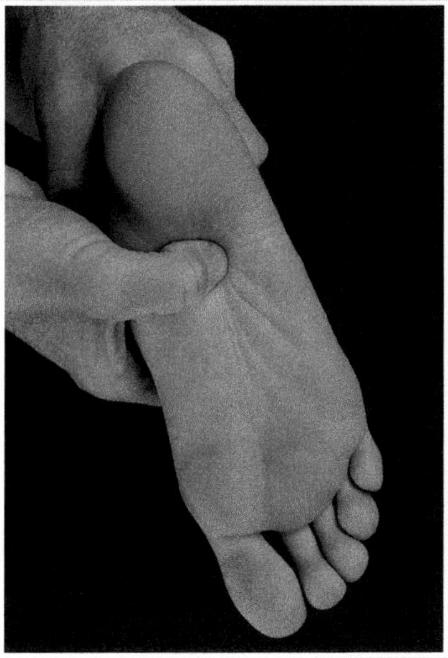

Fig. 12.75 The anterior calcaneal tubercle

MA: The adjacent figure, showing a plantar view of the foot, allows a more precise topographic location of the structure under discussion. If you start from the medial border of the foot, you can use the talar neck as a landmark for positioning your thumb, and then you need only go round the medial border of the foot to reach the structure you are after.

ATTACHMENTS

It gives origin to the plantar calcaneocuboid ligament, which is inserted distally into the cuboid tuberosity and runs deep to the long plantar ligament.

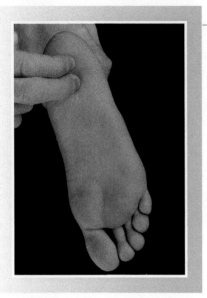

Fig. 12.76 The calcaneal tuberosity

MA: It is also called the posterior calcaneal tuberosity and occupies the posterior third of the bone, corresponding to the part of the calcaneus that rests on the ground. It has two processes: the medial and the lateral.

ATTACHMENTS

Between these two processes arises the long plantar ligament, which is inserted distally into the cuboid tuberosity and into the bases of the metatarsals II and IV.

Fig. 12.77 The medial process of the calcaneal tuberosity

MA: It is the bulkier of the two posteriorly facing processes of the tuberosity.

ATTACHMENTS

It gives origin to adductor hallucis and, more posteriorly, to flexor digitorum brevis. Still more posteriorly is attached the plantar aponeurosis, which is also attached to the entire width of the calcaneal tuberosity.

> **CLINICAL NOTE**
>
> **Medial calcaneal neuritis (Baxter's nerve entrapment)**
>
> Starting from this process, proceed along the posterior and plantar surfaces of the calcaneus toward the big toe and look for any tenderness on palpation with pressure. This condition results from repeated impacts of the foot on hard ground with the calcaneus in the valgus position.

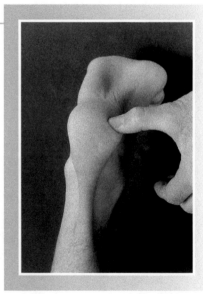

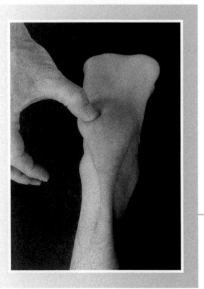

Fig. 12.78 The lateral process of the calcaneal tuberosity

MA: It is the less bulky of the two posteriorly facing processes of the tuberosity.

ATTACHMENTS

It gives origin to abductor digiti minimi.

Other methods of approach

The other methods of approach to palpation described below are meant to make it easier to learn the articular approaches relevant to this region.

Fig. 12.79 The plantar aspect of the base of the fifth metatarsal

MA: While the subject lies prone, the practitioner flexes her knee, takes hold of her foot, and "wedges" the posterior aspect of her calcaneus between the little finger and the ring finger of either his left or right hand. Then he uses the thumb of the same hand to palpate the plantar aspect of the base of the fifth metatarsal and also the tuberosity of the metatarsal. His other hand lies on the dorsal aspect of the subject's foot.

Note: The grip used to clasp the calcaneus can differ from that described here, as it depends on the body types of subject and practitioner. It can be used in all methods of approach to the plantar aspects of the foot, as described farther on.

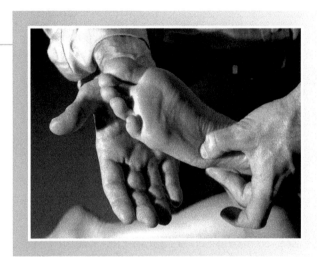

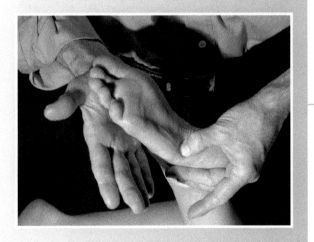

Fig. 12.80 The plantar aspect of the cuboid

MA: The subject and the practitioner adopt the same positions as described in Figure 12.79. The practitioner then places his thumb on the plantar aspect of the cuboid.

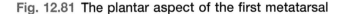
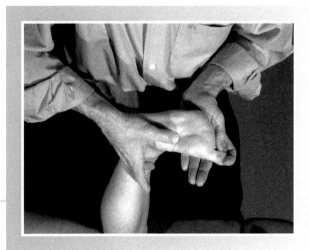

Fig. 12.81 The plantar aspect of the first metatarsal

MA: The practitioner places his thumb on the plantar aspect of the first metatarsal and can palpate its posteromedial tuberosity (medially) and its posterolateral tuberosity (laterally).

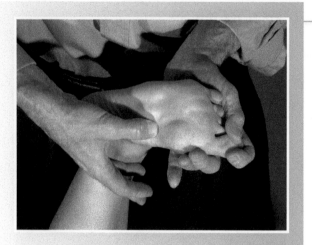

Fig. 12.82 The plantar aspect of the medial cuneiform

MA: The practitioner moves his thumb on the plantar surface of the subject's foot toward the calcaneus until he can palpate the plantar aspect of the medial cuneiform.

Fig. 12.83 The plantar aspect of the tuberosity of the navicular

MA: You have already encountered this structure (1) while studying the medial border of the foot (Figs. 12.37 and 12.38). You can also palpate it using this plantar approach, as shown in the adjacent figure.

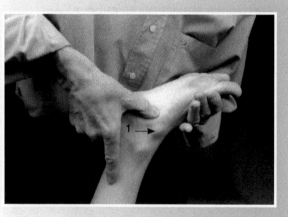

Fig. 12.84 The plantar aspect of the navicular

MA: Starting from the plantar aspect of the tuberosity of the navicular (1), proceed by moving your thumb laterally to reach the plantar aspect of the navicular.

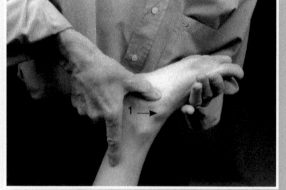

Fig. 12.85 The plantar approach to the ligament-related part or middle part of the talar head

MA: You can palpate the talar head between the navicular (1) and the sustentaculum tali, which lies a finger-breadth distal to the medial malleolus. Your fingers will feel it as a smooth surface.

This structure can be palpated by a medial and a plantar approach, since this part of the talar head is quite "free" on the plantar aspect of the foot.

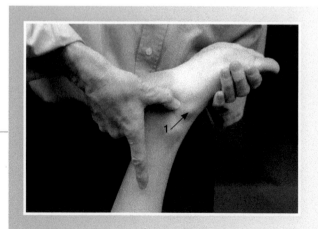

ARTHROLOGY

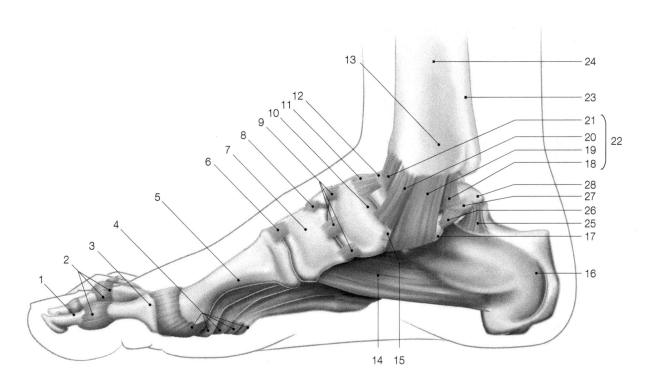

Joints of the foot (medial view)

1. Distal phalanx of the big toe
2. Capsules of the interphalangeal joints
3. Proximal phalanx of the big toe
4. Capsules of the metatarsophalangeal joints
5. First metatarsal
6. Dorsal tarsometatarsal ligament
7. Medial cuneiform bone
8. Dorsal intercuneiform ligament
9. Dorsal cuneonavicular ligaments
10. Navicular bone
11. Dorsal talonavicular ligament
12. Talus
13. Medial malleolus
14. Long plantar ligament

15. Plantar calcaneonavicular ligament
16. Calcaneus
17. Sustentaculum tali
18. Posterior tibiotalar part of deltoid ligament
19. Tibiocalcaneal part of deltoid ligament
20. Tibionavicular part of deltoid ligament
21. Anterior tibiotalar part of deltoid ligament
22. Medial collateral ligament or deltoid ligament
23. Fibula
24. Tibia
25. Posterior talocalcaneal ligament
26. Medial talocalcaneal ligament
27. Posteromedial tubercle of the talus
28. Posterolateral tubercle of the talus

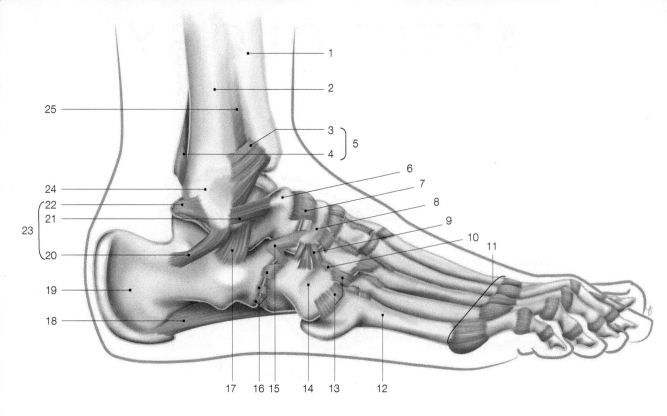

The ankle joint and joints of the foot (lateral view)

1. Tibia
2. Fibula
3. Anterior tibiofibular ligament
4. Posterior tibiofibular ligament
5. Tibiofibular joint (syndesmosis)
6. Talus
7. Dorsal talonavicular ligament
8. Navicular bone
9. Dorsal cuboideonavicular ligament
10. Dorsal cuneocuboid ligament
11. Articular capsules of the metatarsophalangeal joints
12. Fifth metatarsal

13. Dorsal cuboidometatarsal ligaments
14. Cuboid bone
15. Bifurcate ligament
16. Dorsal calcaneocuboid ligament
17. Lateral talocalcaneal ligament
18. Long plantar ligament
19. Calcaneus
20. Calcaneofibular ligament
21. Anterior talofibular ligament
22. Posterior talofibular ligament
23. Fibular collateral ligament
24. Lateral malleolus
25. Interosseous membrane

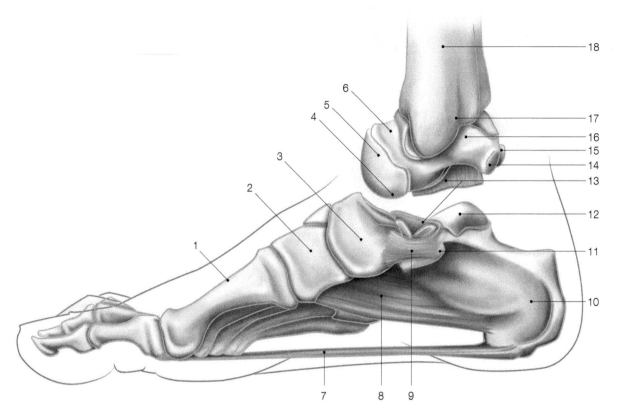

Open subtalar joint (visualization of the interosseous talocalcaneal ligament)

1. First metatarsal
2. Medial cuneiform bone
3. Navicular bone
4. Articular facet of talar head for plantar calcaneonavicular ligament
5. Navicular articular surface of the talar head
6. Talar neck
7. Plantar aponeurosis
8. Long plantar ligament
9. Plantar calcaneonavicular ligament
10. Calcaneus
11. Sustentaculum tali
12. Posterior talar articular surface
13. Interosseous talocalcaneal ligament
14. Posteromedial tubercle of the talus
15. Posterolateral tubercle of the talus
16. Talus
17. Medial malleolus
18. Tibia

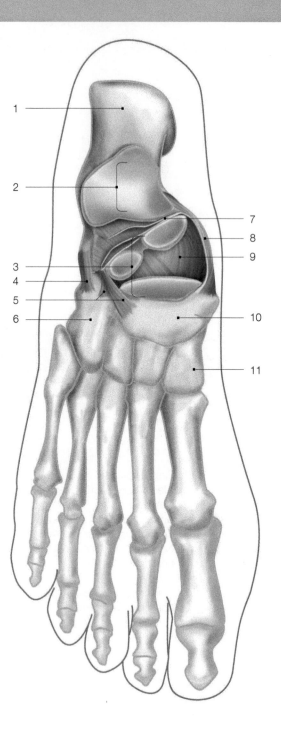

Subtalar and talocalcaneonavicular joints

1. Calcaneus
2. Subtalar joint
3. Talocalcaneonavicular joint
4. Dorsal calcaneocuboid ligament
5. Bifurcate ligament
6. Cuboid bone
7. Interosseous talocalcaneal ligament
8. Free border of the plantar calcaneonavicular ligament
9. Plantar calcaneonavicular ligament
10. Navicular bone
11. Medial cuneiform bone

THE JOINT SPACES AND THE LIGAMENTS

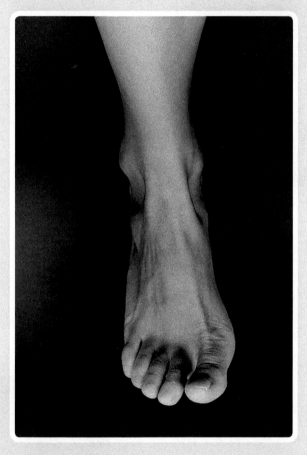

Fig. 12.86 Anterior view of the ankle and dorsal view of the foot

The joints accessible to palpation are (from the tips of the toes to the ankle):
- the interphalangeal joints (Figs. 12.88 and 12.89)
- the metatarsophalangeal joints (Figs. 12.89–12.91)
- the tarsometatarsal joints (Figs. 12.92–12.96)
- the transverse tarsal joint (Figs. 12.97–12.99), including the bifurcate ligament (Fig. 12.98) and the talocalcaneonavicular joint (Fig. 12.99)
- the subtalar joint (Figs. 12.100 and 12.101)
- the ankle joint (Figs. 12.102–12.107)
- the ligaments of the ankle joint (Figs. 12.108–12.113)
- the posterior tibiofibular ligament (Fig. 12.114).

The interphalangeal joints (synovial hinge joints)

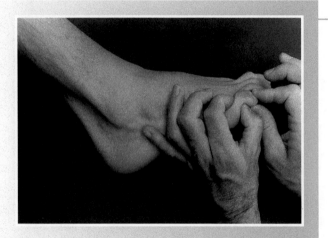

Fig. 12.87 The interphalangeal joints of the little toe

MA: There are two of them, and they are easily identified. In the adjacent figure the practitioner's proximal grip immobilizes the proximal phalanx, while his distal grip plantar-flexes the distal phalanx.

Note: They are hinge joints. Their articular surfaces are these: on the one hand, the articular surface of the distal extremity of the pulley-shaped head of the immediately posterior phalanx; on the other, the articular surface of the base of the immediately anterior phalanx with an ill-defined median ridge as its special feature.

Fig. 12.88 The interphalangeal joint of the dorsiflexed big toe

MA: The big toe has the distinction of having only one interphalangeal joint. In the adjacent figure, the practitioner's proximal grip fixes the proximal phalanx, while his distal grip dorsiflexes the distal phalanx.

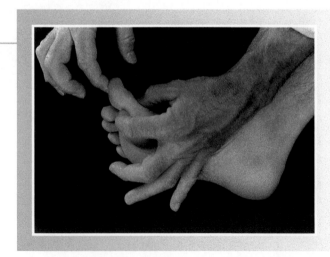

The metatarsophalangeal joints (synovial ellipsoid joints)

Fig. 12.89 The metatarsophalangeal joints: dorsal view

MA: In the adjacent figure, as the practitioner's hands take hold of the subject's toes and plantar-flex them, the dorsal articular surfaces of the metatarsal heads come into view.

Note: The practitioner's fingers will feel the articular surfaces as smooth: the most accessible is obviously that of the big toe.

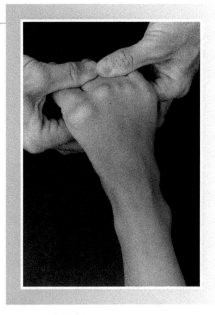

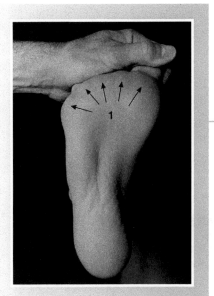

Fig. 12.90 The metatarsophalangeal joints: plantar view

MA: In the adjacent figure, as the practitioner's hand takes hold of the subject's toes and dorsiflexes them, the plantar articular surfaces of the metatarsal heads (1) come into view.

Note: The articular surface of each metatarsal "juts out" considerably on its plantar aspect.

Fig. 12.91 The metatarsophalangeal joint of the big toe

MA: As the practitioner examines this joint, he will feel the sesamoid bones on their plantar aspects (Figs. 12.72 and 12.73).

> **CLINICAL NOTE**
>
> This joint is adversely impacted in the presence of hallux valgus (big toe adducted relative to the axis of the foot passing through the second metatarsal). This deformity is the result of wearing inappropriate shoes: high heels, and forefoot squeezed into a shoe that is too narrow. The problem is worse if the subject has a pes planus valgus.

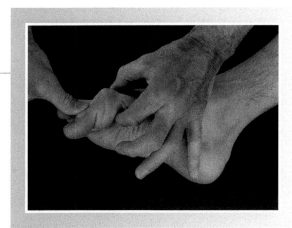

The tarsometatarsal joints

They connect the three cuneiforms and the cuboid to the five metatarsals. There are three such joints:

- one medial joint between the medial cuneiform and the first metatarsal (Fig. 12.96);
- an intermediate joint connecting the intermediate and lateral cuneiforms to the second and third metatarsals (Figs. 12.94 and 12.95);
- a lateral joint connecting the cuboid to the fourth and fifth metatarsals. They are synovial joints of the plane variety (Figs. 12.92 and 12.93).

Though there are three synovial cavities, the intermediate and the lateral joints most often communicate with those of the intercuneiforms and cuneocuboid joints. The medial cuneometatarsal joint is the only independent joint.

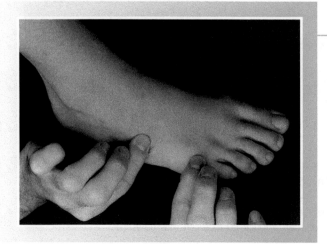

Fig. 12.92 The joint space between the cuboid and the fifth metatarsal

MA: Place the index finger of your left hand on the anterolateral part of the cuboid while staying in contact with the base of the fifth metatarsal. In order to feel the joint space properly, you need only take hold of the head of the fifth metatarsal and move it up and down repeatedly, and your index finger will feel the joint you are after.

Fig. 12.93 The joint space between the cuboid and the fourth metatarsal

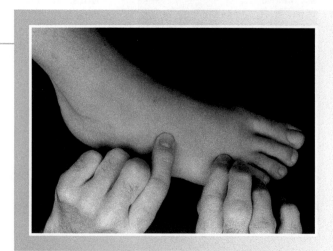

MA: To continue the maneuver shown in the previous figure, just move the index finger of your proximal hand a little medially to face the anteromedial part of the cuboid while staying in contact with the base of the fourth metatarsal.

Note: The two joint spaces described in Figures 12.92 and 12.93 oppose the cuboid to the fourth and fifth metatarsals and constitute the cuboideometatarsal joint, also called the lateral tarsometatarsal joint.

CLINICAL NOTE

The metatarsocuboid joint must be examined in cases of foot sprain associated with inversion and plantar flexion of the foot. Palpation with pressure of the two joint spaces forming this joint will elicit or exacerbate pain. You can also invert the bases of the fourth and fifth metatarsals while stabilizing the cuboid so as to stretch the ligaments of the joint, and this procedure will cause pain.

Caution: The tuberosity of the base of the fifth metatarsal can be fractured.

Fig. 12.94 The joint space between the lateral cuneiform and the third metatarsal

MA: Starting from the position shown in Fig. 12.93, move your index finger about one finger-breadth toward the middle of the foot in order to come into simultaneous contact with the distal border of the lateral cuneiform and with the base of the third metatarsal.

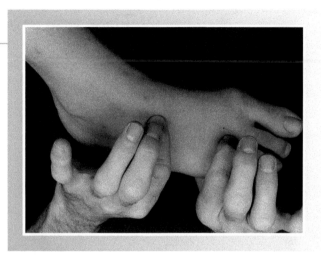

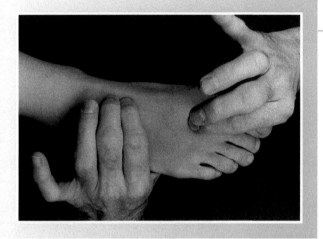

Fig. 12.95 The joint space between the intermediate cuneiform and the second metatarsal

MA: Again using the same contact as that shown in Fig. 12.94, you need only move it about one finger-breadth toward the middle of the foot, while keeping in mind that the distal border of the intermediate cuneiform lies deep relative to the distal border of the other cuneiforms, which flank it, one on either side. Then move your index finger toward the subject's hindfoot to gain contact with the intermediate cuneiform and with the base of the second metatarsal.

Note: The two joint spaces described in Figures 12.94 and 12.95, with the intermediate and lateral cuneiforms facing the bases of the second and third metatarsals, form the intermediate cuneometatarsal joint, which has very limited mobility, unlike its medial and lateral counterparts. It is a plane synovial joint.

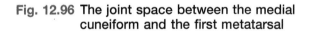

Fig. 12.96 The joint space between the medial cuneiform and the first metatarsal

MA: To locate the medial cuneiform: In the adjacent figure the practitioner uses his proximal hand to grip the joint space in question, while using his distal hand to mobilize the head of the first metatarsal.

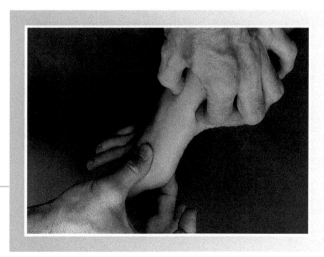

The transverse tarsal joint

It connects the distal tarsus to the proximal tarsus. Functionally speaking it consists of the talocalcaneonavicular joint (a ball-and-socket synovial joint) and the calcaneocuboid joint (a saddle synovial joint). The bifurcate ligament is common to these two joints.

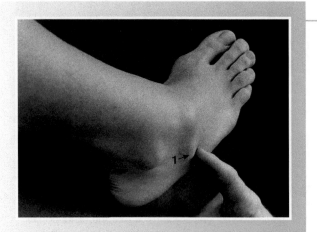

Fig. 12.97 **The lateral part of the transverse tarsal joint**

MA: It corresponds to the calcaneocuboid joint. The practitioner's index finger rests on the calcaneal articular surface for the cuboid, which is the anterior aspect of the calcaneus as it articulates with the cuboid.

Inverting the subject's foot makes it easier to gain access to the lateral part of this aspect, indicated by the index finger.

1. The rostral process of the calcaneus

Fig. 12.98 **The bifurcate ligament of the transverse tarsal joint**

MA: It arises proximally from the dorsal aspect of the rostral process (1) of the calcaneus and divides into two bundles:

• a lateral bundle inserted into the dorsal aspect of the cuboid (2);
• a medial bundle inserted into the entire surface of the lateral border of the navicular (3).

Note: It is deemed to be the key ligament for this joint.

> **CLINICAL NOTE**
>
> This joint can be sprained. Palpation with pressure applied to the bifurcate ligament and the dorsal calcaneocuboid ligament will cause pain, similar to that resulting from a passive stretching of these ligaments associated with immobilization of the calcaneus and inversion of the cuboid.
>
> In cases of torsion of the foot caused by inversion and plantar flexion, this ligament must be investigated, using palpation with pressure along with a replay of the traumatic process. With one hand fix the calcaneus and with the other invert the cuboid: these two clinical maneuvers will elicit pain.

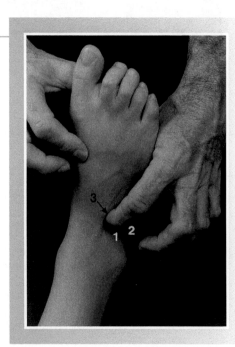

Fig. 12.99 The medial part of the transverse tarsal joint

MA: It corresponds to the talocalcaneonavicular joint. Everting the foot will help to free up the talar head, which articulates distally with the navicular (1).

In the adjacent figure the practitioner's index finger faces the middle part of the talar head, which is related to the plantar calcaneonavicular ligament. It is felt under the index finger as a smooth surface. It is coated with cartilage on its dorsal part.

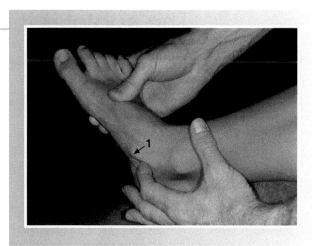

The subtalar joint (a synovial joint of the ellipsoid variety)

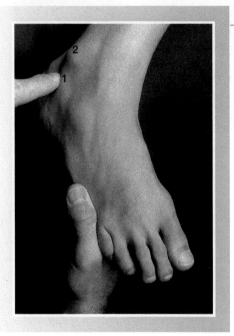

Fig. 12.100 The subtalar joint: lateral view

MA: The practitioner's index finger points to the lateral part of the joint space of the subtalar joint. The bony prominence, facing his index finger, is the lateral process of the talus (1), which "supports" the most lateral part of the fibular facet of the body of the talus.

ATTACHMENTS

The lateral talocalcaneal ligament is attached to the lateral process of the talus.

> **CLINICAL NOTE**
>
> The talocalcaneal ligament can also be sprained or pulled. Palpation with pressure, as well as inverting the calcaneus with respect to the talus, will elicit pain.
>
> The clinical maneuvers used to elicit pain include palpation with pressure and a replay of the traumatic process.
>
> **Beware:** The possibility of a fracture of the lateral process of the talus must be considered.

1. Lateral process of the talus
2. Lateral malleolus

Fig. 12.101 The subtalar joint: medial view

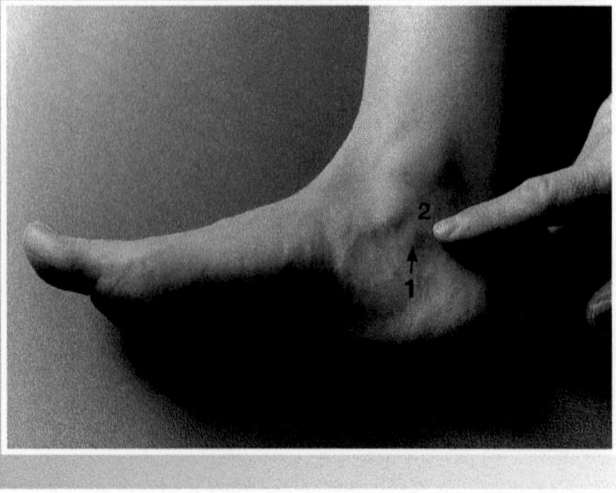

MA: The practitioner's index finger indicates the medial part of the space of the subtalar joint. The bony prominence facing the index finger is the sustentaculum tali (1), which supports the middle talar articular surface of the calcaneus, which is often directly continuous with its anterior talar articular surface.

> **CLINICAL NOTE**
>
> Torsion of the everted foot can pull the medial talocalcaneal ligament, which connects the medial talar tubercle with the posterior border of the sustentaculum tali. Palpation with pressure applied on the posterior border of the sustentaculum tali and on the medial talar tubercle will elicit pain. Causing the joint space to gap at this level by everting the calcaneus with respect to the talus will support or refute this hypothesis by eliciting or failing to elicit pain.

1. Posterior part of sustentaculum tali
2. Medial talar tubercle

The ankle joint (synovial joint of the hinge variety)

Fig. 12.102 The border of the lateral lip of the talar trochlea

MA: Place the index finger of your proximal hand on the anterior border of the distal epiphysis of the subject's fibula with his foot in the neutral position. You need only plantar-flex the foot slightly for your fingers to feel the border you are after.

By slightly adducting the foot while you plantar-flex it, you can get a better feel of this structure.

Note: Despite being smooth, this border is felt as "sharp" because it is coated with cartilage.

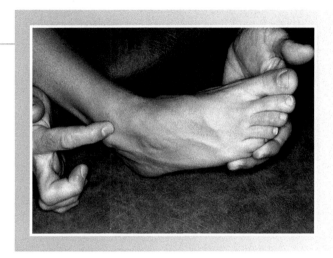

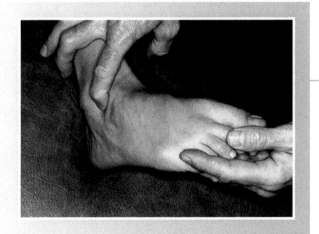

Fig. 12.103 The articular surface of the fibular malleolus

MA: Start by putting the subject's foot in the neutral position and proceed by placing the index finger of your proximal hand just anterior to the anterior border of the inferior extremity of the fibula. With your distal hand invert and slightly plantar-flex his foot simultaneously. The articular facet of interest is felt as a smooth surface under your index finger.

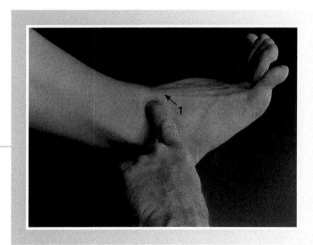

Fig. 12.104 The lateral lip of the talar trochlea

MA: Starting from the lateral border already located (Fig. 12.102) you need only slide your index finger deep to the tendon of extensor digitorum longus (1) toward the medial border of the foot.

Inverting and plantar-flexing the foot will cause the talar trochlea to "jut out" laterally on the foot and ease your access to the articular surface you are interested in.

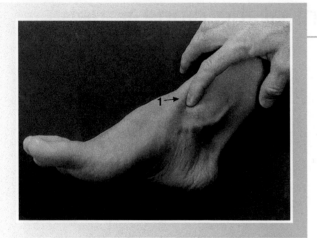

Fig. 12.105 The medial border of the medial lip of the talar trochlea

MA: Place the index finger of your distal hand on the anterior border of the medial malleolus at its junction with the anterior border of the tibial epiphysis. With the subject's foot in the neutral position you need only plantar-flex it slightly to be able to feel this border under your finger. It is better to evert the foot slightly at the same time to avoid any hindrance from the tendon of tibialis anterior (1).

Note: This border, which your finger feels as a smooth surface, is much less prominent on its medial side.

Fig. 12.106 The articular surface of the tibial malleolus

MA: First place the index finger of your distal hand anterior to the anterior border of the medial malleolus and then proceed to "uncover" as much as possible the tibial articular surface by everting and slightly plantar-flexing the foot simultaneously. Your finger will feel this articular surface as smooth.

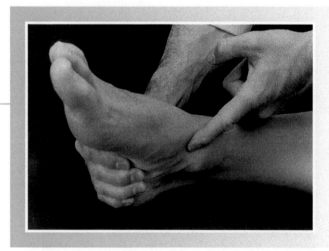

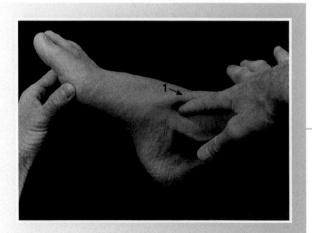

Fig. 12.107 The medial lip of the talar trochlea

MA: Starting from the medial border already located (Fig. 12.105) just slide your finger posterior to the tendon of tibialis anterior (1) toward the lateral border of the foot. From this starting point it is preferable to follow this maneuver with eversion and plantar flexion of the foot, in order to bring out the talar trochlea on the medial border of the foot and thus facilitate your access to the articular surface you are after.

The ligaments of the ankle joint

Fig. 12.108 The anterior talofibular ligament

MA: In order to be able to approach this ligament you must bear in mind its proximal insertion into the middle part of the anterior border of the lateral malleolus and of its distal insertion into the lateral aspect of the talar neck just distal to the lateral malleolar articular surface on the lateral aspect of the talar neck. It is sometimes useful to adduct, supinate, and slightly plantar-flex the foot to obtain better access to this ligament.

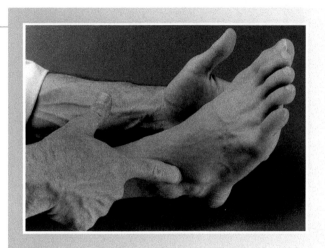

> **CLINICAL NOTE**
>
> It is the ligament most often sprained when the foot is suddenly inverted and plantar-flexed. Palpation with pressure applied along its course elicits or exacerbates pain in cases of sprain or pull of this ligament.
>
> **Caution:** An avulsion fracture of the anterior border of the fibular malleolus is always a possibility. Anterior swelling with or without ecchymosis is associated with this injury to the ligament.

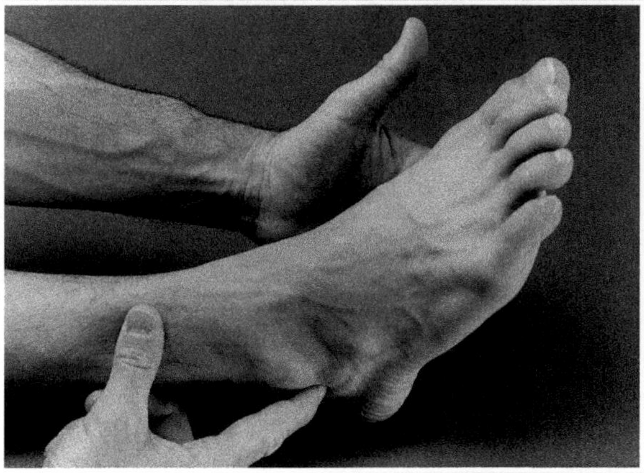

Fig. 12.109 The calcaneofibular ligament

MA: To approach this ligament correctly you must have a clear mental picture of its course, and also of its proximal insertion into the medial border of the lateral malleolus deep to the ligament described in Fig. 12.108, and of its distal insertion into the lateral aspect of the calcaneus.

> **CLINICAL NOTE**
>
> When there is swelling on its anterior aspect with or without a concomitant ecchymosis, this ligament must be investigated following a varus torsion of the foot coupled with plantar flexion. Palpation with pressure at this level, as well as inversion of the calcaneus, will cause pain if the ligament is injured.

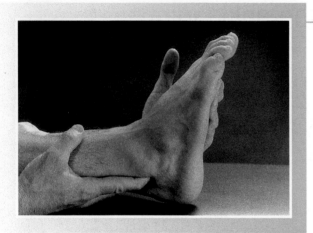

Fig. 12.110 The posterior talofibular ligament

MA: To approach this ligament correctly, it is essential that you have a clear idea in your mind of its proximal insertion into the medial aspect of the lateral malleolus deep to and posterior to its articular surface and of its distal insertion into the lateral tubercle on the posterior border of the talus. It runs virtually horizontally between these two structures.

Note: It lies distal to the posterior tibiofibular ligament of the inferior tibiofibular joint.

CLINICAL NOTE

Palpate the posterolateral tubercle of the talus and the posterior border of the fibular malleolus looking for tenderness.

Caution: Do not forget that the posterior border of the talus lies medial to the calcaneal tendon.

Fig. 12.111 The superficial layer of the medial collateral/deltoid ligament

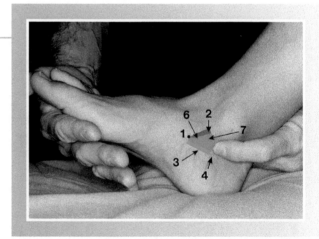

It consists of two bundles:
- a tibionavicular bundle (6), running from the tibial malleolus to the anterior part of the navicular (1);
- a tibiocalcaneal bundle (7), running from the tibial malleolus to the sustentaculum tali (4) and the posterior part of the plantar calcaneonavicular ligament (3).

Note: The practitioner's index finger points to the entire superficial bundle of this ligament.

1. Navicular bone
2. Anterior tibiotalar ligament (belongs to the deep layer; see Fig. 12.113)
3. Plantar calcaneonavicular ligament
4. Sustentaculum tali
5. Posterior tibiotalar ligament (belongs to the deep layer; not shown here; see Fig. 12.113)
6. Tibionavicular ligament
7. Tibiocalcaneal ligament

CLINICAL NOTE

Look for a pain elicited by palpation, with pressure applied at the level of the body of this ligament and of its attachments, as a possible sign of a pulled ligament. Stretching this structure by everting the calcaneus on the talus will confirm or refute this possibility.

Note: A sprain of this ligament is very rare.

Fig. 12.112 The deep layer of the medial collateral/ deltoid ligament: its anterior part

MA: It comprises two bundles:
- the anterior tibiotalar ligament,
- the posterior tibiotalar ligament.

Note: The practitioner's index finger is pointing to the anterior tibiotalar ligament stretching from the tibial malleolus to the talar neck.

1. Tibialis anterior
2. Tibialis posterior
3. Plantar calcaneonavicular ligament
4. Sustentaculum tali

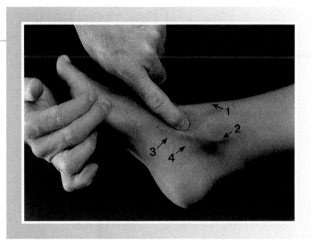

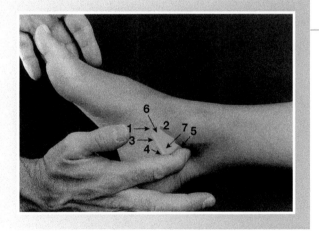

Fig. 12.113 The deep layer of the medial collateral/ deltoid ligament: its posterior part

MA: The posterior tibiotalar ligament (5) is inserted into the medial aspect of the tibial malleolus distal to its articular surface and into the posteromedial tubercle of the talus.

Note: In the adjacent figure the most posterior part of this ligament is being palpated close to its insertion into the posteromedial tubercle of the talus.

1. Navicular bone
2. Anterior tibiofibular ligament
3. Plantar calcaneonavicular ligament
4. Sustentaculum tali
5. Posterior tibiotalar ligament
6. Tibionavicular ligament
7. Tibiocalcaneal ligament

The posterior tibiofibular ligament

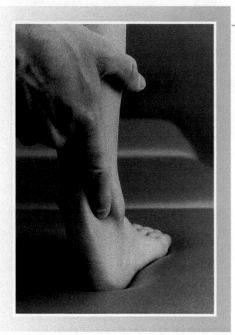

Fig. 12.114 The posterior tibiofibular ligament

MA: As you slide your index finger along the lateral retromalleolar groove, the first ligament felt as you proceed proximodistally is the posterior tibiofibular ligament. Distal to it you come across a bundle of fibers reinforcing the articular capsule and finally, more distally, you come into contact with the posterior talofibular ligament.

Note: This ligament belongs to the distal tibiofibular joint, also known as the distal tibiofibular syndesmosis.

Two other ligaments unite these two bones, i.e., the anterior tibiofibular and the interosseous ligaments.

MYOLOGY

Fibrous and tendinous sheaths of the foot

1. Extensor digitorum longus
2. Fibularis longus
3. Fibularis brevis
4. Superior extensor retinaculum
5. Lateral malleolus
6. Inferior extensor retinaculum
7. Fibularis tertius
8. Tuberosity of the fifth metatarsal
9. Abductor digiti minimi
10. Soleus
11. Tibialis anterior
12. Extensor hallucis longus
13. Medial malleolus
14. Tendinous sheaths
15. Extensor hallucis brevis
16. Extensor digitorum brevis
17. Interossei

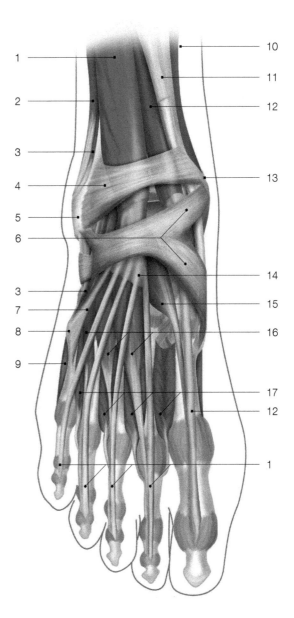

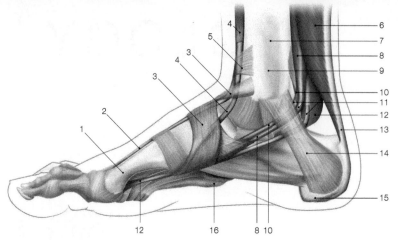

Muscles of the foot (medial view)

1. First metatarsal	9. Medial malleolus
2. Extensor hallucis longus	10. Tibialis posterior
3. Inferior extensor retinaculum	11. Tendinous sheath
4. Tibialis anterior	12. Flexor hallucis longus
5. Superior extensor retinaculum	13. Calcaneal tendon
6. Triceps surae	14. Flexor retinaculum
7. Tibia	15. Calcaneal tuberosity
8. Flexor digitorum longus	16. Tuberosity of the fifth metatarsal

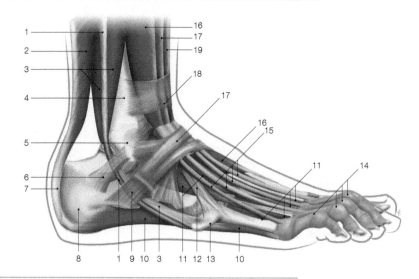

Muscles of the foot (lateral view)

1. Fibularis longus	11. Extensor digitorum brevis
2. Triceps surae	12. Fibularis tertius
3. Fibularis brevis	13. Tuberosity of the fifth metatarsal
4. Fibula	14. Dorsal aponeurosis
5. Lateral malleolus	15. Extensor digitorum longus
6. Superior fibular retinaculum	16. Extensor hallucis longus
7. Calcaneal tendon	17. Inferior extensor retinaculum
8. Calcaneus	18. Superior extensor retinaculum
9. Inferior fibular retinaculum	19. Tibialis anterior
10. Abductor digiti minimi	

Intrinsic muscles of the foot (plantar view)

1. Calcaneal tuberosity
2. Abductor hallucis
3. Plantar aponeurosis
4. Medial plantar septum
5. Flexor hallucis longus
6. Transverse bundles
7. Superficial transverse metatarsal ligament
8. Fibularis longus
9. Abductor digiti minimi
10. Lateral plantar septum
11. Tuberosity of the fifth metatarsal
12. Third plantar interosseus
13. Flexor digiti minimi brevis

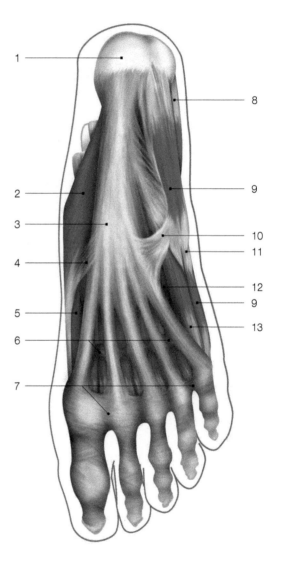

MUSCULOTENDINOUS STRUCTURES OF THE ANKLE AND THE FOOT

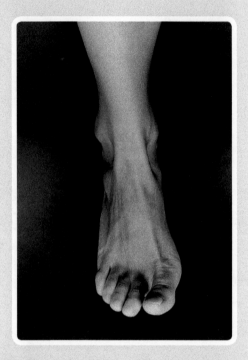

Fig. 12.115 Anterior view of the ankle and dorsal view of the foot

As you go "round" the ankle, you can identify the following structures:

- the tendon of tibialis anterior (Fig. 12.119)
- the tendon of extensor hallucis longus (Fig. 12.120)
- extensor hallucis brevis (Fig. 12.121)
- the tendon of extensor digitorum longus (Fig. 12.122)
- the tendon of fibularis tertius (Fig. 12.123)
- the body of extensor digitorum brevis (Fig. 12.124)
- the tendon of fibularis brevis (Fig. 12.125)
- the tendon of fibularis longus (Fig. 12.126)
- the posterior part of the body of fibularis brevis (Fig. 12.127)
- the calcaneal tendon (Figs. 12.128 and 12.129)
- the tendon of tibialis posterior at the medial malleolus (Fig. 12.130)
- the tendon of tibialis posterior at the medial border of the foot (Fig. 12.131)
- the tendon of flexor digitorum longus at the medial malleolus (Fig. 12.132)

- the tendon of flexor digitorum longus at the medial border of the foot (Fig. 12.133)
- the tendon of flexor hallucis longus in the medial retromalleolar groove (Figs. 12.134 and 12.135)
- the tendon of flexor hallucis longus at the medial border of the foot (Figs 12.136 and 12.137)
- the inferior fibular retinaculum (Fig. 12.116)
- the inferior extensor retinaculum (Fig. 12.117)
- the dorsal fascia of the foot (Fig. 12.118).

MA: Note: This topographical region must not be taken in the strict sense of the term. It is simply a didactic tool used to tackle structures that extend well beyond it at the level of the foot.

ACTIONS AND INNERVATIONS

- The anterior group of leg muscles (see Figs.11.11–11.23).
- The lateral group of leg muscles (see Figs. 11.24–11.37).
- The posterior group of leg muscles (see Figs. 11.38–11.66).

Fig. 12.116 The inferior fibular retinaculum

MA: In this figure clearly visible is the lateral part of the inferior extensor retinaculum (designated by the practitioner's finger), which courses on top of the tendons of extensor digitorum longus (1) and of fibularis tertius (2) before blending with the inferior fibular retinaculum (3) on the lateral border of the foot.

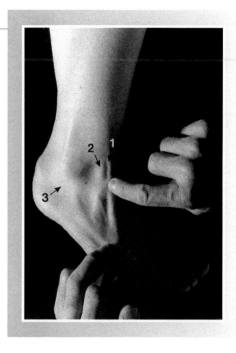

Fig. 12.117 The inferior extensor retinaculum

In this figure the diverging proximal (1) and distal (2) bands of the inferior extensor retinaculum are clearly distinguishable.

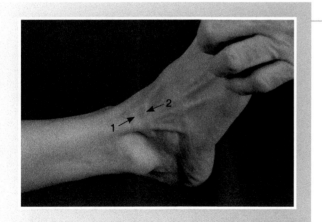

The dorsal fascia of the foot

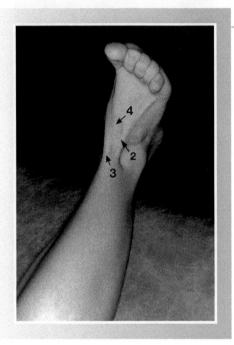

Fig. 12.118 The dorsal fascia of the foot

MA: This figure highlights the dorsal fascia of the foot (2), which overlies the tendons of extensor hallucis longus (4) and tibialis anterior (3).

Fig. 12.119 The tendon of tibialis anterior

MA: This big strong tendon is shaped like a cylindrical cord and comes into view just anterior to the medial malleolus on its way to the medial border of the foot, where it is mostly inserted into the medial cuneiform, while sending a tendinous slip to the posteromedial tuberosity, at the base of the first metatarsal. In the adjacent figure, the practitioner with his left hand keeps the subject's foot inverted and dorsiflexed and asks the subject to maintain this foot position. The index finger now points to the tendinous insertion of the muscle into the medial aspect of the cuneiform.

> **CLINICAL NOTE**
>
> This tendon can be the seat of a tendinopathy and of a total rupture, the latter occurring particularly in athletes engaged in very high-intensity sports.

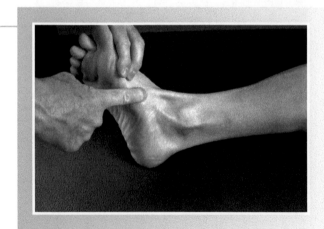

Fig. 12.120 The tendon of extensor hallucis longus

MA: The subject is asked to extend both the interphalangeal and metatarsophalangeal joints of his big toe. The practitioner can place his thumb on the dorsal surface of the subject's big toe in order to resist these movements and make him aware of them. The tendon will stand out just lateral to the tendon located in Fig. 12.119.

Note: The tendon of this muscle also contributes to adduction, supination, and dorsiflexion of the ankle. It is inserted into the dorsal aspects of both phalanges of the big toe.

> **CLINICAL NOTE**
>
> Overuse of the muscles of the anterolateral compartment of the leg (tibialis anterior, extensor hallucis longus, and extensor digitorum longus) can cause a tenosynovitis, manifested by pain on palpation elicited along the length of the tendon, indicated here by the practitioner's index finger, and also through the extensor retinaculum.

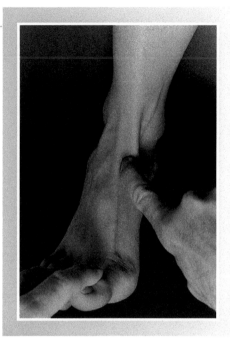

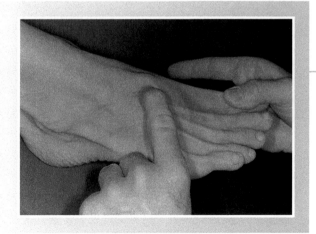

Fig. 12.121 The body of extensor hallucis longus

MA: This muscle is not always present. It is the most medial part of extensor digitorum brevis because it is the part of the muscle meant for the big toe.

Ask the subject to extend her first metatarsophalangeal joint repeatedly to allow you to locate this muscle on the dorsum of the foot just lateral to the tendon of extensor hallucis longus located in the previous figure.

Note: It comes to lie deep to the tendons of extensor digitorum longus and is inserted into the base of the proximal phalanx of the big toe.

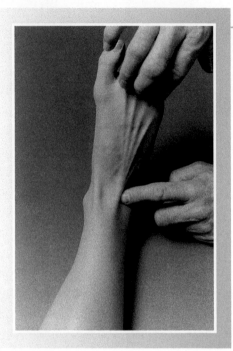

Fig. 12.122 The tendon of extensor digitorum longus

MA: Since it contributes to dorsiflexion of the ankle and abduction of the foot, you need only ask the subject to perform these movements, and the tendon will stand out at the ankle just lateral to the tendon of extensor hallucis longus.

A wide contact placed on the dorsal aspect of the last four toes in order to oppose any extension of the corresponding interphalangeal and metatarsophalangeal joints will bring out the tendons on the dorsum of the foot.

Note: This muscle also contributes to abduction, pronation, and dorsiflexion of the foot.

> **CLINICAL NOTE**
>
> As with extensor hallucis longus, overuse of this muscle can lead to a tenosynovitis, revealed by pain on palpation at the level of the instep, exactly at the spot indicated by the practitioner's index finger and also through the extensor retinaculum.

Fig. 12.123 The tendon of fibularis tertius

MA: Ask the subject to abduct, pronate, and dorsiflex his foot while you may or may not resist these movements by placing your contact along the lateral border of the foot, as shown in the adjacent figure.

The tendon will stand out lateral to the tendon of extensor digitorum longus, which is intended for the fifth toe. It courses toward the dorsal surface of the base of the fifth metatarsal, where it is inserted.

Note: It is not always present.

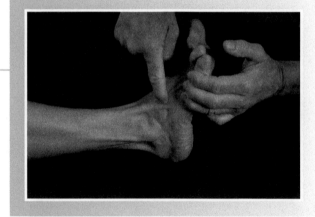

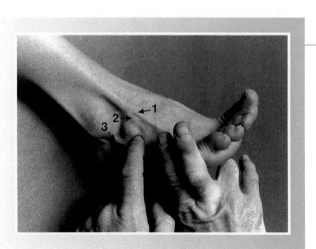

Fig. 12.124 The body of extensor digitorum brevis

MA: Ask the subject to extend the interphalangeal and metatarsophalangeal joints of her toes simultaneously (the fifth toe is not supplied by this muscle).

The body of this muscle will stand out lateral to the tendons of extensor digitorum longus (1) and fibularis tertius (2), anterior to the lateral malleolus and medial to fibularis brevis (3).

Note: Resistance applied to the lateral border of the foot by your distal hand is intended to bring out the tendinous structures that "frame" this muscle, which is indicated by your index finger. Most of the time this muscle has the appearance of a globular structure attached to the anterior segment of the dorsal surface of the calcaneus. It is the only intrinsic muscle on the dorsal aspect of the foot.

Fig. 12.125 The tendon of fibularis brevis

MA: With the subject's foot in the neutral position, ask him to perform a pure abduction of his foot. You can resist this movement with your distal hand resting on the lateral border of his foot.

The index finger of your proximal hand indicates the structure you are after.

Note: This tendon runs dorsal to the fibular trochlea before gaining insertion into the base of the tuberosity of the fifth metatarsal.

> **CLINICAL NOTE**
>
> Rupture of the superior fibular retinaculum causes displacement of fibularis longus anterior to the lateral malleolus. This abnormality can be a congenital malformation.

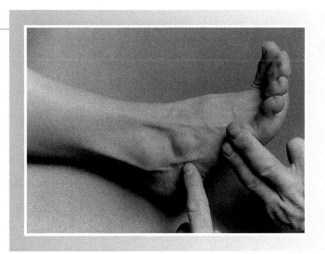

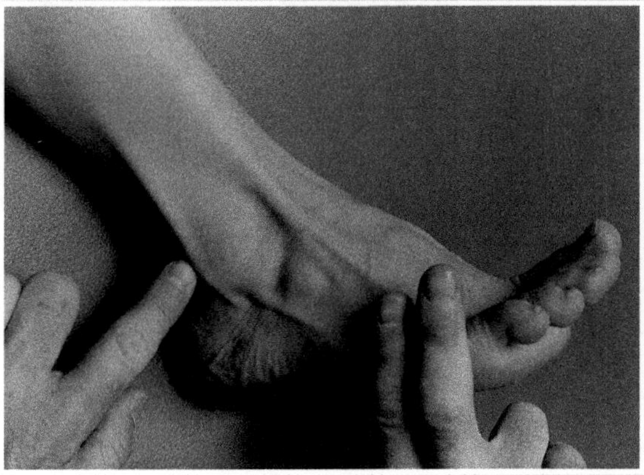

Fig. 12.126 The tendon of fibularis longus

MA: You can ask the subject to perform the same movements as those described in Fig. 12.125. This may be enough to bring out the tendon on the lateral border of the foot before it enters its groove on the cuboid. In addition, you can ask the subject to pronate and plantar-flex his foot.

Note: This tendon passes plantar to the fibular trochlea and is inserted into the posterolateral tuberosity of the first metatarsal. It very often sends out tendinous slips for insertion into the medial cuneiform, the second metatarsal, and the first dorsal interosseus.

> **CLINICAL NOTE**
>
> As in the case of fibularis brevis, a shallow retromalleolar groove can cause problems for these two tendons. Tenosynovitis of the fibular muscles reveals itself as tenderness on palpation of these tendons. The tuberosity of the fifth metatarsal can be painful, and pain can be elicited by passive inversion of the foot and eversion of the foot against resistance.

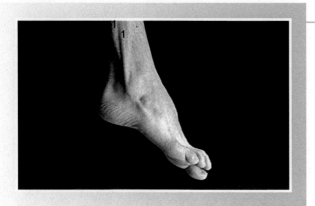

Fig. 12.127 The body of fibularis brevis

MA: The subject is asked to perform the same movements as those described in Figure 12.125. The body of the muscle (1) is accessible where it runs proximal to the lateral malleolus and deep and anterior to the tendon of fibularis longus.

Depending on the subject, the body of this muscle may be more noticeable anterior or posterior to the tendon of fibularis longus.

Fig. 12.128 Posterolateral approach to the calcaneal tendon

MA: This tendon is superficial and easily accessible.

> **CLINICAL NOTE**
>
> This tendon can be affected by a tendinopathy, which can develop into tendinosis, when the tendon undergoes fibrosis and thickening, the latter being visible on palpation, particularly in cases when the patient ignores or underestimates the severity of the lesion and presents after some delay. Partial or total rupture of this tendon can also occur.

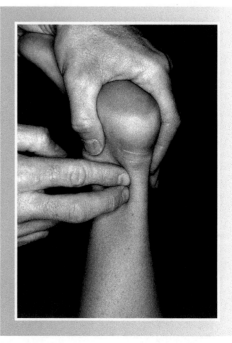

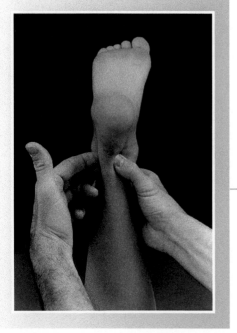

Fig. 12.129 Anterolateral and anteromedial approach to the calcaneal tendon

MA: You need only use your thumb to push the tendon laterally to gain access to its anterolateral part, which you can examine by sliding the pad of your thumb to and fro. Likewise, you can simply push the tendon medially with your thumb to gain access to the anteromedial part of this tendon.

> **CLINICAL NOTE**
>
> With this approach you can detect nodules or microruptures in the tendon, which are signs of a weakened tendon potentially at risk for partial or total rupture.

Fig. 12.130 The tendon of tibialis posterior at the medial malleolus

MA: After placing the subject's foot in the plantar-flexed position, ask him to adduct it against resistance applied on its medial border.

The tendon will stand out on the posterior border of the medial malleolus.

> **CLINICAL NOTE**
>
> An obese middle-aged woman with a pes planus valgus is potentially at risk of rupturing this tendon. For a man with a similar static foot deformity (pes planus valgus) intensive jogging can lead to rupture of this tendon. Any tendon passing anterior to the medial malleolus is also subject to displacement.

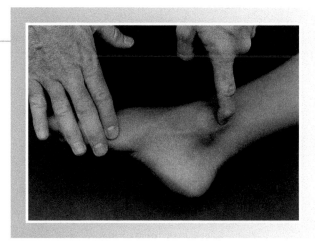

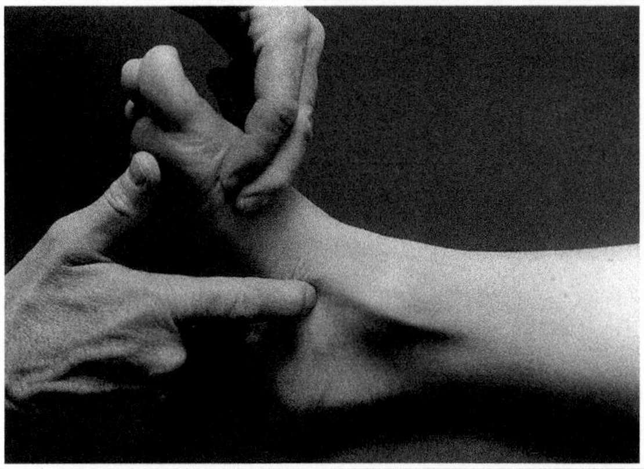

Fig. 12.131 The tendon of tibialis posterior at the level of the navicular bone

MA: The method used to tighten this tendon is the same as that described in Fig. 12.130. After skirting the medial malleolus, the tendon runs along the medial border of the foot and is inserted into the navicular tuberosity (as indicated by the practitioner's index finger in the adjacent figure), into all the tarsal bones except the talus, and into the metatarsals except the two extreme metatarsals, i.e., the first and the fifth.

Fig. 12.132 The tendon of flexor digitorum longus at the medial malleolus

MA: The practitioner places one hand on the plantar aspects of the subject's last four toes and asks him to flex these same toes rapidly and repeatedly. Meanwhile his other hand, placed posterior to tibialis posterior (1), will feel these repeated muscle movements. His index finger is pointing to flexor digitorum longus (2), which also lies posterior to the medial malleolus.

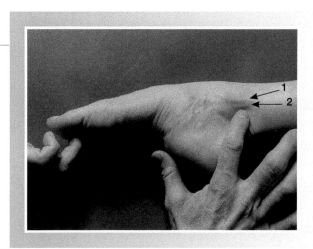

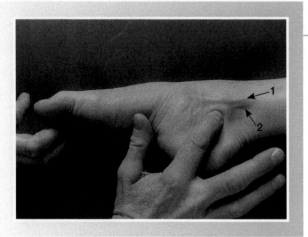

Fig. 12.133 The tendon of flexor digitorum longus on the medial border of the foot

MA: After skirting the medial malleolus inside its own osteofibrous sheath, the tendon crosses the deltoid ligament of the ankle joint and runs along its own groove on the apex of the sustentaculum tali.

In the adjacent figure the practitioner's index finger rests on this groove. Thereafter the tendon (2) comes to lie on the plantar aspect of the foot.

Captions for Figures 12.133 and 12.134

1. Tibialis posterior
2. Flexor digitorum longus
3. Flexor hallucis longus

Fig. 12.134 The tendon of flexor hallucis longus in the medial retromalleolar groove

MA: The practitioner places one hand on the plantar aspect of the subject's big toe and asks her to flex it rapidly and repeatedly. These repeated muscle movements will be felt in the medial retromalleolar groove at a distance from the medial malleolus and quite close to the calcaneal tendon.

Note: The tendon (3) of this muscle, which stands out in the adjacent figure, is not visible in all subjects.

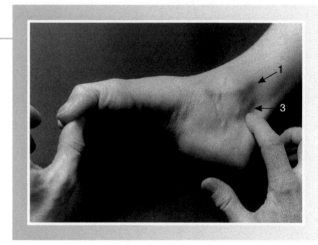

> **CLINICAL NOTE**
>
> Soccer, high jump, and classical dance are all sports liable to produce a tenosynovitis related to this muscle. The risk is higher if an os trigonum (a supernumerary bone) is present on top of the posterolateral tubercle of the talus. Other factors also contribute to this type of injury.

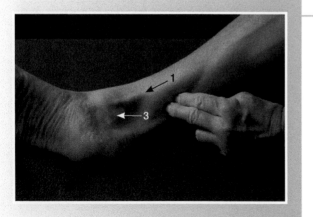

Fig. 12.135 Flexor hallucis longus: close-up of its body

1. Tibialis posterior
3. Flexor hallucis longus

Fig. 12.136 Flexor hallucis longus on the medial border of the foot

MA: Beyond the ankle joint the tendon (2) slides into the groove on the posterior aspect of the talus (between its posterolateral and posteromedial tubercles) and comes to lie deep to flexor digitorum longus (2) as it runs along its own groove on the medial aspect of the calcaneus plantar to the sustentaculum tali.

Note: It may be of interest, as shown in the adjacent figure, to stretch the tendon of tibialis posterior (1), since it serves as a landmark in the search for the tendon in question.

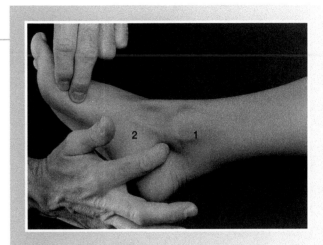

> **CLINICAL NOTE**
>
> The sheath for this tendon starts at the tibial malleolus and ends at the level of the navicular. In cases of suspected tenosynovitis it is necessary to have in mind the full extent of this sheath in order to perform a proper palpatory examination.

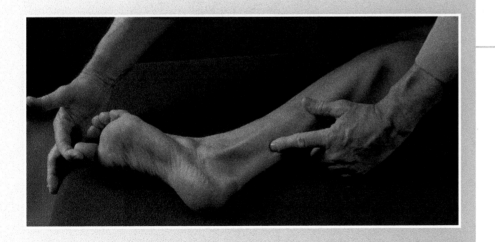

Fig. 12.137 The tendon of flexor hallucis longus: lateral approach

MA: The body of this muscle is also palpable lateral to the calcaneal tendon.

THE INTRINSIC MUSCLES OF THE FOOT

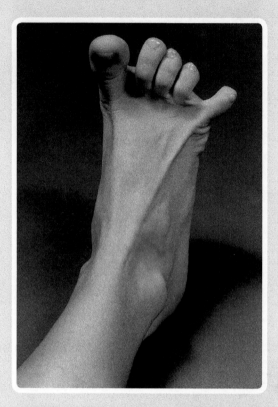

Fig. 12.138 Dorsal view of the foot

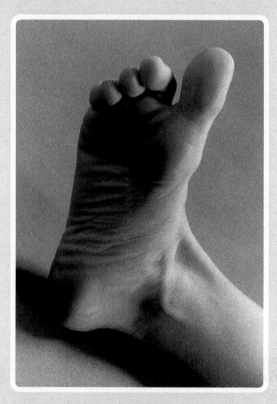

Fig. 12.139 Plantar view of the foot

The muscular structures accessible to palpation are:

- extensor digitorum brevis (Figs. 12.140–12.144)
- extensor hallucis brevis (Fig. 12.142)
- abductor digiti minimi (Fig. 12.145)
- flexor digiti minimi brevis (Fig. 12.146)
- opponens digiti minimi: visualization of its action (Fig. 12.147)
- abductor hallucis (Fig. 12.148)
- flexor hallucis brevis (Fig. 12.149)
- adductor hallucis (Fig. 12.150)
- quadratus plantae (Fig. 12.151)
- flexor digitorum brevis: visualization of its action (Fig. 12.152)
- plantar and dorsal interossei: visualization of their actions (Figs. 12.153–12.155).

ACTIONS

- Extensor digitorum brevis extends the proximal phalanges and flexes them laterally.
- Extensor hallucis brevis extends the big toe.
- Abductor digiti minimi abducts the little toe.
- Flexor digiti minimi brevis flexes the little toe.
- Opponens digiti minimi pulls the fifth metatarsal medially.
- Abductor hallucis:
  - abducts the proximal phalanx of the big toe on the first metatarsal;
  - flexes and abducts the big toe.
- Flexor hallulcis brevis flexes the big toe.
- Adductor hallucis adducts and flexes the big toe.
- Quadratus plantae stabilizes flexor digitorum longus by pulling it medially.
- Flexor digitorum brevis flexes the middle phalanx of each of the last four toes on its proximal phalanx and flexes each proximal phalanx on the corresponding metatarsal.
- The plantar and dorsal interossei flex the proximal phalanges of the toes.
  - The dorsal interossei move the toes away from the axis of the foot, i.e., the second toe.
  - The plantar interossei move the last three toes toward the axis of the foot.

INNERVATIONS

- Extensor digitorum brevis: deep fibular nerve (L4, L5, S1)
- Extensor hallucis brevis: deep fibular nerve (L4, L5, S1)
- Abductor digiti minimi: lateral plantar nerve (S1, S2)
- Flexor digiti minimi: lateral plantar nerve (S1, S2)
- Opponens digiti minimi: lateral plantar nerve (S1, S2)
- Abductor hallucis: lateral plantar nerve (S1, S2)
- Flexor hallucis brevis: medial plantar nerve (L5, S1)
- Adductor hallucis: lateral plantar nerve (S1, S2)
- Quadratus plantae: lateral and medial plantar nerves (S1, S2)
- Flexor digitorum brevis: medial plantar nerve (L5, S1)
- Plantar and dorsal interossei: lateral plantar nerve (S1, S2)

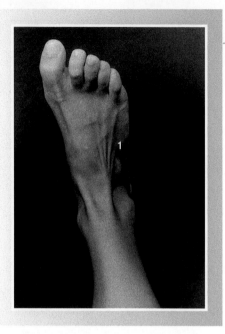

Fig. 12.140 Extensor digitorum brevis: visualization and topographical location

MA: It is the only muscle (1) that belongs to the dorsal region of the foot.

ATTACHMENTS

- It arises from the anterolateral part of the dorsal aspect of the rostral process of the calcaneus.
- It is inserted by four tendons:
  – the first into the dorsal aspect of the base of the proximal phalanx of the big toe;
  – the three lateral tendons into the lateral borders of the tendons of extensor digitorum longus for the second, third, and fourth toes.

Fig. 12.141 Extensor digitorum brevis

MA: You simply have to ask the subject to extend, against or without resistance, the four proximal phalanges of the corresponding four toes. The body of the muscle (1) becomes visible anterior to the lateral malleolus and lateral to extensor digitorum longus (2). Farther on it is more difficult to feel the muscle, since it is overlain by extensor digitorum longus.

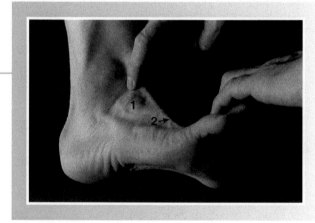

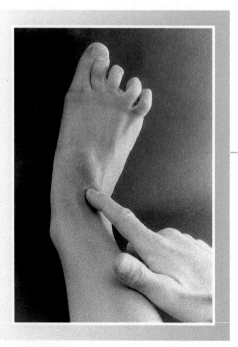

Fig. 12.142 Extensor hallucis brevis

MA: It is part of extensor digitorum brevis. Ask the subject to perform the same movements as described in Fig. 12.141. The body of the muscle becomes visible distal to the inferior extensor retinaculum and medial to extensor digitorum longus.

Fig. 12.143 Termination of the tendons of extensor digitorum brevis on the second and third toes

MA: Ask the subject to perform the movements described in Figure 12.141. Place the pads of three fingers on the dorsal aspects of the toes and gently plantar-flex them in order to make these tendons stand out as follows: the tendon inserting into the tendon of extensor digitorum longus for the second toe (1) and the tendon inserting into the tendon of extensor digitorum longus for the third toe (2).

1. Tendon of extensor digitorum brevis for the second toe
2. Tendon of extensor digitorum brevis for the third toe

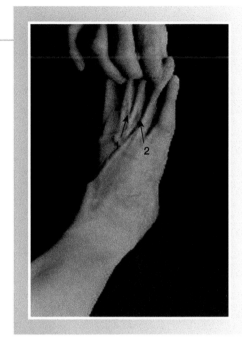

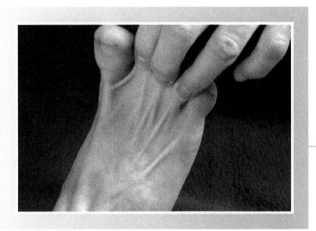

Fig. 12.144 Close-up of the terminations of the tendons of extensor digitorum brevis for the second, third, and fourth toes

Fig. 12.145 Abductor digiti minimi

MA: Place the pads of your fingers widely along the lateral border of the subject's foot and ask her to abduct her little toe repeatedly. As the muscle contracts you can readily feel it under your fingers.

ATTACHMENTS

- It arises from:
  - the plantar surface of the lateral process of the calcaneal tuberosity,
  - the plantar aponeurosis,
  - the tuberosity of the fifth metatarsal.
- It is inserted into:
  - the inferolateral aspect of the base of the proximal phalanx of the little toe.

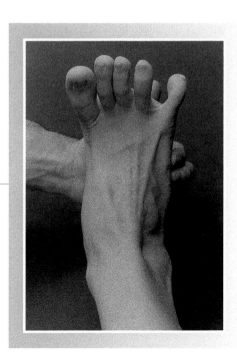

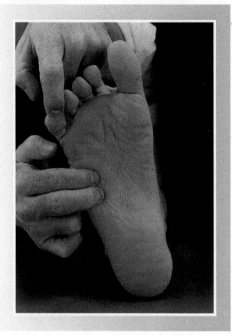

Fig. 12.146 Flexor digiti minimi brevis

MA: Place the pads of two of your fingers on the plantar aspect of the fifth metatarsal while moving them slightly toward the medial border of the foot.

Laterally, the muscle is overlain by abductor digiti minimi.

ATTACHMENTS

- It arises from:
  - the lateral part of the ridge of the cuboid,
  - the fibrous sheath of fibularis longus,
  - the base of the fifth metatarsal.
- It is inserted into the plantar aspect of the base of the proximal phalanx of the little toe.

Fig. 12.147 Visualization of the action of opponens digiti minimi

MA: Its action is to pull the fifth metatarsal medially.

Note: Like the two muscles mentioned in Figs. 12.145-146 it belongs to the lateral muscle group. It cannot be palpated on its own and may be absent.

ATTACHMENTS

- It arises from:
  - the lateral part of the ridge of the cuboid,
  - the plantar fibrous sheath of fibularis longus,
  - the base of the fifth metatarsal.
- It is inserted along the full length of the lateral border of the fifth metatarsal.

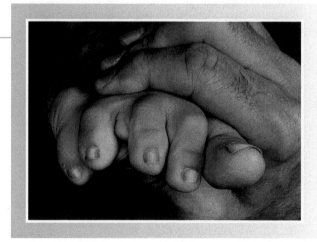

THE INTRINSIC MUSCLES OF THE FOOT

Fig. 12.148 Abductor hallucis

MA: With the pads of your fingers, make a broad contact with the medial border of the subject's foot and ask her to abduct her big toe on the first metatarsal. If the subject is unable to do so, ask her instead to flex her big toe on the first metatarsal. You will easily feel the muscle as it contracts on the medial border of the foot, in particular on the plantar aspects of the medial cuneiform and of the navicular.

ATTACHMENTS

• It arises from:
  – the plantar aspect of the medial process of the calcaneal tuberosity,
  – the plantar aponeurosis.
• It is inserted into:
  – the medial sesamoid,
  – the medial border of the base of the proximal phalanx of the big toe.

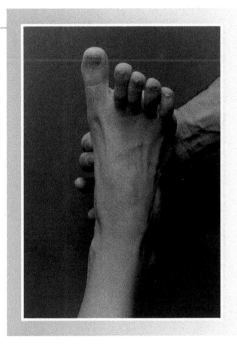

Fig. 12.149 Flexor hallucis brevis

Place the pads of two fingers in such a way as to achieve maximal contact with the plantar aspect of the first metatarsal proximal to the sesamoid bones. Then move them slightly toward the medial border of the foot in order to feel the medial head of the muscle. To feel its lateral head you must move your contact toward the lateral border of the foot, remembering that the lateral head is partially overlain by the tendon of flexor hallucis longus. The subject's contribution consists of flexing her big toe on the first metatarsal.

Note: The layering of multiple muscles will make it difficult to palpate a particular muscle on its own.

ATTACHMENTS

• It arises from:
  – the plantar aspects of the intermediate and lateral cuneiforms,
  – the calcaneocuboid ligament,
  – the tendinous slips of tibialis posterior.
• It is inserted as follows:
  – its medial head into the tendon of abductor hallucis,
  – its lateral head into the tendon of adductor hallucis.

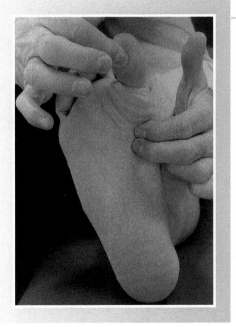

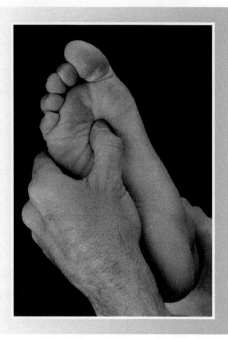

Fig. 12.150 Adductor hallucis

MA: Use a wide contact, with your thumb facing slightly laterally as it presses on the plantar aspect of the first metatarsal space. Then ask the subject to flex her big toe on the first metatarsal so that your fingers can feel the contraction of the oblique head of the muscle, which blends with the lateral head of flexor hallucis brevis. It is difficult to feel the contraction of this muscle.

ATTACHMENTS

- It arises by two heads:
  - The oblique head from:
    - the ridge of the cuboid,
    - the plantar aspect of the lateral cuneiform and the bases of the third and fourth metatarsals,
    - the calcaneocuboid ligament,
    - the tendinous slips of tibialis posterior.
  - The transverse head from:
    - the capsules of the third, fourth, and fifth metatarsophalangeal joints.
- It is inserted into:
  - the lateral sesamoid bone,
  - the lateral border of the base of the proximal phalanx of the big toe.

Fig. 12.151 Visualization of the action of quadratus plantae

MA: As seen in the adjacent figure, the practitioner's fingers rest roughly at the junction of the muscle with the lateral border of the tendon of flexor digitorum longus.

Note: Because of its oblique course, the tendon of flexor digitorum longus tends to impart a certain degree of deviation to the foot and the toes. Hence the raison d'être of quadratus plantae is to correct this deviation.

ATTACHMENTS

- It arises by two heads:
  - the lateral head from the plantar aspect of the calcaneus and the plantar calcaneocuboid ligament;
  - the medial head from the concave part of the medial aspect of the calcaneus.
- It is inserted into the lateral border of the tendon of flexor digitorum longus.

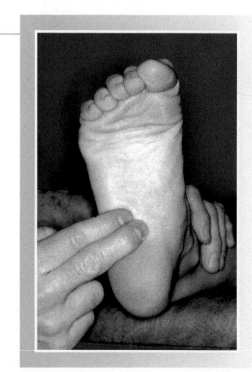

Fig. 12.152 Visualization of the action of flexor digitorum brevis

MA: With your palm take hold of the medial or lateral border of the subject's foot and apply the pads of your fingers over a wide area on the midline of the sole of her foot. Then you need only ask her to flex her toes repeatedly on her metatarsals to allow you to feel the muscle contracting under your fingers.

Note: The tendons of the muscles described in Figs. 12.146–12.151 lie deep to those of flexor digitorum longus.

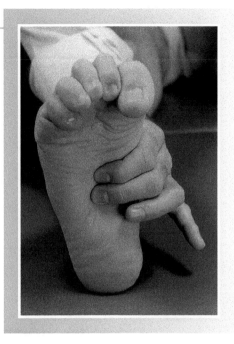

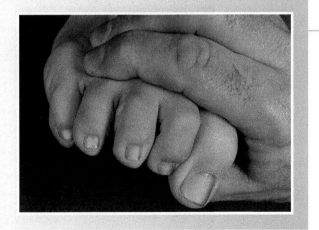

Fig. 12.153 Visualization of one of the actions of the plantar interossei and of the lumbricals

MA: The adjacent figure allows visualization of the proximal phalanges flexing on the metatarsals of the last four toes. Contrary to what is shown in the figure, the big toe is not involved in this movement. The plantar interossei flex the proximal phalanges of the last four toes and move the last three toes closer to the axis of the foot, which passes through the second toe.

The lumbricals flex the proximal phalanges of the last four toes and extend the other two phalanges on their corresponding proximal phalanges.

ATTACHMENTS

- The three plantar interossei arise on the medial aspects and plantar borders of the third, fourth, and fifth metatarsals, and each is inserted into the medial part of the base of the proximal phalanx of the corresponding toe.
- The lumbricals:
  - The four lumbricals arise from both borders of the third, fourth, and fifth tendons of flexor digitorum longus, except for the first lumbrical, which arises from the medial border of the tendon for the second toe.
  - They are inserted into the medial aspects of the bases of the proximal phalanges of the last four toes, and each sends a tendinous slip into the corresponding extensor tendon.

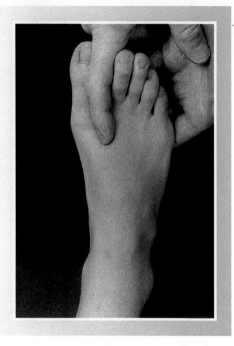

Fig. 12.154 The first dorsal interosseus

MA: The approach to these dorsal interossei is made through the four intermetatarsal spaces.

They are directly accessible to the practitioner's fingers pressed flat on the lateral aspects of the metatarsals.

Fig. 12.155 Visualization of one of the main actions of the dorsal interossei

MA: The adjacent figure shows abduction of the second, third, and fourth toes relative to the axis of the foot, which passes through the second toe and has a special status.

Note: These muscles also flex the proximal phalanges of the last four toes.

ATTACHMENTS

- These four dorsal interossei arise from the lateral and medial aspects of the second, third, and fourth metatarsals, and from the medial aspect of the fifth.
- They are inserted into the lateral aspects of the proximal phalanges of the second, third, and fourth toes (for the second, third, and fourth dorsal interossei). The first dorsal interosseus is also inserted into the medial aspect of the first phalanx of the second toe.
  - The second dorsal interosseus is inserted into the lateral aspect of the base of the first phalanx of the second toe.
  - The third and fourth dorsal interossei are inserted into the lateral aspects of the bases of the proximal phalanges of the third and fourth toes.

Note: It is clear that the various actions of the intrinsic muscles of the foot, when viewed individually, are less important than their overall action when viewed as a functional **indivisible unit.**

If they are viewed from this angle, one can imagine their considerable role in walking and in standing upright, without forgetting their extraordinary ability to adapt when the subject is called upon to move on diverse and extremely variable surfaces, such as sandy or rocky terrain, etc.

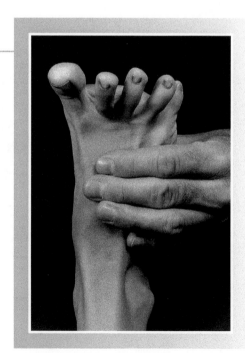

NERVES AND BLOOD VESSELS

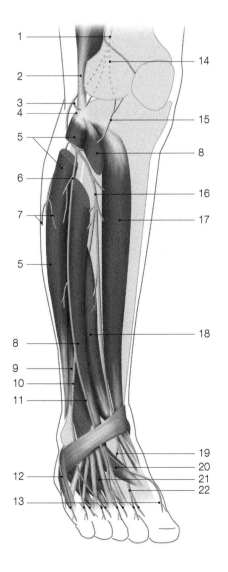

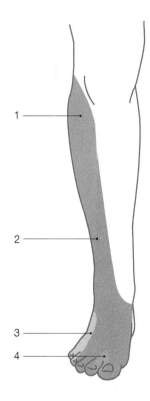

Common fibular nerve

1. Common fibular nerve
2. Tendon of biceps femoris
3. Articular branch
4. Fibular head
5. Fibularis longus
6. Superficial fibular nerve
7. Branches of lateral sural cutaneous nerve
8. Extensor digitorum longus
9. Fibularis brevis
10. Intermediate dorsal cutaneous nerve
11. Medial dorsal cutaneous nerve
12. Lateral dorsal cutaneous nerve
13. Dorsal digital nerves
14. Lateral sural cutaneous nerve
15. Anterior recurrent articular nerve
16. Deep fibular nerve
17. Tibialis anterior
18. Extensor hallucis longus
19. Lateral branch of deep fibular nerve
20. Extensor hallucis brevis
21. Extensor digitorum brevis
22. Medial branch of deep fibular nerve

Common fibular nerve (cutaneous branches)

1. Lateral sural cutaneous nerve
2. Superficial fibular nerve
3. Sural nerve via its lateral dorsal cutaneous branch
4. Deep fibular nerve

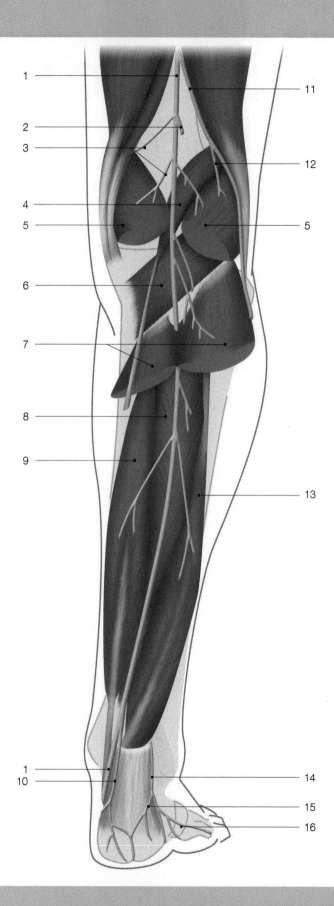

Tibial nerve

1. Tibial nerve
2. Medial sural cutaneous nerve
3. Articular branches
4. Plantaris
5. Gastrocnemius
6. Popliteus
7. Soleus
8. Tibialis posterior
9. Flexor digitorum longus
10. Medial calcaneal branch
11. Common fibular nerve
12. Lateral sural cutaneous nerve
13. Flexor hallucis longus
14. Sural nerve
15. Medial calcaneal branch
16. Lateral dorsal cutaneous nerve

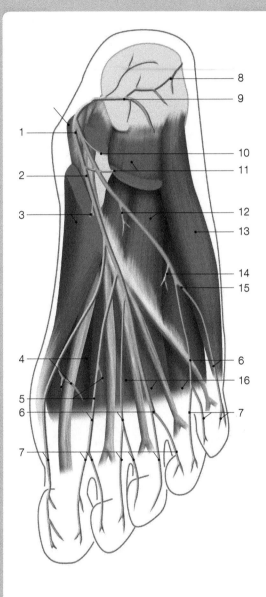

Innervation to the sole of the foot

1. Tibial nerve
2. Medial plantar nerve
3. Abductor hallucis and its nerve
4. Flexor hallucis and its nerve
5. First lumbrical and its nerve
6. Common plantar digital nerves
7. Proper plantar digital nerves
8. Lateral calcaneal branch of sural nerve
9. Medial calcaneal branch
10. Nerve to abductor digiti minimi
11. Flexor digitorum brevis and its nerve
12. Quadratus plantae and its nerve
13. Abductor digiti minimi
14. Deep branch to the interossei
15. Superficial branch to the fourth interosseus
16. Second, third, and fourth lumbricals

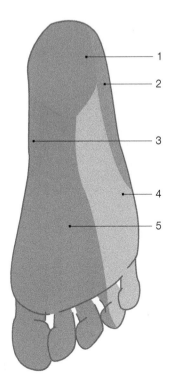

Sensory areas of the sole of the foot

1. Tibial nerve (medial calcaneal branches)
2. Sural nerve via lateral calcaneal and lateral dorsal cutaneous branches
3. Saphenous nerve
4. Lateral plantar nerve
5. Medial plantar nerve

THE MAIN NERVES

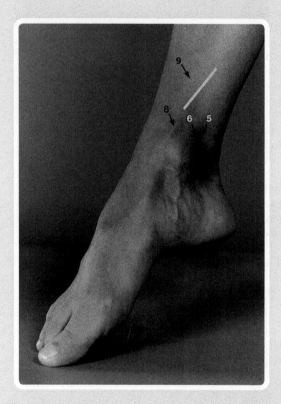

Fig. 12.156 **Medial view of the ankle and foot**

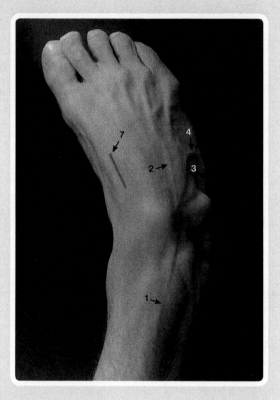

Fig. 12.157 **Anterior view of the ankle and dorsal view of the foot**

1. Superficial fibular nerve
2. Intermediate dorsal cutaneous nerve
3. Collateral dorsal lateral cutaneous nerve
4. Anastomosis between intermediate dorsal cutaneous nerve and dorsal lateral cutaneous nerve
5. Tibial nerve
6. Posterior tibial artery
7. Dorsalis pedis artery
8. Great saphenous vein
9. Saphenous nerve

The notable structures accessible to palpation are:
- Superficial fibular nerve (Fig. 12.158)
- Collateral dorsal lateral cutaneous nerve (Figs 12.159–12.160)
- Saphenous nerve (Fig. 12.162)
- Sural nerve (Fig. 12.163)
- Tibial nerve (Fig. 12.164)
- Deep fibular nerve (Fig. 12.165).

Fig. 12.158 The deep fibular nerve

MA: There are two ways of investigating this nerve:
- either look for it very high in the leg (roughly at the junction of the proximal two thirds and the distal third of the anterolateral segment of the leg);
- or look for it much more distally at the level of the instep.

Note: In the two figures (Figs. 12.157 and 12.158) it becomes subcutaneous after perforating the deep fascia of the leg.

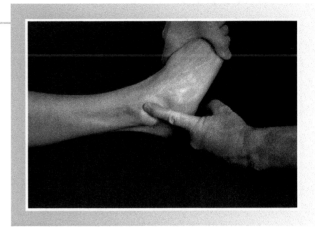

CLINICAL NOTE

If the patient reports pain and/or sensory disturbances on the dermatome of the nerve, proceed by plantar-flexing his forefoot and his toes in order to elicit or exacerbate the pain or the paresthesias. Palpation with pressure can also be used clinically to provoke the above-mentioned symptoms. The etiological factors include:

- a direct trauma inflicted along the course of the nerve (sports injury or car accident);

- an ankle sprain caused by inversion and plantarflexion of the foot, with violent overstretching of the nerve (the nerve can be overstretched proximally at the fibular neck and/or distally at the level of its subcutaneous attachments);

- repeated microtraumas due to the wearing of high heels (which displaces the talus anteriorly) along with laces or straps that compress the nerve along its course.

When the lesion of the fibular nerve is distal and if the medial dorsal cutaneous nerve is involved, the patient will feel pain in the dorsomedial part of the foot; if the lateral dorsal cutaneous nerve is involved, the pain will be felt on the dorsum of the foot.

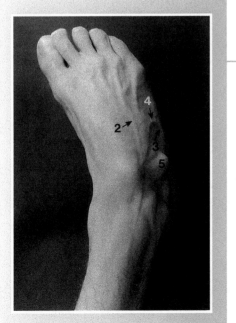

Fig. 12.159 The lateral cutaneous nerve (branch of the sural nerve) (3) and the anastomosis (4) (often absent) between the intermediate dorsal cutaneous nerve (2) and the collateral lateral dorsal cutaneous nerve (3)

MA: In the adjacent figure it is easy to visualize the superficial fibular nerve (a musculocutaneous nerve) in the distal part and the anterolateral segment of the leg. Beyond the lateral malleolus the nerve continues as the intermediate dorsal cutaneous nerve (2), which runs along the third intermetatarsal space.

Also clearly visible in the adjacent figure are the dorsal cutaneous nerve (3), which is the continuation of the lateral saphenous nerve and runs along the lateral border of the foot, and also the anastomosis (4) between the two nerves mentioned above, which extends distally a long way beyond the rostral process of the calcaneus (5).

Note: The anastomosis between the lateral dorsal cutaneous and the intermediate dorsal cutaneous nerves is not always present.

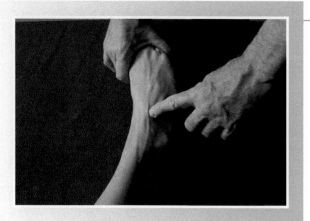

Fig. 12.160 The intermediate dorsal cutaneous nerve

MA: This is a lateral view of the nerve, whose topographical relations with other neural structures in this region have already been described in Fig. 12.159. The practitioner's index finger is seen pointing to the nerve.

Fig. 12.161 The medial dorsal cutaneous nerve

MA: In order to stretch this structure you need only plantar-flex the subject's foot. The nerve is seen running toward the medial border of the big toe and is designated by the practitioner's two fingers.

The same maneuver applies to the search for the superficial fibular nerve.

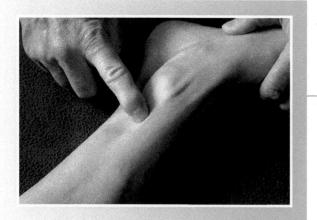

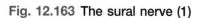

Fig. 12.162 The saphenous nerve

MA: To stretch this nerve, just evert the subject's foot. This nerve is accompanied along its course by the saphenous vein. The practitioner's index finger is pointing at it.

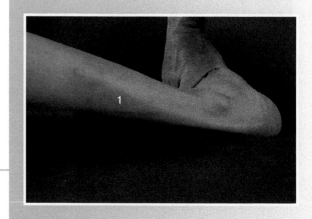

Fig. 12.163 The sural nerve (1)

MA: To stretch this nerve you need only dorsiflex the subject's foot. It can be palpated on the posterior aspect of the calcaneal tendon, i.e., in the distal third of the posterior aspect of the leg.

Fig. 12.164 The tibial nerve

MA: The practitioner's index finger is pointing at the nerve in the medial retromalleolar groove.

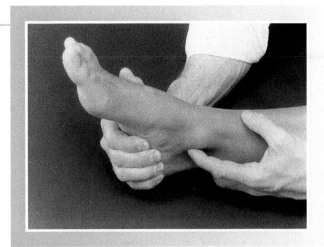

> **CLINICAL NOTE**
>
> **Medial tarsal tunnel syndrome**
>
> This is associated with pain or paresthesias involving the dermatome of the plantar nerves and of the medial calcaneal nerve. The medial retromalleolar region can be swollen and/or distended. Palpation with pressure, applied to the nerves along the medial border of the ankle, will elicit pain and possible paresthesias that can radiate distally and/or proximally into the calf region. Valgus displacement of the calcaneus can exacerbate the symptoms, whereas a varus displacement can attenuate them. The causes of this syndrome can include:
>
> - fracture of the medial malleolus, the talus or the calcaneus;
>
> - the ill effects of hiking, running a marathon, and military marches;
>
> - static problems of the foot (in particular, a severe valgus deformity of the calcaneus);
>
> - forms of mechanical or inflammatory tenosynovitis of the medial tarsal tunnel muscles (tibialis posterior, flexor digitorum longus, flexor hallucis longus);
>
> - venous stasis at the level of the tunnel.

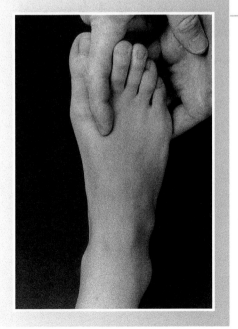

Fig. 12.165 The deep fibular nerve

MA: The nerve runs deep to the extensor retinaculum and divides into two branches:
- a lateral branch supplying extensor digitorum brevis;
- a medial branch consisting of a motor nerve for the first dorsal interosseus and a sensory nerve supplying the patch of skin between the big toe and the second toe.

> **CLINICAL NOTE**
>
> Depending on the site of the lesion, whether proximal or distal to the bifurcation of the nerve into its two terminal branches, there can be motor difficulties with weakness of the extensors of the toes or purely sensory disturbances (pain or paresthesias) when the medial branch is involved. These pains can be elicited or exacerbated by palpation with pressure and/or by stretching of the nerve. The possible causes include:
>
> - direct trauma (fall of a heavy object on the dorsum of the foot, while playing soccer, etc.);
>
> - the wearing of high heels, which projects the talus forward against the extensor retinaculum, along with the use of straps that compress the nerve (a double form of compression from inside and outside).
>
> - The wearing of sports shoes with laces tied too tight can also compress the sensory branch of the nerve.

THE MAIN BLOOD VESSELS

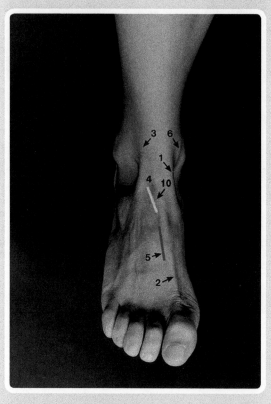

Fig. 12.166 Anterior view of the ankle and
of the foot

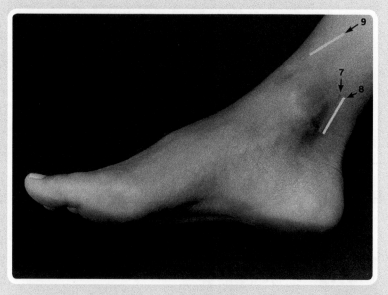

Fig. 12.167 Medial view of the ankle and of the foot

1. Tendon of tibialis anterior
2. Tendon of extensor hallucis longus
3. Tendon of extensor digitorum longus
4. Inferior extensor retinaculum
5. Dorsalis pedis artery (Fig. 12.169)
6. Long saphenous vein
7. Posterior tibial artery (Fig. 12.168)
8. Tibial nerve (Fig. 12.169)
9. Saphenous nerve
10. Deep fibular nerve

Fig. 12.168 Posterior tibial artery and tibial nerve

MA: The artery enters the medial retromalleolar groove between flexor digitorum longus anteriorly and flexor hallucis longus posteriorly.

To make it easier to locate and take the arterial pulse, the foot must first be slightly inverted in order to relax the diverse soft tissues in the region.

The tibial nerve is then felt under the fingers as a solid cylindrical cord just posterior to the artery.

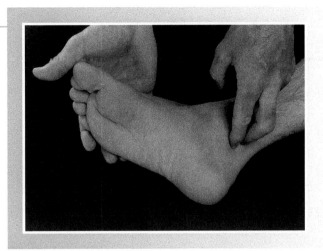

Fig. 12.169 The dorsalis pedis artery and the medial branch of the deep fibular nerve

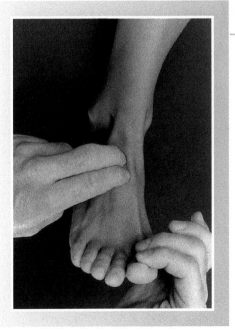

MA: The anterior tibial artery becomes the dorsalis pedis artery where it crosses the inferior extensor retinaculum.

It descends on the dorsal surface of the foot down to the proximal extremity of the first interosseous space, which it crosses vertically to anastomose with the lateral plantar artery.

- The essential landmark on the dorsum of the foot is the tendon of extensor hallucis longus. Using the pads of two fingers, look for the dorsalis pedis arterial pulse on the dorsum of the foot, just lateral to this tendon and medial to the tendon of extensor digitorum longus for the second toe.

The essential landmarks at the level of the instep are the inferior extensor retinaculum and the tendons of extensor hallucis longus medially and of extensor digitorum longus laterally. Using a bi-digital contact you will feel the pulse between these two tendons distal to or through the retinaculum.

- The medial branch of the deep fibular nerve is palpable in the same space as the dorsalis pedis artery, but remember that it lies lateral to the artery.

515

Appendices

Appendix 1

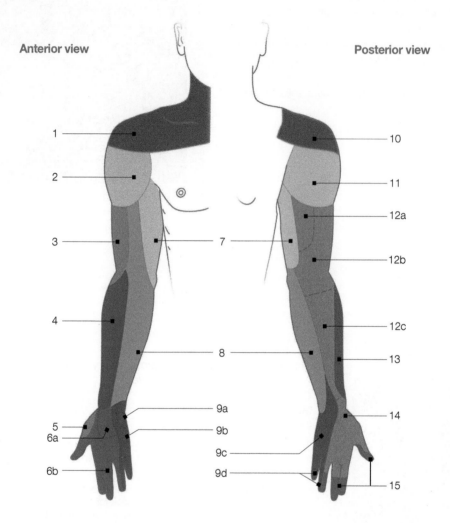

Anterior view

Posterior view

Sensory innervation territories of upper limb

1. Supraclavicular nerves (from cervical plexus – C3, C4)
2. Axillary nerve, superior lateral cutaneous nerve of arm (C5, C6)
3. Radial nerve, inferior lateral cutaneous nerve of arm (C5, C6)
4. Lateral cutaneous nerve of forearm (C5, C6, C7: terminal part of musculocutaneous nerve)
5. Radial nerve, superficial branch (C6, C7, C8)
6a. Median nerve, palmar branch
6b. Median nerve, palmar digital branches
7. Intercostobrachial (T2) and medial cutaneous nerves of arm (C8, T1, T2)
8. Medial cutaneous nerve of forearm (C8, T1)
9a. Ulnar nerve (C8, T1), palmar branch
9b. Ulnar nerve, palmar digital branches

9c. Ulnar nerve, dorsal branch and dorsal digital branches
9d. Ulnar nerve, proper palmar digital branches
10. Supraclavicular nerves (from cervical plexus – C3, C4)
11. Axillary nerve, superior lateral cutaneous nerve of arm (C5, C6)
12a. Radial nerve, posterior cutaneous nerve of arm (C5 to C8)
12b. Radial nerve, inferior lateral cutaneous nerve of arm
12c. Radial nerve, posterior cutaneous nerve of forearm (C5, C6, C7, C8)
13. Lateral cutaneous nerve of forearm (C5, C6, C7), terminal part of musculocutaneous nerve
14. Radial nerve, superficial branch and dorsal digital branches (C6, C7, C8)
15. Median nerve, proper palmar digital branches

Appendix 2

**Cutaneous innervation of upper limb, head, and neck;
anterior view**

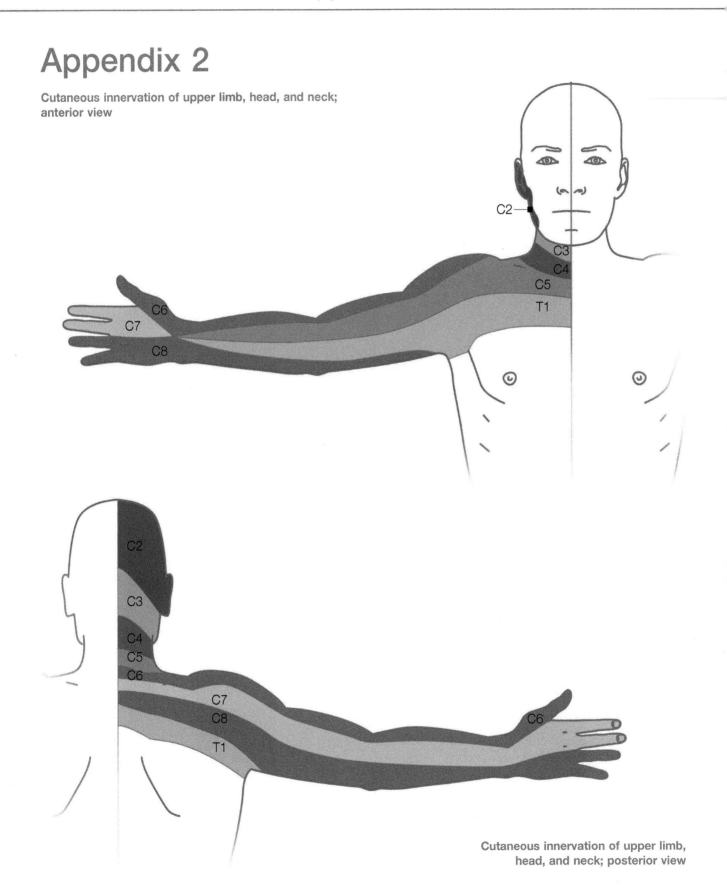

C2

C3
C4
C5
T1

C6
C7
C8

C2

C3

C4
C5
C6

C7
C8

T1

C6

**Cutaneous innervation of upper limb,
head, and neck; posterior view**

Appendix 3

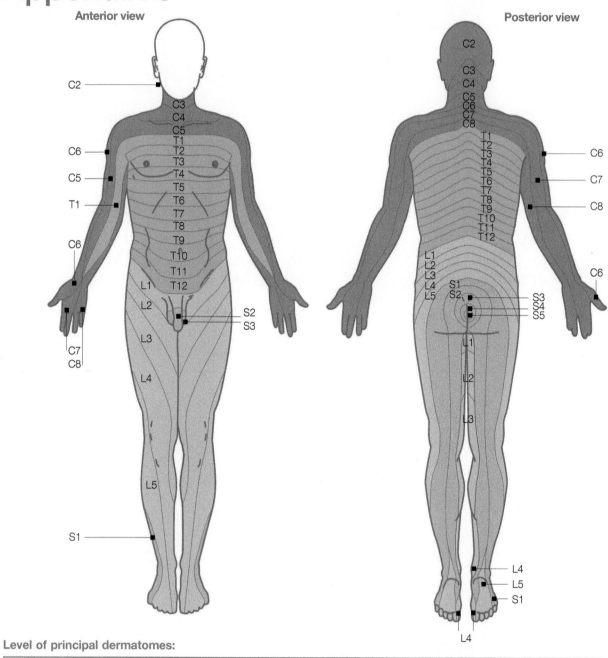

Anterior view

Posterior view

Level of principal dermatomes:

C5	Clavicles	L4, L5, S1	Foot
C5, C6, C7	Lateral parts of upper limbs	S1	Lateral border of foot and little toe
C6	Thumb	S1, S2, L5	Posterolateral surfaces of lower limbs
C6, C7, C8	Hand	S2, S3, S4	Perineum
C8	Ring finger and little finger	T4	Level of nipple
C8, T1	Medial parts of upper limbs	T10	Level of umbilicus
L1, L2, L3, L4	Anterior and medial surfaces of lower limbs	T12	Inguinal region
L4	Medial surface of big toe		

Glossary

Acromegaly

Condition characterized by an unusual noncongenital form of hypertrophy of the upper and lower limbs, of the head and face, of the limb bones, and of their epiphyses (Pierre Marie, 1885).

Anastomosis

Link between two blood vessels and, by extension, between any two similar ducts and between two nerves.

Ankylosis

Total or subtotal loss of movement in a normally mobile joint.

Anteversion

Forward/anterior tilting of an entire organ (cf. **Organ**). In physical therapy the term is used in connection with the pelvis, which is not an organ.

Aponeurosis

A strong whitish membrane of fibrous tissue attached to skeletal muscles. The aponeuroses of insertion are the tendons of flat muscles, and the aponeuroses of investment surround individual muscles or groups of muscles.

Apophysitis

Defective growth of a bony process. It is a form of osteochondrosis (cf. **Osteochondrosis**). Examples: posterior calcaneal apophysitis (Sever's disease) and anterior tibial apophysitis (Osgood-Schlatter's disease).

Archibald's Sign

Shortness of the fourth metacarpal, whose length is less than the lengths of the first and third metacarpals combined; an anomaly observed in Turner's syndrome (cf. Turner's syndrome).

Arthrosis

General term for chronic degenerative and noninflammatory diseases of joints, characterized by a destructive lesion of the articular cartilage coupled with the formation of osteophytes (cf. osteophyte) and of chondrophytes (cf. **chondrophyte**), and presenting clinically with joint pain, creaking noises, reduced mobility, and almost always stiffness but no ankylosis.

Atheromatous plaque

Chronic arterial lesion characterized by the development on the intima (inner coat of a blood vessel) of yellowish plaques made up of lipid (cholesterol) deposits. These plaques, which can ulcerate and release a porridgy material into the bloodstream, represent the initial lesions in atherosclerosis.

Bursitis

Inflammation of a synovial bursa.

Calcification

Deposition of calcium carbonate and calcium phosphate in tissues and organs (cf. **Organs**).

Chondrophyte

An abnormal intra-articular growth of cartilage.

Clinical history

The sum total of the historical information obtained by the physician from the patient regarding his or her sickness.

Cyst

An abnormal cavity separate from its surroundings, containing a soft or rarely solid fluid or a gas. Its lining has no vascular connection with its contents.

Dermatome

A bandlike region of skin supplied by a single spinal nerve. Examination of dermatomes helps in the detection of a lesion affecting one spinal nerve (for example, compression of a nerve by a tumor). The detection of sensitive cutaneous areas allows one to establish whether they coincide with one or more dermatomes. The nerve involved is then identified according to the affected dermatome, thus making it possible to localize the level of the spinal lesion.

Digastric muscle
A muscle with two bellies linked by an intermediate tendon.

Ecchymosis
A violet or black, brown, or yellowish discoloration due to infiltration of a cellular tissue with a variable amount of blood. It can occur in the skin, and in mucosal and serous membranes.

Edema
Serous fluid infiltration of diverse tissues, in particular the connective tissue of the skin or of mucosal surfaces.

Enthesis
The site of attachment of a tendon, a ligament, or a muscle to a bone.

Enthesopathy
A disorder of entheses, i.e., enthesitis, tendinoperiostitis, or rheumatic tendinitis; extra-articular rheumatism (cf. **Rheumatism**) localized at the bony insertions of tendons, ligaments, and aponeuroses.
It is often of traumatic origin, as is epicondylitis.

Epicondylitis
Inflammation of an epicondyle.
Tennis elbow (lateral epicondylitis) is associated with pain in the humeral epicondyle resulting from overuse of the forearm or from a mild trauma followed by a localized periostitis (cf. **Periosteum**).

Etiology
Study of the causes of disease. It is often used as a synonym of *cause*.

Exquisite pain
Sharp pain clearly localized to a very restricted area.

Exudate
A serous, fibrinous, or mucous fluid with a high protein content that infiltrates an inflamed surface.

Fascia
Strong fibrous membrane lining the deep surface of the skin or limiting muscular compartments or anatomical regions (cf. **Aponeurosis**).

Fatigue fracture
Fracture of a healthy bone arising in the absence of any trauma. It occurs in a bone subjected to excessive demands and weakened by advancing age. In sports medicine it involves mainly the lower limbs and recurs after an intense or an unusual bout of physical activity (a very long walk) or as a result of inappropriate footwear.

Femoral trochlea
Also known as the trochlear groove or the patellar surface of the femur. It articulates with the patella.

Foramen
Orifice.

Gerdy's tubercle
Also known as the infracondylar tubercle. It is located on the lateral aspect of the proximal tibial extremity.

Glenoid cavity
Joint cavity adapted to receive the globular condylar head of a bone.

Guyon's canal
Osteofibrous canal (tunnel) on the anterior aspect of the wrist carrying the ulnar nerve and the ulnar blood vessels.

Hypothenar eminence
Elongated muscle mass lying along the medial (ulnar) body of the palm and consisting of the muscles of the little finger.

Ischemia
Reduction or cessation of arterial blood flow to a more or less extensive region of an organ (cf. **Organ**) or of a tissue. Ischemia leads to a reduced supply of oxygen and to metabolic changes.

Glossary

Moderate ischemia, involving a muscle, can only occur during activity when the need for oxygen is increased. Its effects are reversible when it is moderate or transient, but severe or persistent ischemia can result in the death of tissues, known as infarction or gangrene. *Gangrene* is used when the skin is involved and *infarction* when viscera are involved.

Joint

The location at which two or more bones connect. A joint can be immovably fixed (synarthrosis), slightly movable (amphiarthrosis), or very mobile (diarthrosis). The joint is the structure formed by bones covered with cartilage and united by ligaments.

Joint dislocation

Displacement of two bony extremities of a joint with total loss of normal contact between two articular surfaces. It can result from an impact or from a forced movement, more rarely from a malformation (congenital hip dislocation).

Neuralgia

Also called nerve pain. It is a syndrome characterized by spontaneous or induced, continuous, or paroxysmal pain located along the course of a nerve.

Neuritis

Inflammation of one or multiple nerves.
It is included among the peripheral neuropathies, i.e., inflammatory diseases of peripheral nerves in general. The inflammation can be caused by alcoholism, an infection (leprosy, different viruses), a chemical disorder (diabetes), or an injury. Its clinical signs are motor (muscle weakness or frank paralysis) and/or sensory (pins and needles, pains).

Nodule

Cutaneous or mucosal lesion, well demarcated, roughly spherical, and palpable.

Organ

Distinct anatomical structure with a dedicated function. Examples: liver, muscle, cell, tooth, skin.

Osteochondral/osteocartilaginous

Related to a structure containing bone and cartilage.

Osteochondrosis

It is also called osteochondritis. It is a dystrophic process, selectively afflicting some osteocartilaginous areas, e.g., epiphyses, bony processes, small bones, vertebral bodies, as well as some synchondroses (joints where the two bones are linked by cartilage). It also appears to include a group of cases of aseptic necrosis due to some vascular disturbance. Depending on its location it is cured either with no sequelae or with a persistent deformity.

Osteophyte

Exuberant overgrowth of bony tissue from the periosteum (cf. **Periosteum**) along a diseased joint or a focus of chronic osteitis (inflammation of a bone). It can also arise as a result of encroachment of bony tissue on a ligament at its site of insertion.

Palm-up test

Antepulsion of the supinated arm against resistance causing pain along the biceps tendon as a result of inflammation or rupture of the tendon.

Paralysis

The loss of motor function of one or more muscles secondary to an interruption of their nerve supply. When there is only muscle weakness, the condition is known as paresis.

Paresthesia

Abnormal sensation, not painful but unpleasant, felt on the skin. Paresthesia suggests a lesion of nerve fibers and is seen in many neurologic diseases. It presents as spontaneous development

Glossary

of pins and needles, stiffening of the skin (the stiff skin syndrome), and numbness.

Periosteum
Connective tissue membrane that surrounds a bone and mediates its growth in thickness.

Periostitis
Acute or chronic inflammation of the periosteum (fibrous membrane that surrounds a bone and mediates its growth in thickness).

Pes anserinus (Latin: goose foot)
It refers to the three-pronged mode of tibial insertion of the tendons of three muscles, i.e., sartorius, gracilis, and semitendinosus, recalling the foot of a goose. Hence these muscles are known as the anserine muscles and the associated bursa as the anserine bursa.

Plicae
(Latin: plicae, folds) folds, pleats, plications, straps. The plicae in the synovial lining of the knee joint can cause locking of the joint.

Posteromedial/posterolateral tubercles of the talus
The posterior surface of the talus contains a groove with a proximal tubercle lying lateral to it and a less prominent tubercle lying medial to it. The author refers to these as the posterolateral and the posteromedial tubercles.

Posteromedial/posterolateral tuberosity of the metatarsals
The base (posterior extremity) of every metatarsal shows a variable, smooth, rounded protuberance on its medial and lateral aspects, which the author calls the posteromedial or posterolateral tuberosity.

Pronation
Movement of the forearm that leads to an axial rotation of the hand, so that the palm comes to face inferiorly or posteriorly and the thumb medially.

Pronation of the foot
Slight lateral orientation of the sole of the foot, same as eversion.

Pseudarthrosis
Definitive failure of healing of a broken bone leading to the development of abnormal movements of variable range at the site of fracture.

Raphe
Site of junction of two bilaterally symmetrical anatomic structures formed by the intertwining of connective tissue fibers.

Retroversion
Backward/posterior tilting of an entire organ.

Rheumatism
Name given to a wide variety of acute or chronic diseases, characterized by pain and inflammation, occurring mostly in joints and in periarticular soft tissues, but occasionally elsewhere in the body.

Rhizarthrosis
Arthrosis occurring at the root of a finger (thumb), of a toe, or of a limb.

Rostral process of calcaneus
Beak-like (Latin: rostrum, a beak) anterior/distal projection of the dorsal surface of the calcaneus.

Sprain
Lesion of the ligaments of a joint without dislocation of the articular surfaces.
Sprains are due to a sudden movement of a joint beyond its normal range of movements.

Stasis
Severe slowing or stopping of the flow of a liquid in an organism.
Stasis of the circulation in the foot can be due to varices in the lower limbs.

Stenosis
Narrowing with permanent reduction in the caliber of an orifice or of a vessel, coupled with changes in its wall.

Glossary

Subluxation/partial dislocation

It refers to dislocation of one bone of a joint to one side but still in contact with part of the articular surface of the other bone.

Supination

Movement of the forearm that leads to mediolateral rotation of the hand so that the palm comes to face laterally or superiorly.

Supination of the foot

Movement of the sole of the foot so that it comes to face medially.

Synostosis

Fusion of two bones.

Synovial bursa

A synovium-lined sac meant to facilitate the sliding of tendons or muscles.

Synovial membrane (synovium)

Membrane lining the interior aspect of the capsule of mobile joints (diarthroses). It forms pleats or fringes and contains a fluid resembling the white of an egg, known as synovial fluid.

Tendinitis

Inflammation of a tendon.

Tendinopathy

A generic term for diseases of tendons.

Tenobursitis

Inflammation of a tendon and of its associated bursa.

Tenosynovitis

Concurrent inflammation of the tendon and of its surrounding sheath. (cf. **synovial membrane**).

Thenar eminence

Elongated muscle mass in the superolateral part of the palm consisting of the muscles of the thumb.

Thrombosis

Formation of a clot in a blood vessel or in a heart chamber during life.

Trifurcation of the linea aspera

According to the author, the linea aspera of the femur trifurcates or divides proximally into three branches or lips (medial, intermediate, and lateral). According to others, the linea aspera is considered to bifurcate or divide proximally into a medial and a lateral lip.

Tunnel syndrome

Set of peripheral neuralgic disturbances due to compression of a nerve in an inextensible tunnel.

Turner's syndrome

Syndrome occurring in females and characterized by short stature, arrested development, failure of development of the ovaries, and a cluster of anomalies (thoracic, of the face, neck, and limbs; lymphedema; cardiac and renal malformations; and mental deficiency).
It is caused by a chromosomal abnormality.

Valgus

The term refers to a limb or a segment thereof with a lateralward deviation relative to the axis of the body. Examples: coxa valga, genu valgum, talipes equinovalgus.

Varus

The term refers to a limb or a segment thereof with a medialward deviation relative to the axis of the body. Examples: coxa vara, genu varum, talipes equinovarus.

Index by subject area

Page numbers followed by "*f*" indicate figures, and "*b*" indicate boxes.

Index

Page numbers followed by "*f*" indicate figures, and "*b*" indicate boxes.

Index

Index

Index

Index

Index

Index

Index

Index

Index

Index

Index

Index